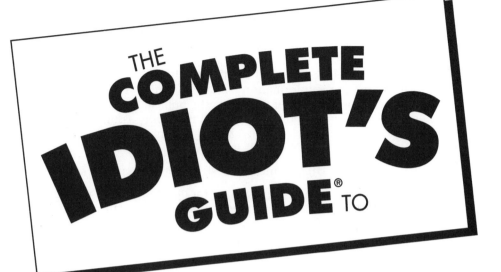

Beautiful Skin

by Marsha Gordon, M.D.,
and Alice E. Fugate

alpha
books

A Division of Macmillan General Reference
A Simon & Schuster Macmillan Company
1633 Broadway, New York, NY 10019

Macmillan Publishing books may be purchased for business or sales promotional use. For information please write: Special Markets Department, Macmillan Publishing USA, 1633 Broadway, New York, NY 10019-6785.

International Standard Book Number: 0-02-862408-4

Library of Congress Catalog Card Number: A catalog record is available from the Library of Congress

00 99   8 7 6 5 4 3 2

Interpretation of the printing code: the rightmost number of the first series of numbers is the year of the book's printing; the rightmost number of the second series of numbers is the number of the book's printing. For example, a printing code of 98-1 shows that the first printing occurred in 1998.

Printed in the United States of America

Note: This publication contains the opinions and ideas of its author. It is intended to provide helpful and informative material on the subject matter covered. It is sold with the understanding that the author and publisher are not engaged in rendering professional services in the book. If the reader requires personal assistance or advice, a competent professional should be consulted.

The author and publisher specifically disclaim any responsibility for any liability, loss or risk, personal or otherwise, which is incurred as a consequence, directly or indirectly, of the use and application of any of the contents of this book.

Alpha Development Team

Publisher
Kathy Nebenhaus

Editorial Director
Gary M. Krebs

Managing Editor
Bob Shuman

Marketing Brand Manager
Felice Primeau

Senior Editor
Nancy Mikhail

Development Editors
Phil Kitchel
Jennifer Perillo
Amy Zavatto

Editorial Assistant
Maureen Horn

Production Team

Development Editor
Mary Russell

Production Editor
Kristi Hart

Copy Editor
Lisa Lord

Cover Designer
Mike Freeland

Photo Editor
Richard H. Fox

Illustrator
Jody P. Schaeffer

Designer
Glenn Larsen

Indexer
Chris Barrick

Layout/Proofreading
Angela Calvert
Kim Cofer

Contents at a Glance

Contents

Foreword

Dear Friend:

You are so lucky. You are about to meet the "secret weapon" of New York women: Dr. Marsha Gordon!

She's certainly *my* secret weapon.

➤ I call her when I'm doing television reports on new skin, hair, or nail treatments or products to get her comments...on-camera and off-camera.

➤ I call her when I'm writing a column about psychology of beauty topics...like "hairanoia" (crying after a bad hair cut), "nail neurosis" (hiding a hand for hours when a nail breaks) or "skin scares" (thinking a blemish is visible from one hundred yards)...

➤ I call her when my friends want to see a dermatologist who *understands*.

➤ I call her when my daughter has a red rash (just last week), my mother has a dry patch (just last month), or anyone else in the family is worried about a bump or a bruise, a mole or a mark, nails, hair, pox, pimples, cold sores, foot funguses, or scalp itch (you get the idea).

➤ And yes, I call her when *I* need a dermatologist, too!

I *used* to call her to suggest she write a book. I wanted her to put *all* her tips and *all* her information and *all* her suggestions on paper. Then I wouldn't have to call her so much. I could just open her book and look up what I need to know. Or start at the beginning and read through and be my own skin care expert. Think of what I would save on phone bills, doctor bills and, of course, on expensive products that I would buy and she'd later tell me were hype.

Well, Dr. Gordon has done it. This is *that* book. *The Complete Idiot's Guide to Beautiful Skin* is really the smart consumer's guide to beautiful skin...and more. It will save us all time and money and worry. I thank her, and you'll thank her, too. Enjoy!

Georgia Witkin, Ph.D.
Assistant Clinical Professor of Psychiatry, Director of The Stress Program, and Assistant Professor of Obstetrics, Gynecology and Reproductive Science at Mount Sinai Medical Center in New York City; author of seven books including *The Female Stress Syndrome*, and *The Male Stress Syndrome*; television health reporter, national talk show host and guest expert on *20/20*, *The Today Show*, *Oprah*, Fox News Channel, and many others.

Introduction

Beautiful Skin: It Shouldn't Be a Secret

Recently, Jessica stopped by my office. An intelligent professional with years of education and work experience under her belt, she had a confession to make: "Dr. Gordon, I just don't know what to do about my skin! I'm starting to get wrinkles, I still get acne, and my jawline is sagging more than I would like. What can I do to make myself look better?"

Does this sound like you? Every day I see dozens of people who ask similar questions. Like Jessica, they are puzzled, even overwhelmed, by all the conflicting information they receive on skin care. Which products work best? Are lasers, facial peels, and plastic surgery safe? What happens if they choose the wrong product—will they damage their skin forever?

Also like Jessica, many are reluctant to bring up their concerns. As she put it: "I feel a bit silly even asking these questions. Am I being too vain?"

"Not at all," I reassured her. "It's normal, healthy in fact, to want to look your best. And certainly the skin-care industry doesn't make it easy."

This is what I tell Jessica and my other patients: When it comes to good skin care, be an informed consumer. Yes, some products definitely work better than others. Some procedures get rid of fine wrinkles but not deep lines; others do just the opposite; still others can do great things for that fold from the nose to the corner of the mouth, but nothing for drooping eyelids or forehead lines. In short, there are many wonderful treatments out there to help you attain beautiful skin, but you have to choose wisely.

That's the goal of this book: to demystify skin care. Beautiful skin shouldn't be a secret, and achieving it need not be a mystery. Sometimes the newest techniques are just what you need, and sometimes time-honored treatments turn out to be the best.

No problem! This book covers all of them.

Your Comprehensive Skin-Care Resource

I recommend reading this book straight through, and then keeping it on hand as a helpful reference.

For instance, look at Chapters 1 through 6 before your next cosmetics shopping spree. Here I discuss the bewildering array of makeup, cleansers, moisturizers, toners, and other skin-care staples, and show you the ingredients that are good and bad for your skin. Check here before spending your hard-earned cash on items you'll never use again.

Is every day a bad hair day? Are your nails so brittle they seem to break when you look at them? Turn to Chapter 7, where you'll learn how to make your hair and nails strong and beautiful.

Medical research reveals that many of the skin changes we call "aging" are not inevitable. In fact, you may be able to prevent them. Chapters 8 through 11 tell what you can do to look younger than your age, no matter how old you are. Chapter 9 discusses factors that age your skin, and Chapter 10 explains how you can cope with your skin's fiercest enemy, sun exposure. Sunscreen is a big help, but only if you select a good one and use it correctly. Chapter 11 shows you how.

Maybe you've heard about tretinoin (the active ingredient in Renova® and Retin-A®) and alpha and beta hydroxy acids. While they can be helpful, the claims made about them are sometimes wildly exaggerated. Chapter 12 examines the hype and reality about alpha and beta hydroxy acids; Chapter 13 looks at how tretinoin really works and whether you are likely to benefit from it.

Wait, there's more:

➤ Pregnancy brings its own joys and skin-care concerns. Chapter 14 discusses what to expect during this special time and how to cope.

➤ Acne, an annoyance for teenagers and adults alike, is one of the most common skin complaints. In Chapter 15, I examine the latest strategies for preventing and treating it.

➤ Treatments for skin conditions—psoriasis, dermatitis, cold sores, and warts, to name just a few—are improving all the time. Chapter 16 offers commonsense advice on recognizing and treating them.

➤ Chapter 17 tells you how to get rid of "other things that go itch in the night," like insect bites, poison ivy, and other pesky stuff.

➤ Suppose you discover a mysterious mark. Is it cancer? Not necessarily. Chapter 18 looks at common "benign bumps" like moles, skin tags, and birthmarks, and discusses ways to get rid of them.

➤ What if it is cancer? Treatments for skin cancer are a medical success story. If discovered early, cure rates are very high. Chapter 19 presents the warning signs and guides you through detecting and getting rid of malignancies.

➤ Don't like the skin you have now? Chapters 20 through 25 look at serious beauty treatments that can make it look delightfully different. Medical science has developed remarkable cosmetic procedures that offer you a wealth of options: chemical peels, laser treatments, collagen injections, fat transplants, sclerotherapy for spider veins. New techniques in plastic surgery can remove fat and "lift" your eyebrows, forehead, neck, or entire face.

Throughout the book, you'll learn what these products and procedures can—and can't—do for you.

How to Make This Book Work for You

Don't have time to read the book straight through? No problem. That's why it's a quick reference as well as a comprehensive resource. For example:

➤ Every chapter starts with a brief preview of chapter highlights. You can see at a glance what it covers.

➤ At the end of every chapter, there's a section called "The Least You Need to Know," which summarizes the most important points in the chapter.

These features help you navigate through the book quickly and find the information you need fast.

As a Bonus . . .

You can never be too rich, too thin, or have too much information, right? That's why, as you read, you'll notice a variety of sidebars. These bonus goodies offer extra background on skin care terms and important issues. They include:

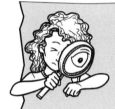

More Than Skin Deep

There's more to your skin than its surface, so these sidebars go below the surface too. They provide background information and a broad perspective.

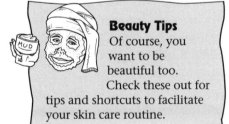

Beauty Tips
Of course, you want to be beautiful too. Check these out for tips and shortcuts to facilitate your skin care routine.

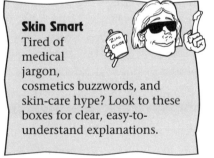

Skin Smart
Tired of medical jargon, cosmetics buzzwords, and skin-care hype? Look to these boxes for clear, easy-to-understand explanations.

Saving Your Skin
What you don't know really can hurt you. These sidebars present cautions and warnings, helpful hints that will keep your skin safe as well as beautiful.

Of course, if you have any questions about your skin, you should always consult your doctor for advice. Reading this book will make it easier to ask the right questions and evaluate your options.

And, to Top Things Off . . .

At the end of the book there's a Glossary that summarizes all the skin-care terms and definitions we covered.

Hungry for still more information? Check out Appendix A, "Bountiful Resources for Beautiful Skin," which gives you lots of additional options. Here you'll find books, articles, and Internet resources, plus contact information for helpful organizations.

Acknowledgments

Special thanks from Marsha: I'd like to dedicate this book to my beloved parents, Rosalie and Alexander Gordon. Their support and encouragement have been my guiding light. And special thanks to my sisters, Helene and Meryl, and to Stephen Bloom, for their love and patience. Thanks to my colleagues Drs. Ron Shelton, Jin Chun, Robert Phelps, Heidi Waldorf, Melanie Grossman, Ed Bottone, and Mark Lebwohl for sharing information and advice. And finally, thank you to my patients, who keep me on my toes and teach me something new every day.

Special thanks from Alice: I'd like to dedicate this book, and give a heartfelt vote of appreciation, to my wonderful husband Steve LoGrasso. Thank you so much for your love and unflagging support—not to mention all the listening! A big thank-you, as well, to my brother and sister-in-law, Warren Fugate and Eileen Kopchik, who kept my computer computing through its darkest hours.

And finally, from both of us: We want to thank our editor, Mary Russell, for her valuable help throughout the development process. We'd also like to thank Nancy Mikhail, Kristi Hart, Maureen Horn, Bob Shuman, Lisa Lord, and the rest of the talented Macmillan staff who worked hard to make this book a reality. Without their efforts, you wouldn't be reading these pages right now.

Part 1
Your Skin: An Owner's Manual

No part of us gets more attention than our skin. We scrutinize, scrub, slather, and lather. We focus on every change, line, and blemish.

A huge industry—make that a multi-billion-dollar industry—has evolved to address our skin concerns. No matter what you're self-conscious about, there are dozens, nay hundreds, of products and practitioners competing for your business. All of them clamor for your money. All claim to be just what your skin needs.

So what does your skin really need, anyway? What's the best way to clean, moisturize, and tone? How can you choose the most flattering cosmetics? What's the best way to care for your hair and nails?

Just keep reading. You'll find answers to all these questions, plus many more, in Part 1.

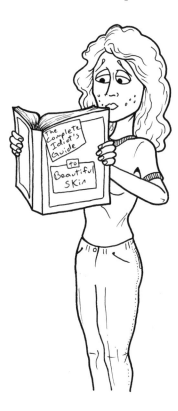

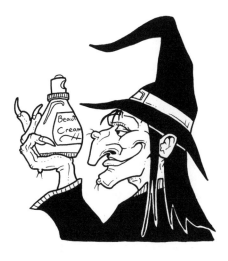

Buying Beauty in a Bottle

Yesterday, my friend Maria stopped by the sales counter of a nationally known brand of beauty products and asked for advice on skin care. The salesperson told her she had extremely dry skin that desperately needed immediate relief.

The salesperson proceeded to demonstrate a night cream, a day moisturizer, an emollient eye cream, a lip balm, a color corrector, and a highlighter for "those dark circles beneath your eyes." All of them happened to be products she was selling, of course.

Not unusual, right? Except that the week before Maria had visited the counter of another well-known company, where the salesperson insisted she had combination skin. The woman recommended a completely different regimen: toner, skin tightener, and cellular renewal lotion, topped off with a preparation of alpha hydroxy fruit acids.

Everything was different, in fact, except for the dark circles beneath Maria's eyes. As she went from one salesperson to another, gathering contradictory advice, those circles got darker by the minute.

Confused? It's Getting Worse!

As Maria would be the first to agree, it's getting harder and harder to find objective, realistic information on skin care. No wonder so many of us feel confused.

The average American adult already uses at least seven different skin care products every day. These include cleansers, moisturizers, astringents, deodorants and antiperspirants, sunscreens, hair care products, and cosmetics for the face, hair, or nails.

This may seem like plenty. You may even be thinking, "Enough already!" But the skin care industry disagrees; it would like to see this list expanded. More than 30 companies compete for space in the toiletries section of your local drugstore. Hundreds of new products debut every year to vie for your attention—and your hard-earned cash.

There's a huge industry out there vowing to beautify your skin. For a price, of course. How big a price? Well, Americans spend $1.3 billion on facial moisturizers every year, plus another billion on antibacterial cleansers and lotions. Drugstores sell $300 million worth of hand and body cream each year; discount outlets sell another $280 million; and these figures don't include the millions we spend in department and specialty stores.

If you decide to investigate cosmetic procedures such as chemical peels, laser surgery, or plastic surgery, be prepared for still more dollar signs. A full-face phenol peel costs between $1,000 and $2,500. A surgeon's fee for a forehead-lift ranges from $1,500 to $5,000, with anesthesia, operating room costs, and related expenses adding another $1,000. Many of these procedures aren't covered by health insurance, so you will pay the tab yourself.

Clearly, it behooves all of us to become informed consumers who know how to get the results we pay for.

My friends and patients often ask me for guidance on how to achieve and maintain beautiful skin. Here are some frequent questions:

➤ Which skin care products really work?

➤ How can you choose the products that are best for your skin type?

➤ What are the best treatments for common problems: skin that is sensitive, oily, dry, itchy, or prone to break out?

➤ Are chemical peels and plastic surgery worth the money?

➤ If they are, which procedures would I recommend?

Saving Your Skin
On a product label, the phrase "patent pending" simply means the company has filed for a patent, but its application has not yet been approved. This does not mean approval is imminent; it's possible the patent might not be granted, period.

Have you, too, wondered how to get the most for your beauty budget? Then this book is for you.

You're Not Getting Older, You're Getting More Products

Louis Harris & Associates recently surveyed more than 1,200 baby boomers (ages 30 to 50) about their feelings on getting older. They must have had a lot to say; their responses filled a report that ran to 74 pages.

More than half the respondents noted that facial wrinkles have a strong influence on how they feel about themselves and their appearance. Most bothersome were the wrinkles around their eyes, with forehead lines coming in a close second. Most admitted they would feel more attractive if they could make those lines disappear.

Do you, too, worry about wrinkles? If so, you have lots of company. It's not surprising we feel uneasy about even the slightest signs of age; America is notorious for equating beauty with youth.

The media reinforce our insecurity by bombarding us daily with negative messages. (You could say we let them get under our skin!) Look at any fashion magazine, and you will see that the models are rarely over 30 (especially the women). How many movies and TV shows star older adults in positive roles? Not many.

Marketers know a bonanza when they see one. In the United States alone, sales of anti-aging creams top more than $1 billion per year. Alpha hydroxy acids, heavily advertised as wrinkle reducers, are used to sell everything from moisturizers to soap.

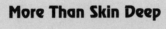

More Than Skin Deep

Anti-aging claims, and the desire to believe them, are not new. Native Americans told the Spanish conquistadors of a fabulous Fountain of Youth—a spring whose water could erase years from all who drank it. In 1513, Spanish explorer Juan Ponce de León sailed to the New World hoping to discover the fountain; instead, he found Florida. Ponce de León drank from every spring he came across in Florida, hoping that one of them would be the legendary fountain, but to no avail. Eight years later he died in battle, no wiser and no younger.

Translating Adspeak

Just how much can you believe of the ads for skin care products? Frankly, not much.

Four of the most popular claims that advertisers make for their products are

➤ "Anti-aging"

➤ "Natural"

➤ "Hypoallergenic"

➤ "Dermatologist-tested"

Let's take a minute to examine each of these claims.

"Anti-Aging" Products

Beauty Tips
Sunscreens contain chemicals that reflect or absorb sunlight. If a sunscreen label lists titanium dioxide or zinc oxide as the active ingredient, it reflects sunlight; active ingredients such as octyl methoxycinnamate or oxybenzone absorb it. Sunscreens in the latter category need to be absorbed into the skin before they become effective, so apply them at least 20 minutes before going outside.

Legally, the only products that can claim to be anti-aging are the ones containing sunscreen. Much of the so-called aging that occurs in skin is actually due to sun exposure, not to getting older. When used properly, an effective sunscreen can indeed help protect your skin from harmful ultraviolet rays. In fact, sunscreens are one of the most important advances in skin care over the past 25 years.

However, not all sunscreens are created equal. Some are far less effective than others, both because of their ingredients and because of the strength of their formulation. Sunscreens are rated with an *SPF* (sun protection factor) number that starts at 2 and goes up. We dermatologists recommend using an SPF of 15 or higher, but many "anti-aging" preparations have an SPF of 8 or lower. In fact, many products touted as "anti-aging" contain so little sunscreen that they are essentially ineffective against sunlight.

You'll get a closer look at sunscreens and how sunlight affects skin in Chapters 9–11. In Chapters 12 and 13 you'll find out about other promising wrinkle fighters like tretinoin (the active ingredient in Renova® and Retin-A®), and alpha and beta hydroxy acids.

"Natural" Products

What does *natural* mean to you? It probably conveys images of Mother Nature, beautiful landscapes, clean air, and pure water. On a product label, the term carries connotations of purity, gentleness, and radiant good health.

You may be surprised to hear there's no FDA definition for the term *natural*. It could mean that a product's ingredients come from nature (whether plant, animal, or mineral). It could also mean that the ingredients imitate natural substances or are chemical precursors of natural substances.

When you consider buying a "natural" product, remember the following:

➤ Even if only one substance in a product is natural, marketers can use this term. Natural ingredients could make up less than 1 percent of the total.

➤ Many items with natural ingredients also contain numerous chemicals, including preservatives, stabilizers, dyes, and fragrances.

➤ At the molecular level, synthetics often resemble natural substances. In fact, chemicals synthesized in a laboratory are often based on natural prototypes. Several laboratory-developed preservatives, for example, are chemically similar to the natural preservative vitamin E.

➤ If a product were truly all-natural, you might not want to buy it anyway. Chemical perfumes, preservatives, and colors make many substances stay fresher and more appealing than they would in their natural state. (You may like that fragrant seaweed extract you bought last week, but would you want to smear the real thing on your skin?)

"Hypoallergenic" Products

"Hypoallergenic" is another claim that sounds meaningful but often isn't. According to the American Academy of Dermatology, only about .021 percent of us experience adverse reactions to skin care products. Most of these reactions are due to irritation, not to allergies.

But you'd never guess this from advertisements, which tout products' "hypoallergenic" properties as all-important. Actually, all *hypoallergenic* means is "less likely to cause an allergic reaction than comparable products." Commercially, this term has little meaning, since companies have a lot of leeway to decide what makes a product comparable. What's more, there are no legal guidelines governing which ingredients can (and cannot) be used in hypoallergenic products.

Certainly you're smart to look for products that will not aggravate your skin. Just remember that products labeled as "hypoallergenic" may still contain potential irritants.

In Chapters 5, "Choosing the Right Toner and Moisturizer," and 6, "At the Cosmetics Counter," I'll provide a closer look at the ingredients most of our skins can do without.

Skin Smart
Hypoallergenic simply means a product is "less likely to cause an allergic reaction than comparable products."

Products That Are "Dermatologist-Tested"

In the meaningless phrase sweepstakes, "dermatologist-tested" is one of my personal favorites. Companies frequently send me samples of products they want me to try or recommend to patients. Some of these products are indeed helpful; others go in the wastebasket.

On a package label, this phrase tells you nothing about how many people tested the item or how carefully and scientifically they tested it. Even if a dermatologist tries a product and doesn't like it, the manufacturer can still say it was "dermatologist-tested," because it was.

So What Can You Believe?

As you've gathered by now, I am skeptical about many product labels and marketing claims. So if you can't always trust them, what can you believe?

In addition to ads, many of us look to two major sources for information and ideas about skin care: the media and the salespeople who sell us the products. What can we expect from them?

The Fashion Media: Fun, but Not Always Factual

The fashion media is a great source for the latest trends in clothing and cosmetics, but it's not always the best source for impartial data on skin care.

> **Saving Your Skin**
> It's not always easy to tell the difference between journalism and advertising. This is especially true on the Internet, where there are fewer restrictions than on print and broadcast media. That helpful home page could be factual, or it could be someone's personal opinion. Always follow your own judgment, especially if it's unclear where posted information came from.

After all, magazines, TV, and radio survive by selling space and airtime to advertisers. Companies buy this space to market their skin care products and services. How long would a magazine stay in business if it angered a lucrative advertiser by publishing articles that praised its competition? How long would a TV show attract advertisers if it broadcast negative ratings of their products?

Not surprisingly, many media pieces tend to favor advertisers' products. Some of the authorities they quote work for these companies, so they may not be impartial.

By all means, enjoy the fashion media for what it does best—informing us about fashion. From time to time, you will also find excellent pieces that present helpful, unbiased information.

Just be aware that when it comes to evaluating skin care products, the media may be constrained by financial considerations. Take its statements about skin care with a grain—make that several large grains—of salt.

Salespeople and How They're (Not) Trained

Many of us look to sales reps for guidance about skin care products. How well informed are they? Just listen to the experience of my friend Alice, who sold cosmetics and toiletries one holiday season in a department store in the St. Louis area.

First off, when Alice applied for the job, the interviewer made no attempt to probe the extent of her knowledge about skin care or cosmetics. She looked presentable, spoke well, and was willing to take a minimum-wage job with odd hours. Apparently this was enough, because she was hired. There was no formal training; she was simply told when and where to show up.

Her first day, she was placed behind a counter to sell products she had never heard of, let alone used. Despite her lack of experience, though, she enjoyed chatting with customers and helping them choose makeup and perfume.

Her favorite customer, she recalls, was a bewildered man searching for a birthday gift for his wife. "I know she's into this stuff," he told Alice, "but I have no idea how to pick out something she'll like." Alice spent a lot of time with him and they investigated a number of products, both in her area and in other brands. Finally he selected a foundation with sunscreen and a scented body lotion, neither of which came from Alice's line.

When he left he was delighted with his purchases, and Alice thought her supervisor would be delighted with her. After all, she'd made a sale, right? Wrong! The supervisor crisply pointed out her mistakes. For starters, she had sold him items from other salespersons' lines; this lowered sales for her brand while depriving them of commissions.

Even worse, she took him at his word when he mentioned his budget and only showed him products in a certain price range. "Always start with your most expensive products," said the supervisor. "Never say you have anything less expensive unless they ask for it specifically."

Alice's major crime was to sell the man exactly what he wanted, without trying to talk him into buying more. "You had the chance to sell him powder, sunscreen, under-eye cream, and moisturizer, but you didn't," the supervisor pointed out.

"But," Alice protested, "the foundation he bought had an SPF of 15, and the sunscreen in my line only has an SPF of 8. Isn't the 15 better?" "That doesn't matter," snapped her boss. "It's all part of the product line. We are here to sell customers a complete line of skin care products."

By recounting this tale, I certainly don't mean to criticize all salespeople. Some cosmetics companies do an excellent job of training their sales representatives, and there are skilled professionals who make a genuine effort to learn their product lines and help customers. There are several whose advice I value, and they have helped me find products I like and have used for years.

However, many salespeople are like Alice was: hired and sent to the sales floor with minimal training. When you ask for advice at the cosmetics counter, you could be speaking with a well-informed representative, or you could be dealing with someone who knows less about skin care than you do.

Saving Your Skin

Here's something to keep in mind at the cosmetics counter. If a product has no SPF number, beware. This means either it contains no sunscreen at all, or it contains so little that it doesn't even qualify for the lowest end of the SPF scale.

While qualified salespeople can be a big help, just remember:

➤ If they are paid on commission, they probably will not refer you to a competing line of skin care products.

➤ Even if they are not paid on commission, they want you to buy their products because they have a sales quota to fulfill.

➤ Supervisors may discourage them from asking too many questions about what's in the products, because the supervisors don't know the answers either.

➤ They may be told to start with the most expensive products in their line and move to less expensive items only if you balk at the price.

Getting Around the FDA

By this point, you may be wondering why there's so much misleading information lurking out there. Aren't there laws about truth in advertising?

Yes, there are. The problem is that it's possible to get around these laws with creative wording.

The Food and Drug Administration, a federal agency, enforces most of the laws involving drugs and personal care products in the U.S. Among other responsibilities, the FDA sets standards for the information that must be shown on packages, such as the list of ingredients, and monitors companies' compliance with these standards.

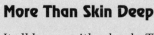

More Than Skin Deep

It all began with a book, *The Jungle,* by Upton Sinclair, which exposed unsanitary practices in the meatpacking industry. Public outcry over the book was so violent that President Theodore Roosevelt wrote to Sinclair and promised to investigate his charges. Sinclair suggested that the investigators work undercover; official visitors, he said, wouldn't get the true story. Roosevelt followed his advice and the investigation confirmed Sinclair's horrifying allegations. The result was the Pure Food and Drug Act of 1906, a landmark in consumer protection and still the basis for FDA regulation today.

Any substance that effects permanent changes in the structure or function of the human body is considered a drug, and drugs must go through years of testing before the FDA approves them for general use. Obviously, this is not a desirable option for a company that wants to get its blockbuster wrinkle cream to market right away.

The FDA does watch for marketing claims that directly state a product will cause a permanent change in your skin. But labels and ads can be carefully worded to avoid assertions that the FDA could interpret as direct promises. Of course, marketers also want to convince us, their customers, that this product will work miracles. Not an easy line to walk, but this is why the skin care industry spends millions on marketing every year.

Watch for these marketing tricks:

➤ Putting words in quotation marks. Words surrounded by quotes do not have to meet a strict definition; they are open to interpretation by the consumer. From the FDA's point of view, a cream that "rejuvenates" your skin is different from one that rejuvenates without any quotation marks.

➤ Using subjective rather than objective terms. Claiming a product makes skin appear, look, or feel smoother is acceptable; claiming it actually makes skin smoother is not.

➤ Claiming the product will benefit superficial lines or wrinkles. Superficial wrinkles may result from overly dry skin, and moisturizing the skin will make them less visible. This is not the same, unfortunately, as getting rid of wrinkles permanently.

➤ Using elegant words that upon closer inspection don't really mean anything. What does it mean to "tone," "enrich," or "strengthen" skin?

➤ In a variant of the above, using elegant synonyms for everyday terms. Would you buy a cream filled with fat? No; but you might buy it if it were "enriched with lipids." Similarly, you might bypass a facial mask made of plant fibers; call them "botanicals" and they sound much more enticing.

More Than Skin Deep

As an example of how marketers bypass FDA guidelines, consider skin-whitening products. Skin whiteners are popular in Asia—in Japan alone, they are a $1.3 billion business—and companies have started to sell them here, too. Many whiteners contain vitamin C derivatives or placental extracts from sheep and cows. However, in the United States, the only FDA-approved skin-whitening substance is hydroquinone, which is classified as a drug. Consequently, marketers position the whiteners as products that brighten and smooth skin, rather than bleach it. This claim makes them cosmetics, not drugs, and avoids time-consuming federal regulations and testing.

Can You Go by Price?

The companies that bring you cosmetics and toiletries are responsible for packaging, distributing, and promoting their products. But guess what? They don't necessarily make them.

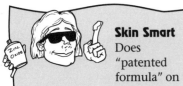

Skin Smart
Does "patented formula" on a label justify a higher price? No. There are millions of cosmetics patents. Often they are granted for unusual formulations, or for combining standard ingredients in a novel way, such as in alcohol rather than oil. While a patent recognizes originality in formulas or procedures, it does not guarantee the product will do anything original or beneficial for your skin.

Many eyeshadows and eyeliners marketed here under a variety of brand names are manufactured by the same firm in Europe. A number of cosmetics are formulated in the same laboratories, either in the United States or abroad, and then packaged and sold by different cosmetics concerns.

Even when manufactured by different companies, products often contain similar ingredients. Look at the labels of several moisturizers, for example, and you will see many of the same ingredients repeated. A lotion that sells for $8.50 at the drugstore may not be all that different from a pricey competitor.

Differences in price reflect the power of brand image and skillful marketing. The price tag on expensive toiletries reflects a tremendous markup above what they cost to make. Like any for-profit firm, a company is only too happy to charge whatever we're willing to pay.

How This Book Can Help

By now, you may be wondering if any skin care treatments are worthwhile! In fact, today we can enjoy a wealth of promising products, not to mention exciting new developments in cosmetic procedures and plastic surgery.

This book will guide you through the maze of products and publicity and help you make decisions you'll be happy with for years to come. It is my earnest hope that, as an informed consumer, you will become the leading authority on your own beautiful skin. Here's to a great new you!

The Least You Need to Know

➤ Legally, cosmetics and toiletries cannot cause permanent changes in the structure or function of your skin. If they could, they would be classified as drugs and subjected to rigorous testing.

➤ Read product labels carefully. Don't rely on salespeople or the media to tell you what a product contains.

➤ Price is not a reliable guide to quality or effectiveness.

➤ If all marketing claims were true, blemishes and wrinkles would be endangered species. Everyone would have gorgeous skin!

➤ Yes, there are products and procedures that can beautify your skin, and they are covered in the rest of the book.

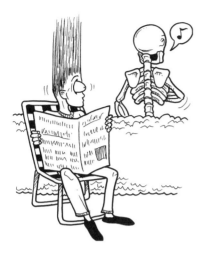

Chapter 2

Your Skin: Don't Leave Home Without It

In This Chapter

➤ Learn how your skin works to keep you healthy

➤ Discover why you're the color you are

➤ See why perspiration is positive

➤ Learn why your skin won't absorb most of the stuff you put on it—and a good thing, too

➤ Find out why products that claim to melt cellulite and shrink pores won't

A sampler of questions from recent ads:

➤ Tired of those unsightly ripples on your thighs? This amazing cream will penetrate your skin and melt that cellulite away. In just three weeks, your thighs will appear softer and smoother.

➤ Embarrassed by those large pores on your face? This astonishing gel will shrink them and return your skin to the smooth, silky appearance of youth.

➤ Is your skin less firm than it used to be? Our cream contains collagen, a natural substance that makes skin supple and strong. Apply it twice daily to supplement your body's own collagen reserves.

Here's my question: Are you tired of products that promise everything but deliver much less?

Many patients ask me whether certain items will melt cellulite or minimize pores. They also wonder whether it's possible to supplement your body's reserves of collagen (or anything else). In fact, is it realistic for any topically applied product to penetrate your skin and improve it from the outside in?

To answer these questions and many more, we need to take a quick look at what skin is, what it does, and how it does it. As you will see, this covering we take for granted is really very complicated—a miracle of design and engineering.

What Has It Done for You Lately?

A pop quiz: What's your largest organ? If you answered "my skin," go to the head of the class—the average person's skin covers about two square yards. Your skin isn't just large; it's also complex. Take a look at this cross section of a piece of it. One square inch of skin contains millions of cells and hundreds of nerve endings, plus lots of muscles, blood vessels, hair follicles, sweat glands, and oil glands.

There's a lot going on in your skin.

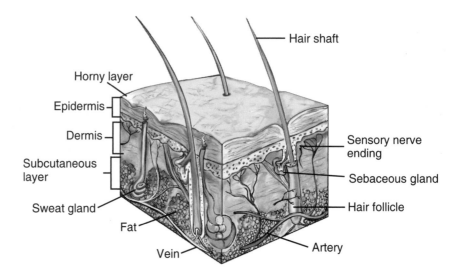

Your skin is far more than a covering that holds you together. It's a dynamic organ that works constantly to keep your body temperature a healthy 98.6 degrees. It cushions your delicate insides and stays on perpetual alert to regulate the proportions of water and salt in your body.

Another benefit: Your skin is an early warning system that helps you respond quickly to pain. Sound like a mixed blessing? But just think what happens when your hand accidentally brushes against a hot stove. Nerve endings in your skin detect the heat and immediately fire emergency signals to your brain, which promptly screams: "That thing you're touching is hot, stupid, so move your hand!" Without your early warning network of skin sensors, you would be badly burned.

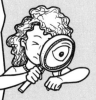

More Than Skin Deep

Vitamin D is crucial for healthy bones; in fact, children who live in parts of the world where the sun is often obscured (deep valleys are a classic example) may suffer abnormal skeletal development. This condition, called rickets, has become rare in industrialized countries since we started adding vitamin D to milk and many other grocery products.

Skin is a barrier that keeps our insides in, even as it keeps unwanted visitors like bacteria and viruses outside. As a final bonus, it even functions as a chemical factory by making vitamin D! Skin cells convert steroid molecules (relatives of cholesterol) in your body to vitamin D when the cells are exposed to sunlight.

Taking It from the Top

Basically, your skin consists of multiple layers of cells. I won't bore you with the names and details of each microlayer; their names come from Latin and Greek, and they're as long and confusing as you would expect medical terms to be.

Instead, I'll focus on the two main layers formed by all these thinner ones: the *dermis* (the inner layer) and *epidermis* (the outer covering). Each plays an important role in keeping your skin healthy and beautiful. Incidentally, even though I refer to them as the "main" layers, both are incredibly thin; the epidermis is one- to two-tenths of a millimeter thick (approximately 0.00394 inch), the dermis is several times thicker.

Skin Smart
The inside layer of skin is the *dermis*. Above it lies the outer layer, the *epidermis* ("upon the dermis"). *Derm* means "skin," and it forms the basis of many medical terms relating to skin, like *dermatologist* (a doctor who treats problems of the skin, hair, and nails).

Scratching the Surface: The Epidermis

Imagine that you're digging a tiny tunnel down through your epidermis. At the bottom you find a skin factory, where specialized cells divide constantly to create new skin cells.

Each new cell starts moving up the tunnel, from the bottom of the epidermis outward. Each starts life as a soft, rounded cell, but morphs along the way into a thin, hardened disc. When viewed under a microscope, older skin cells resemble tiny scales.

By the time they reach the skin surface—a journey of roughly 14 days—the cells are dead. They're also dehydrated, which allows them to fit together tightly and create an interlocked covering called the *horny layer*. (Seriously!)

This is bad for the cells, but good for us. The horny layer makes an effective and durable barrier against the threats of the outside world. Since the cells are deceased, they are also expendable; if you happen to scrape a few off, you're not losing anything you can't replace. Their dry, hardened surface makes an uninviting home for microorganisms, which discourages bacteria and viruses from taking up residence on your skin.

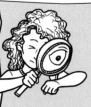

More Than Skin Deep

The thin layer of dead and flattened cells covering the skin surface is the *horny layer*. Okay, stop snickering; the horny layer got its name because it contains *keratin*, a fibrous protein similar to that found in animals' horns and hooves, not to mention your hair and nails. If this term seems too informal, you can impress your friends by using its Latin name, *stratum corneum* (which means—you guessed it—"the horny layer").

As a final safety measure, the cells of the horny layer hang around for only a couple of weeks after reaching the skin surface. Then they slough off, to be replaced by new cells rising from below.

There are a few areas of the skin that do not produce a horny layer, such as the mucous membranes that line the inside of your mouth and eyelids. There's a good reason for this; just imagine how annoying it would be to constantly blink away tiny scales from your eyes! Instead, mucous membrane cells get smaller as they approach the skin surface, and then peel away unobtrusively without hardening.

Digging Deeper: The Dermis

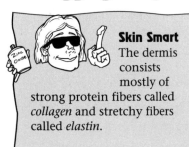

Skin Smart
The dermis consists mostly of strong protein fibers called *collagen* and stretchy fibers called *elastin*.

If you continue your tunnel below the nether regions of the epidermis, you find the dermis, which supports and nourishes the epidermis.

The dermis is a dense layer rich with blood vessels and nerve endings. It consists mostly of strong protein fibers called collagen and stretchy fibers called elastin. *Collagen* is a protein that gives skin its strength and fullness; it also helps repair injured skin by building scar tissue. *Elastin* consists of elastic fibers that give skin its flexibility, enabling it to stretch and contract repeatedly as you move.

Pinch your arm and note how your skin reacts. The firmness you feel comes from collagen. For the skin's ability to resume its original shape, thank your elastin.

Beneath It All: The Subcutaneous Layer

Below the epidermis and dermis lurks another layer of tissue, known by the impressive name of *subcutaneous layer*. While the subcutaneous layer isn't actually part of the skin, it plays a big role in stabilizing skin and protecting the delicate organs underneath. It's also an insulating blanket that slows down the rate at which you lose body heat.

The subcutaneous layer is an extensive network of connective tissue laced with lots of fat cells. When we were infants, it covered our entire body (beneath the skin, that is). Our "baby fat" cushioned us when we fell and provided an abundant energy reserve to fuel youthful high jinks.

As we mature, the subcutaneous layer thins out and redistributes itself in ways that may be all too familiar. Women tend to carry it in their breasts, buttocks, abdomen, hips, and thighs; men accumulate it in their neck, upper arms, abdomen, lower back, and over the buttocks.

The distribution of the subcutaneous layer can definitely have an impact on what your skin looks like. Some of us, for example, develop *cellulite,* a type of fatty tissue which contains constricting fibrous bands of connective tissue. These bands give the skin a characteristic dimpled, ripply appearance. Men rarely develop cellulite, and in women it usually doesn't appear until after age 30. While cellulite is more common in overweight people, even slender folks can have annoying deposits of it.

Skin Smart

The *subcutaneous layer* is an extensive network of connective tissue and fat cells that lies beneath the dermis. While not actually part of the skin, the subcutaneous layer stabilizes it and insulates and protects underlying organs.

Skin Smart

Cellulite is a type of fatty tissue which contains constricting bands of connective tissue. These bands give the skin a characteristic dimpled appearance.

Showing Your True Colors: Melanin

Why do some of us have dark brown skin, while others have very light skin, and still others are somewhere in between? Glad you asked. Skin color comes from a pigment called *melanin*, produced by specialized cells called *melanocytes* in the epidermis and hair follicles. Melanin varies in color from yellowish-brown to brown to black.

All human beings possess roughly the same number of melanin-producing cells. If you are fair-skinned, it's because your melanocytes make less of the stuff than your dark-skinned friends, and what they do make is distributed differently. These differences are

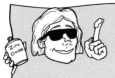

Skin Smart
Melanin is the pigment that gives our skin its distinctive color and protects us against ultraviolet radiation. It is produced by specialized cells called *melanocytes*.

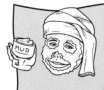

Beauty Tips
Women are often advised to sample foundation colors by trying them on the inside of their wrists; supposedly, this area approximates the color of facial skin. In fact, the skin on your face may be darker because facial skin contains more melanocytes and gets more sun exposure. Be sure to choose a color based on what blends well on your face, not somewhere else.

determined by genetics. If your ancestors were all pale-faced Swedes, you will inherit similar melanocytes—and a similar complexion.

Melanin does more than just create interesting variations in skin color, though. It helps to protect skin against its biggest enemy: the sun. Sunlight contains ultraviolet (UV) radiation, and chronic exposure to UV rays damages cells in the skin. Melanin does its best to help by absorbing UV rays before they can reach the deeper layers of the epidermis and dermis. (For more information on melanin and protecting your skin against the sun and its aging effects, see Chapter 10, "The Sun Is No Fun," and Chapter 11, "Fighting Back Against Photoaging.")

Sweat Glands, Sebaceous Glands, and Other Skin Stuff

I can hear your reaction now: "Sweat? Glands? Why are we reading about this in a book on skin care?!"

Fact is, the specialized glands that produce sweat and other substances are all part of that complex organ, your skin. For that matter, so are your hair and nails. Fingernails, toenails, and hair contain keratin, the same tough protein in the horny layer on the surface of your skin.

In Chapter 7, "Beautiful Hair and Nails," I'll discuss the structure of hair and nails, and what you can do to keep them beautiful. But for now, let's take a look at why these other skin elements are so important.

Perspiration: A Positive View

You may think of perspiration as something that's more annoying than beneficial. But actually sweat glands perform a valuable service by pumping perspiration to the skin surface, where it evaporates, cools us off, and helps maintain a healthy internal body temperature. The flushing action of sweat also helps wash away harmful microbes.

Your skin houses around three million sweat glands. Some parts of the body have especially high concentrations, like your feet and palms; the skin of a typical adult palm harbors about three thousand glands per square inch.

Sweat glands respond to both external and internal factors. Hot weather can make you sweat, and so can strong emotions. If you doubt this, just see how sweaty your palms get next time you have to give a speech.

One of my patients once asked: "If perspiration is so great, why does it smell so bad?" Actually, much of our perspiration isn't really odorous; it's more than 99 percent water. The major culprit behind body odor is a specialized type of perspiration, produced by sweat glands in certain areas of the body, especially the armpits and groin. This fluid is thicker than the other type of sweat, and bacteria on the skin surface break it down into a substance that can only be called—well, let's stick with the term "odorous," shall we?

In many animals, these characteristic odors serve a useful function by signaling identity and sexual interest. (This is why your dog insists on sniffing other dogs' hindquarters when they meet.) Human beings prefer other methods of communication, and we do our best to eradicate these aromas—or at least mask them with others we like better, such as perfume.

More Than Skin Deep

Most of us mask perspiration odor by applying a deodorant or antiperspirant. What's the difference? Deodorants cover the smell with a more socially acceptable fragrance (some also contain antibacterial chemicals to help control odor). Antiperspirants, a more effective strategy, work by plugging the openings to armpit sweat glands, thus blocking perspiration from reaching the skin surface. The chemicals in antiperspirants don't work immediately. To make yours even more effective, try applying it at night so it has several hours to take effect before you need it the next day.

Sebaceous Glands: "Oiling" Your Skin

Another useful component of your skin is *sebaceous glands*. They produce *sebum*, a waxy, oily lubricant that moisturizes and protects your skin.

Sebum may sound unappetizing, but it comes in very handy. For one thing, as it travels to the surface, it carries away dead skin cells and debris from the lining of the pore. It also serves as a natural moisturizer for the skin and hair. If you have "oily" skin, the sheen you see is not actually oil but excess amounts of sebum. While the lubricant may make your face look a bit shiny, it also keeps your skin soft and smooth.

Well, unless you break out. Beneficial though it is, sebum can cause problems when it plugs pores rather than flowing smoothly through them. See Chapter 15, "Acne: An Age-Old Problem," for effective ways to treat this common annoyance.

Skin Smart
Sebaceous glands produce *sebum*, a waxy, oily lubricant that moisturizes skin.

More Skin Stuff

How do perspiration and sebum reach the outside world? They empty onto your skin surface through the tiny openings called *pores*. Sometimes this process gets short-circuited, and your pores fill with dead skin cells and sebum and become dilated and dark. These are called blackheads, and I'll discuss them further in Chapter 15.

Many skin care products promise to "shrink" pores or otherwise minimize them. However, pores are simply openings; they don't have tiny muscles that dilate and contract on demand. There are no substances you can apply to open or close them. You can temporarily shrink the appearance of the opening with toners, however. In Chapter 5, "Choosing the Right Toner and Moisturizer," I'll discuss how.

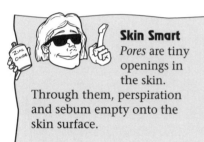

Skin Smart

Pores are tiny openings in the skin. Through them, perspiration and sebum empty onto the skin surface.

Other important components of your skin include small arteries (which supply nourishing blood and oxygen) and veins (which carry away carbon dioxide and other waste products of cellular metabolism). Nerve endings in the skin control blood flow and the activities of your sweat and sebaceous glands. As you saw earlier, they also transmit helpful signals to warn you of pain, pressure, temperature, and touch.

Let's Explode a Few Skin Care Myths!

Okay, now you have an idea of how your skin works. How about those hopeful claims from advertisers who want to convince you they can make it work better? It's time to explode a few myths. Take another look at the ads I cited at the beginning of this chapter. Let's see whether their claims hold up against what you now know about skin.

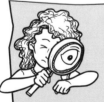

More Than Skin Deep

Skin will absorb some substances, given the right chemistry and conditions. This is the idea behind skin patches, a popular way to deliver medicine into the bloodstream. However, the medications in skin patches are formulated differently from most skin care products: They are highly concentrated and dissolved in an oil base so they can penetrate the epidermis. Furthermore, the substance in a patch is held against your skin for an extended period of time—certainly longer than a cream or lotion is likely to stay around.

Thigh Creams: Can You Melt Cellulite from the Outside?

Many of my patients complain bitterly about cellulite, those dimpled expanses of skin that afflict the upper leg.

Cosmetics companies are rushing to fill the demand by developing thigh creams, topically applied products that claim to trim thighs and smooth cellulite. Already a $90 million market, thigh creams are a hot item and sales continue to soar.

These creams aren't cheap; prices start at around $16.95 for 3 or 4 ounces. A 6-ounce container of some brands retails for $50 or more—definitely a costly proposition!

Thigh creams (as well as many other skin care products) are based on a seductive premise: that rubbing something on the surface will allow your skin to absorb its helpful ingredients. As you've seen, though, skin consists of multiple layers. While a topically applied cream might penetrate the horny layer, the molecules of most compounds are too big to be absorbed much deeper.

This is actually a safety feature since the dermis contains a rich network of blood vessels. If skin readily absorbed anything rubbed on it, foreign molecules would constantly enter our bloodstream and hitch a free ride to other parts of the body. This could have dangerous consequences.

Be wary of any products that vow to "penetrate" your skin. No matter what the ads promise, the molecular structure of most skin care products stops them from reaching the skin's deeper layers. As a general rule, rubbing them on the skin surface will not affect or enhance its underlying structure.

Suppose that a thigh cream somehow beats all these odds and manages to reach your subcutaneous layer. What would it do when it got there? There's no evidence that you can banish fat tissue or fibrous bands by applying these chemicals to it.

Sure, there are effective ways to get rid of fatty tissue, but they involve plastic surgery (see Chapters 24, "Should You Try Plastic Surgery?" and 25, "Popular Choices in Plastic Surgery"). A jar of thigh cream, unfortunately, is not the answer. If all these products slimmed us down like they promise, there wouldn't be a single dimpled thigh in North America. All of us would look like supermodels (from the waist down, at least!).

More Than Skin Deep

Researchers are working to develop topical agents that can penetrate effectively. Scientists at Duke University have packaged vitamin C in a solution of liposomes (synthetic pellets that can penetrate skin's superficial layers). This approach stabilizes the vitamin molecules and allows them to be absorbed by the dermis. While liposomes are promising, they are still experimental. Don't rush out and buy the first liposome cream you see.

Can You "Shrink" Pores?

Last week, one of my patients asked me a question. Barbara, a successful sales rep in her early 40s, felt self-conscious about the texture of her skin. "My pores are so big!" she complained. "Isn't there anything I can do to make my skin look smoother?"

As I explained earlier, pores are simply openings; they don't have tiny muscles that dilate and contract. While we're on the subject, there are no products that will get rid of them, either. You're born with a certain number of pores, and that number remains constant throughout life (barring injury to your skin). For that matter, you wouldn't want it to fluctuate. As you've seen, pores are necessary for normal, healthy skin. Without them, you'd be painfully dry and unable to perspire!

Some people, like Barbara, do have prominent pores. Like skin color, it's a tendency you inherit. Do you think the pores in one part of your face are more noticeable? This is quite common. The center of your face contains more oil glands, so the skin there may look more oily and textured than the skin at the sides of your cheeks and forehead. Sun exposure may also play a role. Over time, sun-damaged skin looks more bumpy and takes on an "orange peel" texture.

If you're concerned about the appearance of your pores, it will help to keep your skin clean so they retain as little dirt and oil as possible. Some companies market products specifically for pores, and some of these items may be helpful. However, one of the most effective ways to clean your pores is that humble remedy, soap and water. (For more information, see Chapter 4, "Clean Living: The Best Way to Clean Your Skin.")

Can You Supplement Your Skin's Collagen and Elastin?

Collagen and elastin are essential components of the skin that help it stay firm and supple. They are also popular components of many moisturizers and skin care products. Some marketers would have us believe that rubbing them on the skin will supplement the body's own built-in supply. This is supposed to reinforce sagging skin and plump out wrinkles.

Beauty Tips
Another approach to cleaning your pores: exfoliating products, which may help keep the superficial portion of the pores clear. You might try a mild toner or an alpha hydroxy acid lotion. For more tips on exfoliants, see Chapter 4.

But, like most cosmetic ingredients, collagen and elastin molecules are too big to absorb into the skin. At the present time, there's no evidence that topical applications can increase the amount of collagen or elastin in the dermis. On the other hand, collagen's large molecules do make it an effective moisturizer. They create a thin film on the skin surface that helps stop moisture from evaporating. (For more on moisturizers, see Chapter 5, "Choosing the Right Toner and Moisturizer.")

As you can see, your skin is a complex, multi-layered organ, and there's a lot more to it than meets the eye. So, the next time you encounter ads for thigh creams, pore shrinkers, and other miracle aids—be sure to read between the lines.

The Least You Need to Know

➤ Your skin is a complex organ—and the largest one you have.

➤ Skin comes in layers—lots of them. Skin cells are born deep within these layers and slowly migrate up to the surface.

➤ Within the lower layer (dermis) is a complex array of glands, blood vessels, and nerve endings. Sweat glands pump perspiration to the skin surface, where it evaporates, cools us off, and helps maintain internal body temperature; its flushing action also washes away harmful microbes. Sebaceous glands produce sebum, a waxy lubricant that moisturizes and protects skin.

➤ Skin color comes from melanin, a pigment that absorbs ultraviolet radiation. When the amount of melanin increases after sun exposure, the resulting "suntan" is your skin's attempt to protect you from dangerous UV rays.

➤ Most over-the-counter products can't be absorbed by skin's deeper layers. Be skeptical of anything that promises to "penetrate" your skin, and keep in mind how your skin works when evaluating product claims.

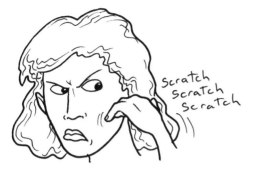

Common Complaints

Scratch Scratch Scratch

Recently a new patient, Susan, came to see me, complaining that her skin felt irritated and dry. "Doctor, I don't know what's wrong!" she said. "Suddenly I'm getting these flaky red patches on my cheeks and my skin feels tight."

As we chatted, I learned several things about Susan:

➤ She had moved from Seattle two months before to start a new job in New York.

➤ She had just celebrated her 54th birthday.

➤ She had just started using a new brand of expensive bar soap, a birthday gift from her daughter.

"Any of these could be responsible for your skin irritation," I told her. "And we'll look at several other possibilities, too. First, we'll find out what's causing the problem, and then we'll find ways to make you feel better."

As she was leaving, Susan thanked me, but still looked puzzled. "I always thought my skin was too oily," she mused, "but it's changed dramatically in just a few weeks, and now it's too dry. What do you think my skin type really is? And is it possible for my skin type to change this much?"

Don't Come Down with the "Too's"

Susan asks good questions. Let's take a minute to tackle this concept of "skin type."

The skin care industry seeks to convince us of two things: 1) there is one ideal skin type, and 2) none of us have it. Of course, the ads promise that we can correct our "faults" and attain perfect skin—if we buy the right products, that is!

If you believe everything the media says, you could end up with what I call a bad case of the "too's." This is a condition in which you start feeling self-conscious and hypercritical of your appearance. You tell yourself: My skin is too oily or too dry. My pores are too big, I have too many wrinkles, and my skin is too bumpy. You get the idea.

In fact, there's no such thing as one "perfect" skin-type. There is no single standard you should work toward achieving. Forget the arbitrary skin-type categories you read about in fashion magazines. You are an individual, and so is your skin. In this chapter, you'll discover ways to make your skin feel beautiful because then it will look beautiful, too.

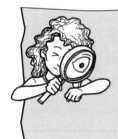

More Than Skin Deep

Depressed from comparing yourself to those gorgeous models in magazine photos? Relax! And remember: Computerized editing techniques allow photographs to be altered in many ways. Features can be transformed, blemishes and wrinkles minimized, colors enhanced. The models may really look like that. Then again, they may not.

News Flash: Your Skin Changes Constantly

As you learned in the previous chapter, skin is a complex organ. And, like your body's other organs, it is dynamic. It's in a state of constant change, adjusting and responding to alterations in its environment.

By "environment," I mean anything that can influence skin's function and appearance. This includes factors both inside and outside your body, such as

➤ Climate and changes in weather

➤ Exposure to the sun

➤ Cosmetics

➤ Moisturizers, cleansers, and other skin care products

➤ Emotions and stress

➤ Hormonal cycles, including your menstrual cycle and menopause

➤ Your overall health

This is just a partial list. Any of these factors, and many more besides, can affect your skin. Like Susan, you could go almost overnight from bemoaning your oily skin to wondering why it's so dry. Since your skin is dynamic, so is your skin type. At various points in your life, you're likely to experience all of the common complaints I discuss in this chapter—dryness, oiliness, combination skin, itching, puffy eyes, and sensitivity.

Saving Your Skin
Ironically, skin care products can cause many skin problems. Cleansers may dry your skin; heavy moisturizers may block pores and cause pimples. Your "skin type" can be a reflection of not just your skin itself, but also what you put on it.

Do You Have Dry Skin?

Like Susan, many women complain of dry skin. Obviously, "dry" is a subjective term. How do you know if your skin really falls into this category?

If your skin

➤ Looks scaly

➤ Has roughened or reddish patches

➤ Feels itchy

➤ Feels tight

➤ Shows tiny (surface) wrinkles that go away when you apply moisturizer

Skin Smart
Xerosis is the term health professionals use to describe epidermis that lacks the usual amount of moisture. Everyone else just calls it "dry skin."

then you may well have dry skin. Naturally, we doctors have a medical term for everything, even dry skin. We call it *xerosis*.

Why Does Skin Become Dry?

Remember in Chapter 2, "Your Skin: Don't Leave Home Without It" when I discussed the horny layer, the covering of hardened flat cells on the skin surface? The horny layer is water-resistant, but not waterproof. We are constantly losing water through our skin, as water from body cells slowly migrates to the surface and evaporates. On an average, we lose about a pint of water daily this way. (This is in addition to the water we lose through perspiration from sweat glands.)

But certain factors can increase the rate at which your skin loses water. If you live in a dry climate, for example, you'll probably experience dry skin because arid air speeds up the evaporation process. Most of us get drier skin during the winter, too, regardless of where we live, because artificially heated air is dry.

Another factor is age. As we get older, the horny layer loses some of its ability to hold water in. Not surprisingly, many of my older patients complain of dry skin.

Pampering Dry Skin

How can you counteract the drying process? Certainly, a mild cleanser and effective moisturizer are important. In Chapter 4, "Clean Living: The Best Way to Clean Your Skin," covers different types of skin cleansers, and Chapter 5, "Choosing the Right Toner and Moisturizer," discusses what to look for in a good moisturizer.

In addition, try these tips:

➤ When it comes to dry skin, cleanliness isn't always next to godliness. Baths and showers strip away skin's natural oils and dry your skin out more. Limit them to every second or third day, if possible. (If you're afraid you won't stay clean, try "spot-washing" just the areas that need it, like armpits, genitals, and feet, rather than immersing your entire body.)

➤ When you do bathe or shower, make it quick. The longer your skin is immersed in water, the more it will dry out.

➤ Keep your water tepid rather than hot. Hot water leaches more oil from your skin.

➤ Bath oils won't do much to combat dryness. Soaking in warm water takes out more of the natural oils and water from your skin than the added oils can keep in.

➤ After bathing, blot your skin with a towel till you're damp but no longer dripping. Then quickly pat moisturizer on your face and body to "seal in" the moisture.

➤ If your home has forced-air heat, consider a humidifier. Just be sure to clean it regularly to avoid problems with mold and bacteria. If you live in a fairly humid climate, simply opening a window a crack will increase moisture in dry heated rooms.

Beauty Tips
Sometimes those flaky areas we call dry skin are really cells in the horny layer that your skin has not shed completely. In this case, a mild exfoliant, such as an alpha hydroxy acid (see Chapter 12, "Help from Hydroxy Acids"), can remove them.

Susan's dry skin, it turned out, resulted from the combined forces of climate, age, and cleansers. Her move from Seattle (a city of temperate climate and abundant rainfall) to New York exposed her skin to drier, colder air. At the same time, natural changes in her skin as she moved through her 50s made it harder for her skin to compensate for the moisture loss.

The final insult, from her skin's point of view, was her daughter's well-meaning gift of fragrant lemon-scented soap. Bar soaps are harsher than some other types of cleansers, and citrus juices, as well as other fragrances, can be irritating.

I advised Susan on new skin care routines and suggested several products. She switched from bar soap to a water-soluble liquid cleanser and bought a creamy, fragrance-free moisturizer.

When I saw her two months later, she was beaming. Her flaky patches had smoothed out and her skin no longer felt tight. "My skin feels great!" she told me.

More Than Skin Deep

If you use a humidifier, be sure to clean it regularly, following the manufacturer's instructions. This is especially important if you live in an area with hard water, since mineral deposits will plug the unit and stop it from working properly. Also, mold and bacteria can collect in dirty humidifiers; you could be inhaling mold spores along with misty air. I want your skin to experience moisture, not mildew!

The Opposite Problem: Oily Skin

Some of my patients would give anything to be in Susan's shoes (or rather, her skin). Their skin is oily, and it drives them crazy.

The term *oily* is a misnomer because it sounds like your skin is coated with liquid oil. In fact, as you saw in Chapter 2, the glossy lubricant on your skin surface is called sebum, and it comes from sebaceous glands deeper in the skin. "Oily skin" simply means your glands produce more sebum than average.

Actually, it can be good to have somewhat oily skin—yes, really! When you produce plenty of sebum, your skin is well moisturized. It feels consistently smooth, and the moisture can reduce the appearance of wrinkles.

The problem, of course, is that oily skin so often breaks out. Sebum has a waxy, rather than liquid, consistency. When it mixes with the skin cells that line the pores, it may make them stick together. This sebum and skin-cell mix can plug the pores. As more sebum flows into the plugged pore, the pore stretches and sometimes breaks, leading to the characteristic blemishes and nodules we call acne.

Chapter 15, "Acne: An Age-Old Problem," offers a complete discussion of acne and acne treatments. But for now, here are some general guidelines on caring for oily skin:

➤ Don't irritate your skin. Yes, I know, people with oily skin are often advised to wash with extremely strong soaps and abrasive scrubs. However, making your skin red and irritated is not what you want either.

➤ Experiment with different kinds of cleansers to see what works best for you. Don't automatically reach for strong antibacterial soaps. You'll probably want to avoid "lipid-rich," "fatted," or "moisturizing" soaps, though. They can aggravate oily skin problems.

➤ Unlike your dry-skinned pals, you can go ahead and bathe every day if you wish. However, don't wash your face more than twice a day, no matter how many pimples you have. Use tepid water (not hot or cold), and avoid bath oils because they can be gummy. After washing, blot gently dry with a clean towel.

➤ Should you use moisturizers? Not necessarily. Some of my patients actually give themselves pimples by applying heavy lotions that their naturally-lubricated complexions don't need. Leave off all moisturizers for a week or so to see how your skin reacts. If you do feel you need a moisturizer, try an oil-free brand.

➤ You'll probably have the best luck with an oil-free foundation that contains no vegetable or mineral oil (note that some oily skin products do contain silicone oils; see Chapter 6, "At the Cosmetics Counter," for more tips on cosmetics).

➤ After your foundation dries completely, smooth on a light-textured oil-free powder. Choose one that's matte rather than shiny because your oily skin has a natural glow. Some foundations and powders actually have oil-absorbing ingredients. They are usually advertised as "oil-control" or "oil-regulating" products.

➤ Another option is a powder-based foundation that dries to a powdery finish. If you go this route, you may not need any powder at all.

If your skin does break out, don't pick or squeeze. Torturing your skin will only inflame blemishes further, and could damage or scar your skin. If you really want to have a pimple squeezed, ask your dermatologist for help.

Coping with Combination Skin

Your nose and chin are oily; they look shiny all the time, and they break out frequently (usually right before an important event). Meanwhile, the sides of your forehead and cheeks are dry. The skin there tends to be rough and flaky, and sometimes your soap makes it burn.

Does this sound like you? Welcome to the joys of combination skin. You feel like you have all the problems of each skin type but none of the advantages, and the products that help one type hurt the other.

All of us have combination skin to some extent. The center of your face contains more oil glands (see the diagram), so you may have what's sometimes called an oily "T zone" on the forehead, nose, and chin. This is perfectly normal, no matter what some cosmetics salespeople tell you.

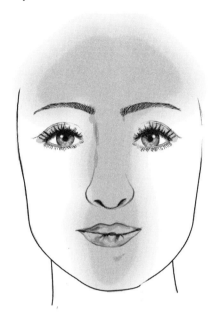

Combination skin often shows a characteristic pattern of oily and dry areas.

However, some people experience wildly differing symptoms, like acne and extreme dryness, at the same time. Frustrating though combination skin can be, there *are* things you can do about it:

➤ First, take a good look at your current skin care routine. Could it be drying out your skin or making it break out? Maybe you should stop applying toner (many toners contain alcohol, which is very drying), or switch to an oil-free moisturizing lotion rather than cream (heavy moisturizers are a frequent cause of pimples). Experiment! You may find that your face is objecting to what you put on it.

➤ Use gentle products; gear your overall face care to the needs of your dry, sensitive skin. If you really want to use stronger measures on the oily areas, apply them locally to the oily areas only and keep them away from your dry skin.

➤ Don't abrade your skin. Rubbing your skin too vigorously with washcloths, scrub pads, and loofahs can scrape it, leaving it red, rough, and irritated. It also pulls and stretches your skin.

➤ Think twice about using alcohol on your skin. Yes, I know, many products for oily skin contain alcohol. The theory seems to be that alcohol cuts oil, so it will work well at "de-oiling" your face. This is okay for some people with very oily skin.

However, it may irritate sensitive skin, even if that skin is oily. And alcohol doesn't do anything about the sebum still in the pores, which is where pimples begin.

As a guiding principle, think twice about doing anything to irritate or overdry your skin, period. Dry, irritated skin is no more attractive than oily skin. And who needs that?

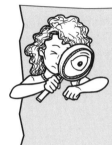

Saving Your Skin

If any skin problems persist for more than three weeks, consult your doctor. Stubborn patches of dry, itchy, or reddened skin, or acne that refuses to go away, could indicate a number of health conditions. Possibilities include allergies, dermatitis, infections, psoriasis, even skin cancer. Prompt diagnosis is the fastest path to a cure.

"Doctor, It Itches!"

In ancient China, they had a proverb: "Only kings and queens should itch, because it feels so good to scratch." You may feel less positive about scratching, particularly if itchy skin is driving you crazy.

Itches are a common complaint, especially in winter. Try to notice where you itch and when. If you consult your doctor about the problem, a detailed description of your itching may help him or her devise a solution.

Dry Skin: Usually the Culprit

In most cases, itching is a harmless, if annoying, symptom of dryness. Refer to the tips in this chapter for soothing and moisturizing dry skin.

Whatever you do, don't scratch. Scratching will stimulate the nerve endings in your skin and make the itching worse. Also, don't use topical antihistamines or medications that claim to stop itching to treat dry skin. They work well on poison ivy or insect stings, but may dehydrate dry skin even more.

Could You Have Allergies?

Does your itching get worse at certain times of the year? Or, maybe it really heats up after you've been around your boyfriend's cat or your mother's perfume.

If so, the itching could be due to allergies. An *allergy*, or *allergic reaction*, is an abnormal reaction of your immune system to a substance that doesn't bother most people. About 10 percent of Americans suffer from allergies. Our reactions include such delightful symptoms as skin rash, intense itching, hives, nasal congestion, and watery eyes.

Here are some of the most common causes of allergies:

➤ *Plant pollens*. If your itching gets worse at certain times of the year, or after you've spent time outdoors, this may be why. Trees usually pollinate in April and May, followed by grasses in May and June, and ragweed and goldenrod in August and September.

➤ *Dust mites*. Dust mites are tiny, eight-legged critters, less than one-twentieth of an inch long, that like to live in household dust. (There's no accounting for tastes, is there?) Actually, much household dust—prepare to be disgusted—consists of the mites themselves and their drop-pings. (Other major players are the dead skin cells shed from your horny layer.) Your itching could be triggered by fragments of dust mites and their feces.

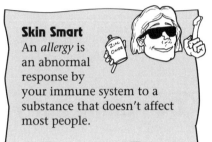

Skin Smart
An *allergy* is an abnormal response by your immune system to a substance that doesn't affect most people.

➤ *Cats and dogs*. Most people with this allergy think it's caused by animal hair. In fact, what sets off your immune system is *dander*, tiny flakes shed from the animal's skin and hair. (On human scalps, this shedding produces dandruff.)

➤ *Feathers in bedding*. Some people are sensitive to the feathers used to stuff pillows and mattresses. If you itch less on synthetic stuffing, this may be why.

➤ *Other common culprits* include perfumes, smoke, cleaning solutions, chemical fumes, deodorants, hair spray, nail polish, and hair dyes. Sometimes these substances can provoke an allergic reaction that affects far more than just the site of application. One of my patients suffered an allergic reaction to hair dye that made her entire face swollen and sore.

If you think you may have allergies, consult your doctor about getting allergy tests. Usually, this testing involves placing small amounts of different chemicals on your skin to see if any of them trigger an allergic reaction. You might also have a blood sample drawn to test for proteins that the immune system produces to fight allergy-causing intruders.

Generally, you can control allergies by taking medications and avoiding whatever sets off your immune system. If you're allergic to dust mites, it will help to keep your home as dust-free as possible. Fabrics—carpeting, curtains, upholstered furniture, bedding, pillows—harbor more dust than hard surfaces do.

Before leaving the subject of itches, I must mention that on rare occasions itching can be a sign of something more serious, like a hormonal abnormality, a blood condition, or even cancer. If your itching does not respond promptly to the pointers in this book, consult your doctor.

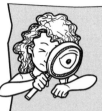

More Than Skin Deep

Your immune system protects you by recognizing "foreign" proteins, like those found in bacteria and viruses, and then organizing the body's defenses to surround and destroy the intruders. Sometimes your immune system forms a grudge against a substance that isn't really harmful, like pollen, and it goes on a rampage every time you're exposed to it. This makes you "allergic" to pollen.

De-Puffing Puffy Eyes

Some of my patients complain that their eyes look puffy, especially in the morning. What, they ask, can they do about it?

Often, puffiness is caused by water retention. If this is the case, gravity is on your side. After you arise in the morning, your body will gradually reabsorb the body fluids that have pooled overnight in the tissues around your eyes.

Hormones can play a role; some women retain water at certain points in their menstrual cycle. Women going through menopause can experience water retention, too. Poor circulation and kidney problems can also cause puffy eyes. And puffy eyes get worse as you age because the tissues get looser, allowing more water to accumulate.

If you're having trouble with puffy eyes, here are some suggestions:

➤ Cut back on salt, which makes you retain water. In particular, watch your salt intake at dinner and during the evening. Incidentally, some soft drinks and other beverages contain sodium; you could be taking in salt without realizing it.

Saving Your Skin

If you wake up every morning with puffy eyes for more than a week, consult your doctor. Persistently swollen eyes could indicate an allergy or, in rare cases, a thyroid, circulatory, or kidney condition.

➤ Keeping well hydrated is great, but don't overdo water or other fluids at bedtime.

➤ Once you're up, stay up. Help gravity do its work. Better still, get moving: Take a walk or do some housework. The more you move around, the more efficiently your body will reabsorb pesky fluids.

➤ Splash a little cool water on your (closed) eyes or apply a cool washcloth.

➤ Try a time-honored remedy: Cut two slices from a refrigerated cucumber. Sit comfortably, lean your head against a supportive headrest, and place one slice on each closed eye. Relax for 10 minutes.

Above all, be gentle with your eyes. Avoid extremes of hot or cold, and don't put harsh or unknown substances on or around your eyes. If you have any doubts about a remedy, don't use it.

Soothing Sensitive Skin

Do you have sensitive skin? So do I. In fact, so do most people. By this, I mean that all of us have the potential to develop skin irritations. As I mentioned earlier, skin is not static; it changes constantly in response to everything around (and inside) it. Even if you've never considered your skin especially sensitive, it could start acting up tomorrow.

The list of potential skin irritants is as varied as we are. Some of them, unfortunately, are common in skin care products. See Chapter 5, "Choosing the Right Toner and Moisturizer," for more details on ingredients to avoid, and follow these tips to reduce your risk of problems:

➤ Look for products labeled "fragrance-free" or "without perfume." According to the American Academy of Dermatology, fragrances cause more skin reactions than any other ingredient. And here's a discouraging fact: More than 5,000 different fragrances are used in skin care products.

➤ Fragrances can show up in items where you least expect them, like toilet paper, laundry detergents, fabric softeners, and household cleaners. Any of them can aggravate your skin.

➤ After fragrances, preservatives are the most common cause of skin reactions. You can't get away from preservatives, since all products that contain water must also contain substances to slow down spoilage. If they didn't, they would quickly become so contaminated that they would be worse for your skin than any preservative. Experiment with products that contain different preservatives to find the ones that don't annoy your skin.

Saving Your Skin
When it comes to product labels, "unscented" is not the same as "fragrance-free" or "without perfume." Products labeled "unscented" may still contain fragrance. Usually these perfumes are added to mask the unpleasant odor of preservatives and other chemicals.

➤ Don't apply cosmetics or any skin care products over broken skin or a skin rash. Give your skin time to heal first. (Topical antibiotic ointments or corticosteroid preparations made to help rashes or broken skin are the exception to this rule.)

➤ Don't pick at, pinch, or otherwise torture your skin. A useful rule to follow is: Don't do anything to your own skin that you wouldn't do to a baby's.

➤ If a product bothers your skin, return it to the store where you bought it and ask for your money back. It's not your fault that it irritated your skin, and you shouldn't be penalized for it. In any case, returning the product provides useful feedback to the store and the manufacturer; if their products are causing skin reactions in consumers, they want to know.

In general, use gentle products on your skin and avoid vigorous scrubbing and scraping. Even the toughest exterior can benefit from babying. Your skin has to last a lifetime, so be good to it!

More Than Skin Deep

Sometimes our skin has a right to get mad at us. One of my patients got so annoyed with a persistent pimple near his eye that he took a needle to it—literally. He cleaned a needle and tried to "burst" the pimple, figuring that would make it go away. Surprise! He woke up next morning with a face that was red, swollen, and painful. By puncturing the pimple, he had introduced bacteria and released irritating sebum into the surrounding tissue. He had to be hospitalized for two days and receive intravenous antibiotics to control his raging skin reaction. Moral: Don't try this at home!

The Least You Need to Know

➤ There is no such thing as "perfect" skin. Even people with gorgeous complexions have trouble from time to time.

➤ Skin is a dynamic, ever-changing organ. At various times in your life, you could have skin that is dry, oily, combination, or sensitive.

➤ Sometimes we are our skin's worst enemy. Many skin problems result from washing too much or using irritating products and cosmetics.

➤ Persistent skin complaints could be caused by health conditions or allergies. Treating the real problem will also help your skin.

➤ When it comes to skin care, the key word is *gentle*. Regardless of your skin type, use mild products and don't overdo. Your skin will thank you!

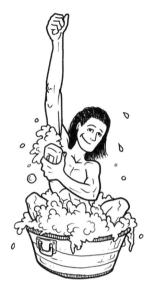

Clean Living: The Best Way to Clean Your Skin

Last year, American women spent almost $2.7 billion on products to clean their skin. Among those women was Dorothy, a real estate agent and grandmother of three.

Dorothy consulted me about her dry skin. "It started gradually, about four years ago," she said. "And it's just been getting worse all the time. Now it's really dry, and to make things worse, I've started breaking out too. Pimples! At my age!"

I reassured Dorothy that her situation isn't that unusual; skin can break out at any age. "Tell me," I asked, "how do you clean your skin?"

"Well, I use soap, of course," she replied. "Otherwise, it just doesn't feel like it gets clean."

To Soap or Not to Soap?

Do you wash your face with soap? Many of us do, for precisely the reason Dorothy mentions: It's the only way we feel really clean.

As kids, we were taught to scrub ourselves with soap. As teenagers, we used more soap—sometimes in extremely strong formulations—to combat acne and oily skin. Now that we're older, many of us continue to follow the same skin care regimen, even though our skin has altered considerably. We may no longer need quite as strong a cleanser, but we use it anyway.

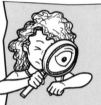

More Than Skin Deep

As a nation, Americans are really into soap. We shower or bathe daily, sometimes several times daily, and spend big bucks on a wide variety of products to scrub and "de-germ" our skin. This is a big contrast to Europeans, many of whom think that Americans overdo it just a bit. Some believe that a certain amount of exposure to germs strengthens one's immunity to disease. Who knows? It could be true.

How Soap Does Its Dirty Work

How do cleansers cleanse, anyway?

All soaps, whether fancy bars for your face or no-nonsense detergents for your floor, function the same basic way. They contain *surfactants*, substances that persuade oil and water to mix so they can be washed away. The stronger the surfactant ingredient in a soap, the more oily residue it can remove.

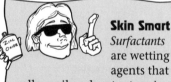

Skin Smart
Surfactants are wetting agents that allow oil and water to mix so they can be lifted off the skin. They are what give soap—any soap—its cleansing action.

As you saw in Chapter 2, "Your Skin: Don't Leave Home Without It," healthy skin is constantly secreting sebum, a waxy lubricant, from pores onto the skin surface. Ideally, an effective soap washes undesirable oils off your face while leaving enough sebum behind to moisturize your skin.

If a soap leaves your skin feeling dry, it is removing too much of this natural moisturizer or altering your natural pH. If it leaves your skin feeling greasy, either it isn't removing enough oil or it contains heavy lubricants of its own that could clog pores.

The pH Problem

In ads for soap and shampoo, you'll hear references to a product's "pH." The *pH* of a substance is a measure of its acid or alkaline content. We rank pH on a scale ranging from 0 to 14, with 7 being neutral. The further below 7 a pH value is, the more acidic the substance; the higher above 7, the more alkaline.

Why am I boring you with chemistry? Because soap has a built-in problem of incompatibility with skin: Its pH is generally too alkaline. Our skin is slightly acidic, with a pH of about 5 to 6, but the pH of most bar soaps hovers around 10 (although some are neutral, and a few are acidic). This change in the skin's pH can leave us with a tight, uncomfortable feeling.

> **Skin Smart**
> The *pH* scale (0–14) is a measure of how acid or alkaline a substance is. The pH of healthy skin is around 5–6. Dermatologists refer to the skin's acid pH level as its "acid mantle"; the acidity helps repel microorganisms from the skin surface.

A Survey of Soaps, or, A Soap by Any Other Name . . .

If you look in any drugstore, you'll face a bewildering variety of soaps, each claiming to do wonders for your skin. What type of soap is best for you? Here's a rundown:

➤ Deodorant soaps are stronger than many others because they contain an antibacterial ingredient to get rid of odor-causing bacteria. Use them on your body if you like that squeaky-clean feeling, but I don't recommend them for the face.

➤ Acne soaps are also strong, with drying ingredients or exfoliants.

➤ Beauty bars often have synthetic detergents, which (as you'll see) can be less drying and irritating to the skin than their natural counterparts. They often include moisturizers.

➤ Superfatted soaps contain extra fatty substances (such as cocoa butter, cold cream, petrolatum, or lanolin) to make them less drying.

➤ Transparent soaps, which contain fat and glycerin, are less harsh than some other soaps. They also don't lather quite as well as opaque soaps and tend to melt faster.

➤ Castile soaps, named for the region of Spain where they were first developed, are prepared from olive oil and come in both liquid and bar forms. Olive oil is a good moisturizer, although another component in many castile soaps, sodium hydroxide, may irritate some skins.

If it seems like there's no perfect soap—well, that's true. By its nature, soap offers a tradeoff: clean versus demoisturized. As with all skin care products, experiment to determine what works best for you.

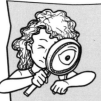

More Than Skin Deep

Soap is the oldest cleaning agent, dating back thousands of years. According to legend, the soap-making industry was born on Sapo Hill near ancient Rome, where peasants offered animals as burnt sacrifices to the gods. Fat from the animals overflowed the altar and soaked down through the wood ash into the clay soil. Quite by accident, someone discovered that this soapy clay was great for washing clothes. By 100 A.D., soap was a hit throughout the Roman Empire. Fittingly, the modern word *soap* comes from Sapo Hill, where it all began.

Do You Need an Antibacterial Soap?

In recent years, Americans have gone on an antibacterial binge, buying antiseptic facial soaps, body soaps, household cleaners, even pretreated germicidal sponges. Do you really need to use such a strong soap at home?

Probably not. Most antibacterial soaps on the market contain triclosan or other compounds that do kill bacteria and some viruses more effectively than regular soap. However, most regular soaps also get rid of most of the microbes we worry about.

Many doctors believe that it's overkill (so to speak) to use antibacterial soaps in the home. Some of these cleansers can be harsh and may irritate your skin. Unless your home situation requires hospital-quality disinfecting or you have a particular problem with infection, you probably don't need them.

What About Natural Soaps?

Many of my patients ask about soaps containing natural ingredients, like avocado, oatmeal, and citrus juice. They expect these soaps to be milder and less drying than synthetic products.

Ironically, however, synthetic cleansers may be far more gentle than their natural counterparts. Why? Because their pH can be custom-crafted in a laboratory to match the skin's own pH as closely as possible. Soaps with a similar pH are easier on your skin, since they clean with less impact on the skin's natural pH level. This leaves your skin feeling less "dry" after washing.

In my opinion, there's a lot of hype surrounding natural skin care products in general, and natural soaps in particular. Many natural soaps contain the same basic ingredients: animal or vegetable fat (such as lard, tallow, or coconut oil) and an alkaline surfactant. In addition, many claim to have nutrients that "nourish" the skin and promote good health, including vitamins, herbs, flowers, vegetables, and fruits.

Just be aware that you cannot absorb these nutrients through your skin, and you can't nourish your skin from the outside. Using a vitamin E soap won't supplement your body's supply of that particular vitamin, and sudsing with a vegetable-based cleanser doesn't count toward your daily quota of veggies.

Having said that, I realize that many people do enjoy experimenting with natural products. If that includes you, go for it.

Some of the most popular ingredients in natural soaps include:

➤ Oatmeal, a mild abrasive usually intended for oily skin. Marketers claim it's less irritating and can absorb oil better than some of the other soaps made for oily skin.

➤ Avocado, which is rich in oil.

➤ Aloe vera, the sap from the aloe vera plant, a traditional remedy for skin irritation and burns.

➤ Essential oils, which are highly concentrated extracts of oils from plants (lavender, sandalwood, patchouli, and so forth).

➤ Peppermint, balm mint, wintergreen—depending on your skin, "minty" ingredients can feel refreshing or they can burn and sting. Consider saving them for your feet instead of your face.

If you experience skin irritation from any of these ingredients, switch to a milder cleanser immediately.

Saving Your Skin

If you tend to have allergic reactions to plants, you're more likely to have problems with plant-based soaps and natural skin care products in general.

Getting the Most from Your Soap

No matter what soap you prefer, here are some tips for using it effectively:

➤ Always use the mildest cleanser you can. Even if your skin is very oily, using a highly alkaline soap that strips a lot of your natural oils could irritate your skin.

➤ Try a liquid cleanser, such as a moisturizing body wash or body shampoo. Bar soaps are often more harsh than liquids.

➤ Wash your face by using your fingertips to work up a lather, and then rinse by splashing water on your face with your hands. Rinse well (at least a dozen splashes); soap film will irritate your skin if you don't get it off completely.

Beauty Tips

It's easy to forget that bubble bath is a type of soap. Soaking in a bubbly tub, especially in hot water, will strip the oils from your skin and dry it out. In addition, some people react to the heavy perfumes and bubble-making agents in these products.

➤ Even if your skin is oily, don't wash your face more than twice a day. Instead, use an oil-control lotion under your makeup, or carry blotting papers with you to remove shine throughout the day.

➤ Be flexible. Your skin changes constantly in response to a lot of different variables: the seasons, hormonal cycles, lifestyle, and emotions, just to name a few. Be prepared to adjust your cleaning routine as necessary. The soap that seems just right during a hot humid summer may be too harsh during the winter.

Saving Your Skin
How do you know if your current cleanser is too strong? Try washing your face, blotting it dry with a towel, and waiting 20 minutes. Then smile. Does your skin feel tight, like it's being pulled? If so, it's time to find a milder cleanser.

Be careful if you use a washcloth on your face; it can be abrasive and hard on your skin. Make sure you rinse your washcloth thoroughly after you use it, since soap residue left on the cloth will irritate your skin the next time you use it. Also, let the washcloth air-dry completely between uses; keeping it constantly damp is unsanitary.

Water-Soluble Cleansers

If your skin feels dry, especially after you wash with soap, consider trying a *water-soluble cleanser*. These products, which come in liquid form, dissolve in water. You can splash them off or wipe them away. Some also contain a light emollient to leave the skin feeling moisturized.

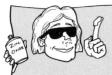

Skin Smart
Water-soluble cleansers are non-soap lotions that dissolve in water. They don't clean quite as well as soap, but are less drying.

Water-soluble cleansers represent a tradeoff: They don't clean quite as well as soap, but their ingredients are milder and often they are less drying. A good product can do an effective job of cleaning your skin and removing makeup, without stripping away as much oil as soap would.

As with all skin care products, it's important to comparison shop. Any company can label its cleanser "water-soluble," but some of them definitely clean better and rinse away more easily than others.

When using a water-soluble cleanser, follow these tips:

➤ Wash your hands first, then wet your face thoroughly. If you're doing this at the sink, use your hands to splash water on your face. Use tepid water, rather than hot or cold.

➤ Rub the cleanser gently over your face. If you like, you can also pat it lightly around your eyes to take off eye makeup.

➤ Use your hands in preference to a washcloth; washcloths can be rough-textured and abrasive. If you really don't want to use your hands, choose a soft, smooth-textured fabric for your washcloth, and be gentle.

➤ Rinse by splashing lots of tepid water on your face with your hands.

➤ If your face doesn't feel quite clean, or if there are remnants of makeup left, repeat these steps.

➤ Your skin should feel clean and moisturized, but not greasy. If one cleanser doesn't seem to do the job, try another.

Most water-soluble cleansers don't lather, but some do. The lathering products tend to be a little stronger and more drying (although still less drying than soap), and some women with oily skin prefer them. If this sounds good to you, look for terms like "gel," "foaming," or "face wash" on the label.

Lathering cleansers may not be appropriate for washing off eye makeup, since they may be too drying for your eyelids. A good compromise might be a non-lathering cleanser around your eyes, and a foaming variety on the rest of your face.

Remember Dorothy, my patient with the double whammy of dry skin and pimples? I advised her to switch from bar soap to a water-soluble cleanser, and her dry skin improved almost immediately. It turned out that she had been applying a heavy cream moisturizer (to compensate for her soap-induced dryness), so I recommended a lighter moisturizing lotion instead.

So effective was her new cleansing regimen that within a few weeks her pimples had disappeared, even as her skin felt more supple. She was delighted with the results.

Wipe-Off Cleansers

Wipe-off cleansers include cold creams and liquid makeup removers. They tend to be heavier than water-soluble cleansers and harder to remove. Often they require repeated wiping, which pulls at the skin.

I'm not a big fan of these products myself. However, cold cream remains popular with many women for removing makeup. Certainly modern cold creams are a big improvement over their greasy forebears, and they wipe off much more easily.

Saving Your Skin
Most facial cleansers that cause problems don't cause them immediately. It may take as long as six months before pimples, dry skin, or other reactions appear. Don't assume that your current cleanser is okay just because you've been using it for a month or so. Persistent problems call for an assessment of every product you put on your skin.

Skin Smart
Wipe-off cleansers are not water-soluble so they must be removed, as their name says, by being wiped off. They can leave an oily residue on the skin that may block pores and make you break out.

Look for one with a light texture that wipes on and off easily; if you have to rub and tug at your skin to get it off, it's too heavy. Remove the cleanser with a soft clean cloth or soft, high-quality facial tissues (bargain-brand tissues can be rough and irritating). It should leave your skin feeling pleasantly moisturized, but not greasy.

Try a sample of a product, or buy a trial size rather than a magnum container. Before you invest a lot of money in any wipe-off cleanser, make sure it won't block your pores and cause pimples.

If you have extremely dry skin, wipe-off cleansers may be your best choice. However, many women have better luck with the water-soluble cleansers described earlier.

Shedding Your Skin: Exfoliants

As you saw in Chapter 2, your skin cells are born deep in skin's lower layers, migrate to the surface over a period of about two weeks, and then form part of the horny layer before being shed. Sometimes the cells in the horny layer don't shed as evenly or regularly as they should. Skin cells may clump together after they reach the surface and not slough off like they're supposed to. The old cells, enduring greater exposure to the elements, become dry, cracked, and uneven.

Often these developments are caused by natural changes that occur in the skin as you get older. You may also see similar changes in acne-prone skin, where clumps of sticky skin cells plug up the pores. Whatever the cause, the result is skin that looks dull, rough, even flaky (the flakes are those dead horny layer cells hanging around after they're no longer wanted). Another result can be acne, if excess cells block pores and interfere with the normal secretion of sebum.

How can you get rid of old skin cells? You might try an *exfoliant*, a product that removes excess cells from the skin surface.

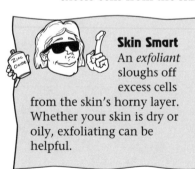

Skin Smart
An *exfoliant* sloughs off excess cells from the skin's horny layer. Whether your skin is dry or oily, exfoliating can be helpful.

A word of caution here: Advertisers would have us believe there's a fabulous new skin lurking just underneath the outer layer, and exfoliating a few cells will unveil it in all its glory. But remember, all the horny layer cells are dead anyway; the difference between the ones on top and those just below is subtle, to say the least.

Shedding your outer microlayer will not magically clear up all skin problems. It won't stimulate your skin to produce new cells, nor will it give you the gleaming epidermis of your favorite model or movie star (sorry).

So what can exfoliants do? They can make your skin look a little smoother because they rub off beat-up surface cells and expose the newer ones underneath. They also help your skin absorb moisturizers better because the hard, dead surface cells have been removed. And they can minimize acne by removing the clumps of sticky cells that block the surface of the pores. Pretty good, when you find a product that does something beneficial for both dry and oily skin!

Exfoliants come in many forms: abrasive sponges, pads, and brushes; cosmetic scrubs; facial masks; toners; alpha and beta hydroxy acids; tretinoin; and skin peels. Toners are covered in Chapter 5, "Choosing the Right Toner and Moisturizer," alpha and beta hydroxy acids in Chapter 12, "Help from Hydroxy Acids," tretinoin in Chapter 13, "Tretinoin and Antioxidants: Age-Tamers?" and skin peels in Chapter 20, "Make Your Skin More A-Peeling." In this chapter, you'll learn how to use the rest of these products most effectively.

Abrasive Sponges, Pads, and Brushes

Several companies market special pads and brushes for exfoliating your skin. I don't recommend them as a rule. Many are too abrasive and irritating. They're also hard to keep clean, and you certainly don't want to scrub your face with a rough, dirty pad.

If you really want to try one of these items, here are some tips:

➤ Choose the softest brush you can find.

➤ Start by using it no more than once a day, at bedtime.

➤ Wet your face and the brush thoroughly, and rub the brush very gently on your skin. You may want to apply a creamy moisturizer to your face first, to reduce the abrasive action.

➤ Rinse your face thoroughly by splashing with water.

➤ Gently blot your face with a clean towel until it's damp but not completely dry, then apply moisturizer.

➤ Go easy the first several times you use the brush, to make sure your skin won't get irritated.

➤ Always clean the brush with soap and water every time you use it, and allow it to air dry before you use it again.

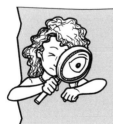

More Than Skin Deep

When using any exfoliant, be gentle! Hard scrubbing will hurt your skin, not help it. At best, you could end up with irritated skin; at worst, it could become inflamed or even infected. If you wouldn't do it to your best china, for heaven's sake, don't do it to your face.

Cosmetic Scrubs

I sometimes advise patients to use cosmetic scrubs rather than brushes or pads. Remember that they too must be used with extreme care to avoid irritation. Cosmetic scrubs are creams or lotions containing small particles. When you rub them on your face, the particles scrub horny layer cells from your skin, to be washed away when you rinse off the cream.

There are a number of good cosmetic scrubs available. Here's how to find one that works well for you:

➤ Choose a product with a light texture and fine, even particles. Scrubs with large or irregularly shaped particles can scratch and irritate your skin. Products that are too heavy or waxy will be hard to rub on and wash off. Some scrubs contain oils that may actually clog pores.

➤ Natural abrasives aren't necessarily better than synthetics. Fragments of peach pits, almond pits, sea shells, and other natural substances are often irregular and sharp-edged. They can nick skin and do more harm than good.

➤ Start slow by using the scrub no more than once a day, at bedtime. Exfoliation can make your skin more sensitive to sunlight, so let it recover overnight. And, as always, use a sunscreen in the morning.

➤ Always wet your face thoroughly before using the scrub. Dab it on your face and massage gently with upward strokes. Use your hands, not a washcloth, brush, or pad. Avoid pulling and stretching your skin.

➤ Rinse off by splashing tepid water on your face.

➤ Blot your face gently with a clean towel, and apply moisturizer while your skin is still damp.

This is not a case of "no pain, no gain." If any scrub feels uncomfortable or painful while you're using it, or if it leaves your skin feeling sore or scraped, try a different one. But not immediately; apply a soothing moisturizer and wait several days to give your skin time to recover. If irritation persists, call your doctor.

Facial Masks

A third exfoliant option is a *facial mask*, a product that you rub on your face and leave in place for awhile. When you remove the mask, it can lift old skin cells and impurities off your skin.

There are four main types of masks:

➤ Wax-based masks go on warm, then are removed after they cool. They help moisturize the skin.

➤ Earth-based masks (the familiar "mud packs") contain clays that can absorb skin oil. They are most popular for acne and oily skin.

➤ Hydrocolloid masks are water-based pastes, often with added ingredients like honey, avocado, or vitamin oils.

➤ Vinyl and rubber masks come in a tube or pouch, which you squeeze to apply directly to your face. The mixture dries, leaving a thin film on your skin that removes surface oil and cells when you strip it off.

Beauty Tips
As with all exfoliants, I recommend using a mask in the evening, not in the morning before an important meeting. That way, if your skin reacts badly, it will at least have several hours to recover before being exposed to sunlight and the scrutiny of co-workers.

Masks can feel soothing, moisturizing, and refreshing. On the other hand, they can also be irritating and drying. It all depends on the ingredients and how your skin reacts to them.

A mask should not hurt or sting. If you experience any discomfort while it's on, remove it immediately and splash your face with tepid water. If your skin still feels uncomfortable, wash with a mild soap, preferably a water-soluble cleanser, and rinse thoroughly.

Then (I bet you know what I'm going to suggest next) blot your face gently dry, apply moisturizer—and find a different product!

The Least You Need to Know

➤ Skin changes constantly, and so should the way you wash it. The soap you use during summer may parch your face in winter.

➤ Although it's the most popular cleanser, soap can be harsh and drying. Explore alternatives, like water-soluble cleansers and mild exfoliants.

➤ Exfoliants, which remove dead skin cells, can benefit a wide variety of skin types.

➤ No product should burn or sting your skin. If it does, it's not for you.

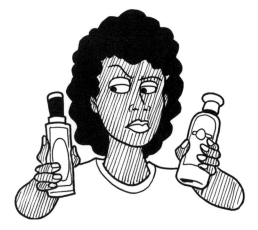

Choosing the Right Toner and Moisturizer

In Chapter 1, "Buying Beauty in a Bottle," you met my friend Maria, who was searching for the perfect line of skin care products. She's still searching!

Over a recent lunch, Maria produced her latest purchases: attractively packaged toner and moisturizer made by a well-known company. "They smell wonderful," I commented. "But I know your skin tends to get dry. Why did you buy the toner? Why not just the moisturizer?"

"Well, the salesperson said they really should be used together for a complete skin care program," she replied. "I put the toner on first to tighten my pores, and then I use the moisturizer to make my skin less dry."

Over dessert, I admitted I was skeptical. "Toners can be very drying," I pointed out. "I'm afraid that you might need that moisturizer just to counteract the toner."

"Then why do companies sell them together, and tell you to use both?" she asked.

Good question. Often the reason may be simple: They make more money that way.

Does Your Skin Really Need "Toning"?

What are toners, anyway? You may see them sold under a variety of names: astringents, fresheners, clarifying lotions. No matter what they're called, *toners* are solutions or lotions designed to remove surface skin cells, soap residue, and oils from skin. They're often heavy on water and alcohol, and sometimes contain other ingredients like salicylic acid, witch hazel, or propylene glycol.

When you put toner on your face, your skin tingles. In fact, this is why many people buy it; they enjoy the sensation of coolness and find it refreshing.

If you enjoy the tingle, go for it. Be aware, though, of the real reason your skin tingles: Something in the toner is irritating it. Generally, it's ethyl alcohol, a topical antiseptic and solvent.

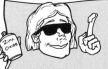

Skin Smart
Toners are solutions or lotions that remove surface skin cells, soap residue, and oils from the skin. Some can be irritating, especially those with a high alcohol content.

Beauty Tips
While toners don't really shrink pores, sometimes they can give that impression. For instance, if oils and dead skin cells clog the outer portion of a pore, they will make it stretch slightly. Removing these residues with a toner can allow the pore to return to normal size.

While some people enjoy that tingling sensation, others say that toners make their skin burn, sting, or itch. Not surprisingly, they also find toners drying. This is just as true for expensive products as it is for discount brands.

Let's look at some of the claims that marketers make for toners:

➤ Can toners close your pores? As we saw in Chapter 2, "Your Skin: Don't Leave Home Without It," pores don't have muscles, and they can't open and shut on command. Therefore, toners won't close or tighten them. Some toners may give the appearance of minimizing pores, but that's because they irritate your skin and make it swell slightly. This does shrink pore openings, but only temporarily.

➤ Can they deep-clean your skin? Well, that depends on what you mean by "deep." A toner can remove surface oils and debris, which may be helpful for oily or acne-prone skin. They can also clean the outermost area of a pore, but they don't go any deeper than that.

➤ Do toners make your skin produce less oil? No. Some marketers would have you believe their products can lower the skin's oil output, but this isn't true; the toner cuts surface oil only.

Using a Toner

You are most likely to benefit from a toner if you have oily skin and want a little extra help removing surface oil and cosmetics that your cleanser leaves behind.

Follow these steps:

➤ Wash your face thoroughly and gently; rinse by splashing tepid water on your face with your hands. (See Chapter 4, "Clean Living: The Best Way to Clean Your Skin," for guidelines on cleansers.)

➤ Pat your face gently with a clean, soft towel until it's damp, but not completely dry.

➤ Soak a clean cotton ball with toner. Rub it gently over your entire face (be careful not to tug or stretch your skin). Then splash off with water.

➤ If you see any makeup left on the cotton, soak a new cotton ball in toner and repeat the process.

➤ Apply your moisturizer.

Look for a toner that leaves your skin feeling smooth, not dry. Any tingling you experience should feel pleasant and pass quickly.

The Case for Irritant-Free Toners

Some companies have come out with toners that are advertised as "irritant-free." Before accepting this label at face value, check the product's ingredient list. If you notice any ingredients that bother your skin (see "Ingredients to Avoid" later in this chapter), find another toner.

For most of my adult patients, I recommend sticking with a good, mild cleanser followed by a moisturizer. Toners may be used occasionally to remove dead surface skin cells. Generally, I recommend more frequent use in the hot humid summer months than in the winter.

Teenagers with oily or acne-prone skin may benefit from the daily use of toners because they remove surface oils and dead skin cells that can clog the outermost portion of pores. But no one should use a toner to make up for inadequate cleaning. If your cleanser isn't removing makeup and surface oil effectively, maybe you should think about looking for another cleanser.

Saving Your Skin
As with all skin care products, don't use any toner that makes your skin burn, sting, redden, swell, flake, or break out. Nor should the toner leave your skin feeling dry, tight, and irritated. Return it to the store where you bought it and try a different product. If any skin reaction lasts longer than three weeks, consult your doctor.

Why Use Moisturizers?

Unless your skin is extremely oily, you'll need a moisturizer. In fact, a good moisturizer is one of your skin's best friends.

As you saw in Chapter 3, "Common Complaints," water constantly evaporates through our skin into the air, at a rate of roughly one pint per day. The more water our skin loses, the drier it gets. This evaporation rate can vary based on a number of factors, including genetics (we inherit a tendency toward dry or oily skin), climate (if the air around us is very dry, we lose water faster), and age (over time, the horny layer becomes somewhat less effective at holding water in).

How do moisturizers help? They form a film on your skin that functions as a barrier, helping to hold the water in longer. This is a good thing, but not necessarily for the reasons advertisers would have you believe.

Sometimes moisturizers are advertised as preventing wrinkles. However, moisturizers applied to the surface of the skin do not change the physiology of the dermis. Therefore, in and of themselves they don't prevent wrinkles from forming. (Certain additions to moisturizers, such as alpha hydroxy acids and sunscreens, may help in this regard. See Chapters 11, "Fighting Back Against Photoaging," and 12, "Help from Hydroxy Acids.")

That said, it's true that the very fine lines caused by facial tightness when the skin is dry can be eased by applying a moisturizer, and a moisturized wrinkle tends to look softer than a dry one.

Stalking the Perfect Moisturizer

An effective moisturizer should contain an oil or oil-like substance that spreads out smoothly to create an even layer over the skin surface.

You'll find four main types of oils in moisturizers:

➤ *Vegetable oils.* A staggering number of plants contribute moisturizing oils: almond, avocado, basil, carrot, coconut, corn, jojoba, macadamia, olive, palm, rice bran, safflower, sandalwood, soybean, sunflower seed, and wheat germ (to name just a few). Many vegetable oils can be absorbed into the skin, allowing them to moisturize the epidermis. Generally, one moisturizes about as well as any other in this list; exotic specimens from faraway lands aren't necessarily more effective.

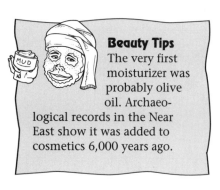

Beauty Tips
The very first moisturizer was probably olive oil. Archaeological records in the Near East show it was added to cosmetics 6,000 years ago.

➤ *Animal oils.* Generally, this means fish oils or lanolin (derived from sheep's wool). Sometimes you will see other animal fats (lipids), such as cholesterol, glycolipids, or phospholipids. Like plant-based oils, animal oils can be absorbed into the skin.

➤ *Mineral oils*. This category includes substances derived from petroleum (the familiar "mineral oil" and Vaseline) and silicone oils derived from sand or rock (cyclomethicone, phenyl trimethicone, dimethicone). They may sound less appealing than plant oils, but they're great moisturizers. Petroleum derivatives are heavy, and some people find they cause pimples; silicone oils are lighter. The molecules of mineral oils are too large to be absorbed by the skin, but this isn't necessarily bad. The oils stay on the skin surface and form an effective barrier against water loss.

➤ *Vitamin E*. Usually listed on labels as *tocopherol*, its chemical name, vitamin E makes a good moisturizing oil. Some companies would have you believe that it can "nourish" your skin, but as you've seen, you can't nourish skin from the outside in. There are also a lot of claims made about its antioxidant properties, but these may be overblown. (For more on antioxidants and vitamins, see Chapter 13, "Tretinoin and Antioxidants: The Age-Tamers?")

Remember, any moisturizer that contains oils may aggravate acne-prone skin. Does this mean people with acne-prone skin shouldn't use a moisturizer at all? No, it doesn't.

Some products contain other substances that aren't oils but can also moisturize effectively—for instance, collagen, a protein component of the skin's dermis layer. Spreading it on your skin won't supplement or strengthen your own collagen, but it does create an effective film that guards against water loss. Collagen molecules are too big to be absorbed, but as you saw for mineral oils, this can be a plus for blocking evaporation.

Other moisturizing ingredients include *humectants*, which may draw water to the skin from the environment or from the dermis. Humectants may be used in "oil-free" preparations, which are recommended for acne-prone skin. Some examples of oil-free moisturizers include the following:

➤ *Mucopolysaccharides and hyaluronic acid*. Like collagen, mucopolysaccharides, including hyaluronic acid, are natural components of skin, with large molecules that can't be absorbed. They form a good water-binding film on the skin surface.

➤ *Glycerin*. A water-attracting humectant, glycerin has long been used to hydrate chapped skin.

> **Saving Your Skin**
> Petroleum jelly can make a great facial moisturizer if you have very dry skin which is not at all acne prone. Massage it into the skin for two or three minutes at night before bed (it's too greasy for daytime use). Then gently wipe off the excess. What remains will hydrate the skin.

> **Skin Smart**
> A *humectant* is a substance that draws water to the skin from the environment or from the dermis, helping the skin retain moisture.

53

➤ *Propylene glycol.* In terms of its action on skin, propylene glycol has similar properties to glycerin. In high concentrations, propylene glycol may be irritating.

Which ingredient is best? All of those I've discussed can do a good job of holding in water, and a typical moisturizer contains several. If you have dry skin, you might look for a blend of an emollient that sinks into the skin (such as vegetable or animal oil) and one that remains on the skin surface to bind in water (like mineral oil or collagen). Experiment to find the combination that works best for you.

If your skin is naturally oily, you may not need a moisturizer. Try cutting back on toners and switching to a milder cleanser to make sure you're not drying out your skin with harsh products. If you still feel you need a moisturizer, try one labeled "oil-free." Note that some "oil-free" moisturizers do contain silicone oils, which tend to be lighter-textured than vegetable and animal oils, and better tolerated by many oily complexions. For more information, see "Ingredients to Avoid" later in this chapter.

Another choice for people with oily skin is an "oil-controlling" moisturizer. These products contain ingredients such as talc, clay, or special polymers that absorb oil. Their moisturizing components prevent them from drying the skin too much, while their oil absorbers soak up excess oils.

More Than Skin Deep

Lanolin, a popular moisturizer, comes from a greasy coating found on sheep's wool (which explains its other name, "wool wax"). People have appreciated lanolin's lubricating properties for centuries, ever since someone noticed that shepherds' hands became remarkably soft and smooth after handling lambs. In addition to skin care, lanolin is used as a dressing for leather goods, a base in shoe polish and grease paint, and a protective coating for metals. Some people are sensitive to it, and their skin may become red, swollen, and itchy after contact with lanolin-based products. Often they're the same people who itch from wearing wool clothing.

How Many Moisturizers Do You Need?

Until recently, moisturizers came in two basic categories: those for the face, and those for everywhere else. Traditionally, women spent 90 percent of their time and money on the facial products, and only 10 percent on the rest.

Scenting a huge potential market, companies began introducing specialized moisturizers for different areas of the body. First came eye creams, and then foot creams. These days you can find a moisturizer for just about every body part—thighs, legs, elbows, neck, lips, you name it.

Do you really need this many moisturizers? Probably not. There's no reason you can't apply your regular facial moisturizer around your eyes, on your neck, or anywhere else. Any product that hydrates the skin on your face will do the same for the rest of you. The only limitations may be price (facial moisturizers are probably too expensive to lavish on your entire epidermis) and texture (many are creamy and could stain clothing).

You could also use many body products on your face. However, some might not be ideal because they contain alcohol, fragrance, or other potentially irritating ingredients. In my opinion, you need two basic moisturizers: one for your face and one for your body.

If your lips are persistently dry, you could also try a lip moisturizer. You can find a wide choice of brands in cosmetic departments and drugstores. Or, try a petroleum jelly—like Vaseline, which is highly effective and a lot cheaper. You can apply lipstick right over it. If dryness or chapping persist, you may be reacting to your lipstick or lipliner. Stop using the product for a few weeks, and see if that clears up the problem.

Tips for Applying Moisturizer

Whatever moisturizer you choose, remember the following:

➤ Wash your hands first, then your face.

➤ Always apply moisturizer while your face is still damp. Put it on first thing after you step out of the shower or after you wash your face.

➤ Dab moisturizer on each cheek and on your nose, chin, and forehead.

➤ Use your hands to lightly spread the moisturizer over your face with gentle, upward strokes. Don't worry about rubbing the moisturizer in; let your skin absorb it naturally.

➤ Never rub hard or tug at your skin. If your moisturizer is so thick that it's difficult to rub gently, it may be too cold; try placing the container near a lamp or in a warm area before applying it. If it's still too stiff, try a different product.

➤ If your moisturizer doesn't contain sunscreen, apply sunscreen or makeup with sunscreen after the moisturizer dries during your daytime application.

Always wait until your skin is completely dry before exposing it to wind or cold. Otherwise, your skin could become chapped.

Beauty Tips
Some companies market special types of water: sterilized, ionized, European, spa, mineral, or glacier water. They are added to cosmetics or packaged separately in atomizers for misting the skin. As far as your skin is concerned, there's no difference between fancy water and the stuff that emerges from your bathroom tap. Save your money.

Ingredients to Avoid

My patients frequently ask if there are certain ingredients they should avoid in skin care products.

Yes! But which ones they are depends on your skin type, since what bothers oily skin may not irritate dry skin and vice versa. Below, I cite frequent offenders for each skin type. Keep in mind, though, that everybody's skin is unique. You may have no problem with these items, or you may be sensitive to an ingredient that's not listed here.

Dry Skin

If you have dry skin, use caution with the following:

➤ *Acetone.* Removes oil from the skin surface.

➤ *Alcohol.* Can be very drying. Note, however, that some ingredients, like alcohol esters and cetyl alcohol, sound like alcohol but lack its irritating effects.

➤ *Benzoyl peroxide.* A disinfectant and drying agent that's often used for acne. Can be very irritating to dry skin.

➤ *Camphor.* Found in many acne products; can be irritating.

➤ *Citrus juices* (lemon, orange, grapefruit, lime, tangerine). Citrus fruit smells and tastes wonderful but has a high acid content and can irritate the skin.

➤ *Eucalyptus.* A potential irritant found in some acne products.

➤ *Menthol.* Can be irritating.

➤ *Mints* (peppermint, balm mint, wintergreen, and so on). Can feel cool and refreshing, but may irritate the face. Consider saving them for your feet (see "Beauty Treatments to Try at Home," later in this chapter).

➤ *Salicylic acid.* This beta hydroxy acid (see Chapter 12, "Help from Hydroxy Acids") and mild exfoliant can irritate the skin.

Saving Your Skin

Witch hazel, found in some toners, is a compound that combines an extract from the witch hazel shrub with alcohol and water. Note that some products advertised as alcohol-free contain witch hazel.

Remember that labels list ingredients in sequence from highest to lowest quantities. The earlier something comes in the list, the more of it the product contains. Keep this in mind when you evaluate products; something that irritates your skin in high quantities may be fine in lower concentrations.

Oily Skin

Earlier, I noted that ingredients that annoy dry skin may not do the same to oily complexions. Be aware, however, that this isn't always the case; even if an ingredient doesn't dry your skin out, you could still find it irritating or sensitizing.

Oily-skinned folks have other concerns as well when it comes to ingredients. In particular, you need to watch out for the oils in skin care products. Many acne-prone people have trouble with petroleum-based oils (mineral oil and Vaseline, for example), which can be great moisturizers for dry skin but tend to leave a greasy film.

Lanolin, a common ingredient in moisturizers, may also be too heavy for you. Check the product label, since lanolin could appear in several forms (lanolin alcohol, lanolin oil, acetylated lanolin, or hydroxylated lanolin).

Always look for oil-free products, but be aware that many products labeled "oil-free" aren't always, well, oil free. They may lack vegetable, animal, and petroleum derivatives, but some do contain silicone oils (cyclomethicone, dimethicone, or phenyl trimethicone). While they are lighter than other oils and are likely to be well tolerated, they could still cause problems if your skin has a very strong tendency to break out.

I also recommend going light on products with alcohol. Alcohol is drying for almost everybody. Only people with extremely oily skin are likely to be able to tolerate it.

More Than Skin Deep

You've probably seen product labels that claim something is "non-acnegenic" or "non-comedogenic." Supposedly, these terms mean the product won't block pores and cause pimples (*comedo* is the medical term for the familiar blackhead). There are no FDA guidelines governing which products can and cannot call themselves non-comedogenic; some products live up to the label and others don't. Several of my patients have suffered impressive outbreaks of acne after trying non-comedogenic products.

Beauty Treatments to Try at Home

When it comes to beauty treatments, what better place to experiment than at home? Get someone to watch the kids for a couple of hours and indulge yourself. Here are some ideas to get you started.

➤ Unless you have very dry skin, nothing beats a warm (not hot) bath for unwinding after a tough day. Pour in your favorite bath oil. Dim the lights, or light the bathroom with candles. Play your favorite relaxing music.

➤ If your skin is rough or flaky, rub it gently with a clean washcloth, loofah (dried plant fiber with an abrasive texture), or Buf-Puf® (a polyester fiber sponge). Avoid using a loofa or Buf-Puf® on your face, though; they're too harsh for most people. Make sure to dry them thoroughly between uses to prevent bacteria growth.

Beauty Tips

If you have a whirlpool tub, this is the time to enjoy it. Remember, you can't use bath oil in a whirlpool (it will gum the pump mechanism) or bubble bath (your tub will become a bubble machine!) Instead, try a half-cup of apple cider vinegar (check your owner's manual first, of course). It's invigorating, with a pleasantly clean aroma.

Saving Your Skin

If you have a problem with rough skin on your elbows, knees, or feet, salicylic acid ointments can help. Massage these exfoliating ointments in at bedtime; they're too greasy for daytime use.

Beauty Tips

Are your hands and feet very dry? Try smoothing a thin layer of Vaseline or mineral oil over them in the evening. Put on gloves and socks before going to bed. The next morning, your skin will feel soft and super-moisturized.

➤ If you're annoyed by dead skin or calluses on your elbows, feet, or knees, try a pumice stone, a super-cooled piece of rough volcanic lava. Wet both your skin and the stone before using it, then rub it gently over the problem areas only. The key word here is *gently*—don't leave your skin feeling abraded or sore. You can always do it again tomorrow if the first time wasn't thorough enough.

➤ When you're done soaking, blot—don't rub—yourself partly dry with a clean towel, then apply moisturizer to your face and body. Now's the time to try that fancy new lotion you got for your birthday.

➤ Some of my patients ask about using pure oils (such as olive, mineral, or vitamin E oil) as moisturizers. If your skin is very dry, these oils can be effective. This is something you'll want to save for evenings when you have privacy, though, because pure oils look greasy—no amount of powder will cover that shine—and you can't wear makeup over them. Smooth a small amount gently over your clean damp skin. Allow at least a couple of hours before bedtime so the oil has time to soak in. (Remember, these oils are not for acne-prone skin.)

Some pure oils lack preservatives. This is good, because some people are sensitive to preservatives, but also bad because the oils can become rancid. Always use fresh oil that's room temperature, not refrigerated. Rather than olive or peanut, which have strong odors, try a milder-smelling oil, such as sesame or canola, or break open a couple of vitamin E capsules.

➤ Products with mints such as peppermint, balm mint, and wintergreen may be too strong for your face, but they can feel great on your feet. If your feet sometimes feel hot and tired, try massaging them with mint or menthol lotion. Enjoy the tingle!

Finish off your pampering with a nice cup of tea, a time-honored remedy for stress and fatigue. If the caffeine won't bother you, try a cup of green tea; recent studies show it contains cancer-fighting chemicals. If you're gearing down for the evening, though, skip the caffeine and opt for a relaxing herbal tea like chamomile or peppermint.

The Least You Need to Know

➤ Toners remove surface skin cells, soap residues, and oils from the skin. Some tend to be drying. Unless you have very oily skin, you may not need to use them regularly.

➤ Almost everyone will benefit from an effective moisturizer. Regardless of brand and price, all moisturizers work by slowing down water evaporation from the skin surface.

➤ Look for a moisturizer that suits your skin type: those with oils for dry skin, and oil-free moisturizers for acne-prone skin.

➤ Be a smart consumer: Always read the list of ingredients before buying a skin care product and avoid those that don't suit your skin.

➤ Okay, you've done your homework. Now take some time off and pamper yourself.

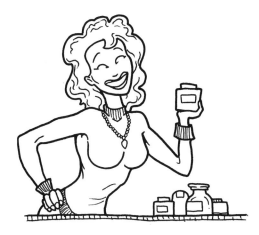

Chapter 6

At the Cosmetics Counter

In This Chapter

➤ Learn to determine your true skin tone

➤ Discover how to choose and use foundation, powder, and blush

➤ Learn about selecting eye and lip products, and how to apply them

➤ Discover how to use cosmetics to emphasize your own natural beauty

Remember my friend Maria, who was having trouble deciding on a line of skin care products? After I persuaded her to return the expensive toner she'd bought, she asked me to help her select some new foundation.

"I don't really like this color," she explained. "It looked great in the store when I bought it, but now my son says it makes me look orange!"

Feel like you have a hard time choosing the right cosmetics? Certainly, feedback from other people can be a big help (although we'd prefer them to be more tactful than this!). Salespeople aren't always the best or most impartial guides to what looks good, and store lighting can be deceptive.

In this chapter, let's look at points to keep in mind during your next visit to the cosmetics counter.

What's Your Skin Tone?

What color is your skin? Which colors will look best on it? These may sound like simple questions, but just wait till you try to choose from all the possibilities in the makeup rainbow.

Certain words are used to describe skin tone, the underlying color of your skin. When you go cosmetics-shopping, you're likely to encounter these terms:

➤ *Porcelain* (pale, even-toned skin color). This skin tone, sometimes nicknamed "peaches and cream," has been upheld as an ideal for many women. It's more common in fashion magazine photos, however, than in real life.

➤ *Ruddy* (undertone of pink or red in the skin).

➤ *Sallow* (yellow or golden undertone; little or no pinkness).

➤ *Olive* (green or ashy undertone).

These concepts are largely independent of race. A fair-skinned redhead may have ruddy skin, but so can a Native American or African American. Some Caucasian women have the golden undertones of a sallow complexion, and so do some Asian and African-American women. There's nothing inherently good or bad about any of these skin tones. Beauty comes in all colors.

You'll have an easier time choosing makeup if you already have a firm sense of what your skin tone is. Don't rely on salespeople to analyze it for you. They may be knowledge-able, with a good eye for color; on the other hand, they may not. And, to be fair, the lighting in most department stores is terrible and makes skin look more yellow or green than it would in natural light.

To determine your true skin tone, ask a friend to evaluate your color in natural light. (Leave off your makeup, and don't do this on a day when you're sunburned.) Keep in mind that skin looks pinker if it's irritated or enduring an outbreak of acne.

> **Skin Smart**
> Standard terms for describing skin tone include *porcelain* (pale, even-toned skin color), *ruddy* (undertone of pink or red), *sallow* (yellow or golden undertone), and *olive* (green or ashy undertone).

> **More Than Skin Deep**
> While a porcelain skin tone is unrealistic for most of us, this hasn't stopped both Western and Eastern cultures from considering it a hallmark of beauty. In old Japan, wealthy women and geishas wore rice powder to lighten their complexions; in traditional Japanese paintings, notice how light-skinned the women are compared to the men. As for Western society, on your next trip to the drugstore take a look at the names cosmetics companies give their foundations. You'll find quite a few with names like "ivory," "porcelain," "bisque" (a type of porcelain), and "shell."

Choosing the Right Foundation, Powder, and Blush

Now that you know what your true skin tone is, it's time to select a foundation that matches it. Notice I said "matches." Sometimes we are advised to buy foundation that's a different shade from our skin, the idea being to "correct" our natural color and make it more beautiful. This goes back to the old notion that we should all appear to have porcelain skin, regardless of our true skin tone.

Some women purchase a lighter shade of foundation, hoping it will make their skin tone look more even. Others choose a darker or rosier shade, hoping it will make them appear suntanned; still others smooth on bronzing gels or powders for the same reason.

Here's my advice: No matter what your natural skin tone, love it and live with it. Don't let the fashion media foist narrow interpretations of beauty on you; let your own beauty show through. From a practical standpoint, applying a foundation that doesn't match your skin doesn't really make you appear a different color, anyway. Frankly, it just looks like you applied the wrong color of foundation.

What if you have great skin and don't want to cover up a thing? You may still find a thin layer of foundation useful. It helps the rest of your makeup adhere better to your skin; it also makes it easier to blend powder and blush.

For more detailed advice and evaluations of specific brands, you may want to consult the helpful books by Paula Begoun, a consumer reporter who specializes in covering the cosmetics industry. See Appendix A, "Bountiful Resources for Beautiful Skin," at the end of this book for more information.

Finding a Good Foundation

There are four basic types of foundation:

➤ *Oil-based.* If oil comes first in the list of ingredients (and water comes second or third), it's an oil-based foundation. This type tends to be rather thick and greasy. If your skin is very dry, you may like this consistency, but many women find these foundations too heavy. One option is to moisten your makeup sponge with water before using it to apply foundation. This will make the foundation go on thinner, although it can be streaky and difficult to blend smoothly.

> **Saving Your Skin**
> Look for a foundation with a built-in sunscreen; this will save you from having to apply foundation and sunscreen separately. For advice on good sun-blocking ingredients, see Chapter 11, "Fighting Back Against Photoaging."

➤ *Water-based.* If water is the first ingredient listed, it's a water-based product. This doesn't mean there's no oil at all (oil may be listed second or third), just that there's less than in the oil-based variety. These foundations are easy to blend on your face; coverage tends to be lightweight and fairly sheer. They lend a slight sheen to the face, which some women like and others don't. Water-based foundations work best for normal to dry skin; if you have oily or acne-prone skin you'll probably prefer an oil-free product.

➤ *Powder-based.* Some powder-based foundations resemble pressed powder, except they offer slightly more opaque coverage. Others, called cream-to-powder, have a creamy texture that dries to a powder finish on the face. Powder-based foundations tend to be sheer, especially the pressed-powder form. They can be great for normal to slightly oily skin. If you have dry skin, you may feel the powder base makes your skin feel even drier, and if your skin flakes at all, these foundations will quickly show it.

➤ *Oil-free.* These foundations are indeed free of vegetable and mineral oils, although some do contain silicone oils. They come in three forms: alcohol-based, glycerin-based, and creams or lotions. I recommend the creams and lotions to patients with oily or acne-prone skin; the other two types can be too irritating. Oil-free foundations go on smoothly but dry fast, so blend them quickly or you won't get even coverage. It's a little harder to blend powder and blush over them compared to water-based foundations.

> **Beauty Tips**
> Always ask for a sample of foundation that you can try at home on a clean face. Many cosmetics lines offer free samples on request. If they don't have prepackaged samples, make your own. Buy a small empty plastic container (available in the travel accessories section at discount stores), and ask the salesperson to put two days' worth of foundation in it.

Like Maria, many women find that the foundation they loved in the store looks orange or pink when they get it home. Whatever type of foundation you prefer, try it on before you buy and check out the color in daylight. The color should blend into your natural complexion without being obvious. If it's at all visible, it's not your color.

Ideally, you should wear a foundation for several hours before making your decision. After it's been on your skin for a while, the color could change, or it could reveal an annoying tendency to settle into facial lines and accentuate them. Wearing it is the only way to know for sure whether the color and texture are right for you.

Getting Powder Down Pat

If you like to use powder, choose one that matches your foundation (which means, of course, that it matches your natural complexion). Face powder comes in two forms: loose and pressed. Each has its advantages: Loose powder can give a lighter, more sheer look, but pressed powder is easier to use. (I don't know about you, but I always seem to get loose powder grains in my eyes.)

Remember that powders (loose and pressed) may contain oil; women with oily or acne-prone skin should stick to oil-free powder. Just as you did with your foundation, try a sample of powder before buying. You need to wear it over your foundation for several hours and check out the color in daylight.

Wait until your foundation is completely dry before applying powder. Go light on powder; too much, and it will cake and crease in facial lines. Apply it gently in the same direction that you put on your foundation to get a smooth finish.

Blushing Beautifully

Blushes come in three basic forms: liquids and gels, cream-to-powder, and pressed powder.

Liquid and gel blushes can be hard to blend evenly. They may also sink into pores and leave tiny colored dots that look like little pinpricks—not the look you want, I'm sure! On the other hand, they are often oil free, which is important for people who tend to develop acne on the cheeks.

Like cream-to-powder foundation, cream-to-powder blush starts creamy and dries to a powder finish. This type can be beautiful on someone with normal to slightly oily skin, but may be too drying and powdery on dry skin and too oily for acne-prone complexions.

The third category, pressed powder, is the most common type and generally works well for everyone. Pressed-powder blushes come in oil-containing and oil-free formulas. Oil-free formulas are, as always, recommended for acne-prone users. I recommend applying pressed-powder blush with a brush.

One of the most common cosmetics questions is the best way to apply blush. Check out the diagram for one suggestion. Many makeup artists recommend starting at a point on your cheekbone below the center of your eye. Using a series of light downward strokes, apply the blush along your cheekbone. Don't stroke in the same direction as your cheekbone, or you could end up looking striped.

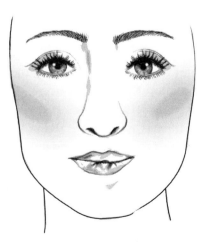

Apply your blusher along the cheekbone with downward strokes.

Follow up by brushing the edges gently with a soft clean sponge to blend the blush into your foundation. Never leave an obvious boundary between the two.

Saving Your Skin
Invest in high-quality makeup brushes with soft, well-shaped bristles. Hard, scratchy brushes with loose bristles will irritate your skin and make colors look streaky.

What about color? Opinions vary. Some makeup artists have strong ideas about which colors look best with each skin tone. Others advise you to adjust blush color to the shade of your lipstick, eye makeup, and even your wardrobe. In my opinion, soft and subtle colors generally work best. Avoid overly bright, deep, or harsh shades that will stand out on your face.

Some salespeople tell you to put blush on your forehead, chin, or nose as well as cheeks. I don't advise this technique because it could make you look too ruddy. Also, don't apply blush too near your eyes; if it gets trapped in laugh lines, it accentuates them, and the powder could irritate your skin.

Cosmetics for Women of Color

While choosing the right cosmetic colors is no picnic for Caucasian women, it can be even worse for Asians and African Americans. Until recently, many major cosmetics companies did not even sell products for darker skin.

Fortunately, things have improved a lot in the last few years. There are companies that specialize in darker shades, and most firms have broadened their color spectrum to include a wider variety of products. Still, there's no denying that it can be a challenge to hunt down the perfect color for your skin.

In addition to the preceding suggestions, the following tips may help:

➤ Dry skin can make dark skin look grayish and ashy. If this is a persistent problem, make sure your moisturizer is hydrating your skin effectively. Experiment with several different brands to find one that works for you.

➤ Some women of color have an uneven distribution of pigment, which makes some areas of the skin darker than others. Match your foundation to the shade that predominates, unless there is a significant color difference. In that case, look for a foundation shade that falls between the two extremes.

➤ If you're really, really frustrated with finding the right shade, look for companies that custom-blend foundation colors. As with any foundation, try to obtain a sample before buying the whole container. Take it home and try it on your face in daylight. Custom-blending foundations can be expensive and time-consuming. I recommend it only if you've tried lots of brands without success.

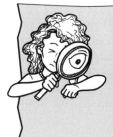

More Than Skin Deep

Some women of color find that areas of their skin grow darker after they've cut or scraped it. Outbreaks of acne can also darken affected skin. These patches may fade on their own, although it can take months or years. Medications can help to fade them faster; consult a dermatologist.

Eye Makeup Without Tears

In eye makeup, as with foundation, I think there's too much emphasis on "correcting flaws" that aren't flaws at all—they're distinctive attributes that make you a unique individual with your own brand of beauty.

Don't think your eyes are too close together, or far apart, or small, or large. Some of the world's most beautiful women have features that are asymmetrical or irregular. The feature you hate may actually give your face interest and character.

Think in terms of accentuating, not hiding, your natural beauty.

Eyeing Eyeshadows

When it comes to eye makeup, the more subtle the better. After all, you want the focal point to be your eyes, not what's painted on your lids. Bright colors around your eyes will also distract from the color on your lips and cheeks.

I recommend subtle neutral shades, at least for daytime. You can stay neutral and still enjoy a range of options: from pale beige to smoky brown, from light gray to charcoal and black, and in-between blends, such as taupe and cinnamon. If you really want more color, look for subtle shades that combine a neutral with a color—slate blue, smoky violet, sage green.

There are a lot of different ways to apply eyeshadow, and I don't have space to cover them all here. This drawing summarizes three variations that are practical and efficient.

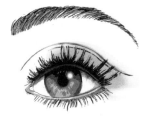 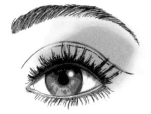 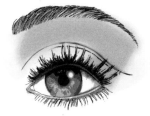

The amount and placement of eyeshadow depends on how dramatic a look you want.

Beauty Tips
Does your powdered eyeshadow get in your eyes? Be sure to knock excess powder off your brush before applying it to your lids.

For a minimally made-up look, shade only the outer portion of your upper eyelid and blend the color into the crease. A second approach, for slightly more color, extends the shaded area into the area beneath your browbone. (Make the color deepest on your eyelid, then soften it above the crease so that it tapers off before reaching your eyebrow.) For more drama, extend the shading forward to fill in the area above the inner corner of the eyelid.

Some general tips about eyeshadow:

➤ Always blend eyeshadow well; don't leave an obvious edge. You want it to look subtle instead of painted on.

➤ Use a good-quality makeup brush rather than a sponge-tip applicator, which pulls on your skin and leaves streaks of color.

➤ Buy single eyeshadows, not sets. Too many eyeshadow sets include colors you won't wear, which wastes your money.

Go for powdered eyeshadows, not creams. Cream eyeshadows are harder to apply and tend to collect in your eyelid crease as the day goes by.

Using Eyeliner

You can buy eyeliners in liquid or pencil form. Liquid eyeliners (which you apply with a thin brush) create the most dramatic, obvious line; pencil lines vary from defined to smudgy. Self-sharpening pencils are more convenient than those you have to sharpen. Yes, they cost more, but it's worth it when you consider how much pencil you lose every time you sharpen it.

Some makeup artists recommend lining your eyes with a dark eyeshadow instead of eyeliner. The eyeshadow can be applied either wet or dry. If you try this, be sure to use a very thin brush that comes to a neat point. Otherwise the color could fill your entire eyelid, and you could end up with a strip of unlined eyelid along your lashes.

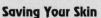

Saving Your Skin
The skin on your eyelids is very sensitive, so treat it gently. Stick with matte-finish eyeshadows; shiny eyeshadows contain tiny light-reflecting particles that can irritate.

Whatever type of eyeliner you choose, follow these guidelines:

➤ Don't apply eyeliner inside your eyelashes. It will smear and flake into your eyes.

➤ Make the line along your lower lashes softer than the line along the upper lashes.

➤ Some eyeliner pencils come packaged with a sponge tip on one end for "smudging" the line. I don't recommend these because the sponge becomes unsanitary with repeated use. Instead, wash your hands thoroughly and smudge the eyeliner gently with a fingertip or cotton swab. Be careful not to pull on your skin.

➤ Avoid lining the eye completely, above and below, from inner to outer corner. Many makeup artists suggest limiting eyeliner to the outer half of the eye. Start the line very thin, and broaden it slightly and gradually to the outer edge.

As with eyeshadows, I recommend a neutral color (brown, black, or gray) for daytime wear. Save the wilder, brighter shades for evenings and parties. Harmonize eyeliner with your mascara, so that it frames your eyes and makes your eyelashes look thicker. A very bright, pastel, or frosted color will draw attention to the eyeliner rather than your eyes.

Saving Your Skin
Liquid eyeliners cause more skin reactions than other types of liners. If your eye area is sensitive, opt for an eyeliner pencil.

Mascara: The Most Popular Cosmetic

Even women who don't wear any other cosmetics generally wear mascara. This handy stuff comes in two forms, waterproof and water-soluble.

Waterproof mascaras, obviously, don't dissolve in water. Great as this sounds (and it's handy for swimmers), it can also cause problems. You remove these mascaras with solvents that you wipe around your eyes. This wiping action may pull at eyelashes, sometimes breaking them, and may drag at the delicate skin around your eyes. These solvents can also leave an oily film in your eyes.

Most of my patients have better luck with water-soluble mascara, which is easier to remove because it does dissolve in water. Be aware, though, that some of these mascaras are more water-soluble than others. Experiment to find a brand that works for you.

As with other eye cosmetics, my personal opinion is that neutral shades of mascara (black and brown) work best. The most popular mascara color sold is black, which works well for most people. If you're a blonde or redhead with very fair skin, however, black may look too harsh; consider a brown mascara instead.

To apply mascara, hold the wand parallel to your lashes. Brush on color from the base of the lashes outward, but don't get it so near the lid that it bleeds into your eyes.

Beauty Tips
Never add water to mascara. It may make the product last a little longer, but it also contaminates it. Remember that you wear mascara very close to your eyes, so don't take chances.

69

For Lasses with Glasses (and Contact Lenses)

Patients who wear glasses and contact lenses often ask me for makeup tips. Traditionally, women who wear glasses have been advised to apply extra eye makeup. This advice may be good if you're nearsighted because the lenses make your eyes look smaller. You can get by with wearing darker colors, and applying them more dramatically, than you could if you didn't wear glasses.

If you're farsighted or wear bifocals, however, the lenses make your eyes look larger. Be careful not to overdo your makeup. Avoid bright, harsh colors and sharply edged eyeliner because your lenses will magnify the result.

Regardless of your prescription, check your blush with your glasses on to make sure it shows below your frames.

If you wear contact lenses, I recommend avoiding any powder around your eyes. My patients have better luck using eye pencils rather than powdered eyeshadows, and pressed rather than loose powder. Nothing is more annoying than finishing your makeup only to feel like you have sand in your eyes.

Saving Your Skin
Never share your cosmetics with other people, and please, don't use anyone else's makeup. It's unsanitary and exposes your skin to whatever may be on theirs.

Some contact lens wearers prefer waterproof mascara so their mascara won't run if their eyes water. Others like water-soluble mascara because, if it does get in their eyes, at least it dissolves. Try both to see which works best for you.

Be aware that makeup removers for waterproof mascaras can leave an oily film that soft lenses will absorb. Don't use an oily makeup remover around your eyes while wearing your lenses.

Tips for Lips

Whatever color you covet, there's a lipstick to supply it. As a general rule, creamy lipsticks go on more smoothly and are better for moisturizing your lips. The catch is that they come off more easily and are more apt to bleed into the lines around your mouth.

Longer-wearing lipsticks tend to be drier and stiffer; they don't feel as good on the lips, but they're less likely to leave lip-prints on your coffee cup. Some women like the precision and control of a lipliner, and it can be used to add subtle color to the lips when you're not wearing lipstick.

Some tips for applying lipstick and lipliner:

➤ Harmonize your lip color to the rest of your makeup. If you're wearing a rosy blush, for instance, a coral lipstick will look too orange. Many cosmetics companies organize their products into color families to make these decisions easier.

➤ When reapplying lipstick, make sure you get all the old stuff off first. Applying new over old can make the color look patchy and uneven.

➤ Do your lips feel dry even with lipstick? Apply a thin layer of a petroleum jelly like Vaseline, then put on lipstick over that. (If your lips still feel chapped, you may be reacting to your lipliner or lipstick. Stop using it for a while, and see if the problem clears up.)

➤ Does your lipstick feather into the lines around your lips? Try switching to a less creamy lipstick and powdering your lips lightly with loose powder before applying it. Some women find that a lipliner also helps.

➤ If you use lipliner, make sure its color matches your lipstick. Some salespeople advise you to outline lips in a darker color. My personal opinion is that a thin dark line around the mouth looks harsh and unflattering.

A final word of advice: Don't try to reshape your mouth with lipstick. If you apply lipstick outside your lipline in an effort to achieve that full-lipped pouty look, it will simply look like you missed your mouth. Magazine photos may get away with this technique, thanks to skillful lighting and camera angles, but in real life it doesn't fly.

Beauty Tips
When using a cosmetics brush, pick up powdered makeup by stroking the flat side of the brush against it. Don't grind the brush against the makeup. This splays the bristles, breaking them and ruining the shape of the brush.

What You Don't Need

In their zeal to sell as many products as possible, some salespeople may suggest that you need some or all of the following items. Some can be useful, some I'm skeptical about. If they appeal to you, great. But don't buy them unless you're convinced, in your own mind, that you will benefit from them.

➤ *Premoisturizers.* Some lines market "premoisturizers" (or submoisturizers) that are supposed to prepare your skin to absorb moisturizer better. Frankly, your skin doesn't need any help with the absorption process. If it feels dry, you may need a richer moisturizer, but you certainly don't need a premoisturizer.

➤ *Color correctors.* These products often simply appeal to women's anxiety about their skin tone. If your skin is ruddy, a salesperson may suggest a green color corrector to balance your natural complexion before applying foundation, or a pink color corrector if your tone is olive or sallow.

Color correctors may be helpful for people who have post-surgical redness after dermabrasions, laser peels, or chemical peels. They may also help people with very ruddy skin caused by rosacea or other skin conditions. But for everyone else, my advice is to be comfortable with your skin color and buy products that enhance it, not fight it.

➤ *Eyelid foundations.* Let's face it: Eyeshadow always wants to end up in your crease. These products are marketed to prevent that. However, you can accomplish the same goal by applying your regular foundation to your eyelids (pat lightly, don't rub), then applying loose powder over it.

➤ *Shiny makeup.* Shiny makeup may look great in magazine photos, but it doesn't do most of us justice. Iridescence catches the light and emphasizes everything you'd rather not draw attention to. Shiny eyeshadows make eyelids look wrinkled even if they're not. Glittery powders emphasize facial lines, and frosted lipsticks highlight lip cracks. If you really enjoy the shimmering look, fine, but save it for evening and incandescent lighting, which softens the effect.

Saving Your Skin
Avoid using blusher or lipstick as an eyeshadow. The eyelid is so sensitive that eye makeup has to be formulated accordingly. Blushers and lipsticks may not be as gentle and may cause reactions.

Now that you've learned all the dos and don'ts, let's go back to what's really important: cosmetics are supposed to be fun. Don't think in terms of employing them to "hide" or "correct" something. Instead, use them to accentuate the features that give your face character and individuality—in short, the qualities that make you beautiful!

The Least You Need to Know

➤ Know your own skin tone and color preferences; don't rely on salespeople to advise you.

➤ Look for foundation and powder that matches your natural skin tone.

➤ The lighting in most stores is terrible. Whenever possible, obtain product samples, try them at home, and evaluate the results in daylight. Wear them for several hours before deciding whether to buy.

➤ When in doubt, go for subtlety. Save shiny cosmetics, bright colors, and outrageous effects for evenings and special occasions.

➤ Attractiveness comes in all designs and colors; the attributes that you consider "flaws" contribute to your unique brand of beauty. Cosmetics are a fun way to enhance it, so enjoy!

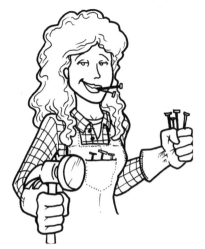

Beautiful Hair and Nails

Juanita consulted her primary care doctor because she was worried about losing her hair. For about six weeks, every time she shampooed she discovered a handful of hair around the drain.

To her surprise, she was referred to me. "I never thought of seeing a dermatologist about my hair," she told me, politely but frankly. "I thought dermatologists dealt with skin." "We do," I replied, "and believe it or not, that includes your hair and nails. Their good health is related to the health of your skin."

At some point, many of us worry about thinning hair. As it turns out, I was able to reassure Juanita about her hair loss and treat it effectively. Read on and I'll tell you about it.

Funny, Hair Doesn't Look Like Skin!

As you saw in Chapter 2, "Your Skin: Don't Leave Home Without It," hair and nails are skin appendages, part of the complex organ that is your skin. Nails and hair develop from specialized cells that work like the cells that produce the skin's horny layer. Like the horny layer, they contain a type of *keratin*, a durable protein that makes them more rigid than cells in the rest of your skin. Keratin reinforces hair strands and makes your nails hard.

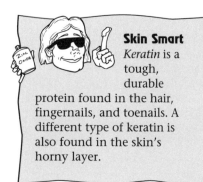

Skin Smart
Keratin is a tough, durable protein found in the hair, fingernails, and toenails. A different type of keratin is also found in the skin's horny layer.

Like everything else in your skin, hair and nails are there for a reason. Hair, for instance, shields us from sunlight and abrasions, and helps hold in body heat. Nails help us grasp objects and protect the delicate edges of our fingers and toes.

Each hair is born in a hair follicle, a tiny complex structure in the dermis or subcutaneous layer. Each follicle manufactures specialized cells that grow into a single hair. This drawing shows a cross-section of a hair. As you can see, it consists of a central core surrounded by a layer of long thin fibers, packaged in an outer layer of overlapping cells. At the root of each follicle is a tiny rounded area of tissue (called the bulb) that supplies the hair with keratin. When you yank out a hair, the small pale bump you see is the bulb.

Each hair consists of a central core surrounded by a layer of long thin fibers, packaged in an outer layer of overlapping cells. Each hair is actually an outgrowth of dead cells and keratin growing upward from a hair follicle.

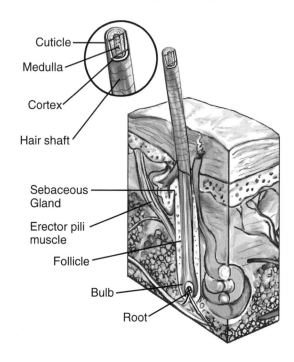

Cuticle
Medulla
Cortex
Hair shaft
Sebaceous Gland
Erector pili muscle
Follicle
Bulb
Root

Remember all those ads for products that promise to "nourish" and "revitalize" your hair? Aside from basic nutritional needs that benefit your entire body, your hair doesn't need nourishment. You can't feed it or improve its structure with topical applications of vitamins or chemicals. (There are ways to damage it, though, as well as ways to protect it, and I'll get into them later in this chapter.)

You have 80,000 to 120,000 hair follicles on your scalp alone, not including the follicles everywhere else. We humans carry hair follicles all over our bodies except on the mouth, the palms of the hands, and the soles of the feet.

If we have so many follicles, why aren't we covered with hair? Actually, we are, but it's not always visible. Humans grow two types of hair: terminal and vellus. *Terminal hairs* are coarse and thick; they are the familiar strands that sprout from scalp, eyebrows, armpits, pubic area, and legs. *Vellus hairs*, which are fine, short, and colorless, grow almost everywhere else. The only thing that saves us from looking as hairy as chimpanzees is that much of our body is covered by vellus, rather than terminal, hairs.

> **Skin Smart**
> *Vellus hairs* are fine, pale, downy hairs that cover much of the body. *Terminal hairs* are longer, coarser, and more pigmented; they form the visible "hair" of the scalp, eyebrows and eyelashes, armpits, genitals, and extremities.

Doctor, What's Wrong with My Hair?

Like Juanita, some people consult me because they're worried about changes in their hair. Many common hair problems result from how we treat our hair. Others may reflect changes in hormones, nutrition, or overall health.

In this chapter, you'll get a look at some of the most frequent hair complaints: hair that is limp, oily, dry, or brittle. But first, let's start with the most common worry of all—hair that doesn't stick around.

Are You Really Losing Your Hair?

As one of my patients said wryly the other day, "I guess this is a case of hair today, gone tomorrow!" Well, not necessarily. Often, what people perceive as hair loss is actually part of hair's normal growth cycle.

This growth cycle, as shown in the following diagram, alternates between an active phase, lasting two to five years, and a resting phase, lasting several weeks or months, during which the hair follicle becomes inactive. At any given time, approximately 15 percent of hairs are in the resting phase. During the active phase, the hair grows roughly a third of a millimeter (about one hundredth of an inch) each day; during the resting phase, it doesn't grow at all. Eventually a new active phase begins, and a new hair is formed which pushes out the old one.

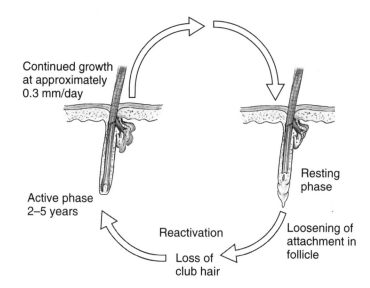

All hair goes through a normal cycle of growth followed by a resting phase. When a new active phase begins, you shed the old hair and replace it with a new one.

Continued growth at approximately 0.3 mm/day

Resting phase

Active phase 2–5 years

Reactivation

Loss of club hair

Loosening of attachment in follicle

The length of your hair's active phase is preset by genetics. The longer the phase lasts, the longer your hair can grow; women with waist-length hair enjoy protracted active phases. As we get older, active phases get shorter and resting phases get longer. If you think your hair doesn't grow as long as it used to, this may be perfectly normal.

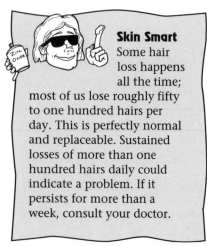

Skin Smart
Some hair loss happens all the time; most of us lose roughly fifty to one hundred hairs per day. This is perfectly normal and replaceable. Sustained losses of more than one hundred hairs daily could indicate a problem. If it persists for more than a week, consult your doctor.

Most of the time, hair growth cycles aren't synchronized. One hair may be starting an active phase while its neighbor is in a resting phase, and a third is in the middle of active growth. This usually prevents massive shedding episodes and obscures the entire cycling phenomenon.

Occasionally, many hairs decide to embark on a resting phase together, and then shed simultaneously as a new active phase begins. This may be a sign of an underlying problem. Factors that can cause this include hormonal changes, pregnancy, illness and high fever, stress, poor nutrition, radiation, and medications. If you notice sustained hair loss for more than a week, talk to your doctor. It will take approximately three months for new hairs to sprout at the scalp after you correct the cause of the condition.

Like Juanita, many people panic when they notice more hair than usual collecting around the bathtub drain or on their hairbrush. In many cases, what they're shedding is their old hair, as their hair prepares to enter a new active phase. In this case, a period of increased shedding can be a good sign: Healthy new tresses are on the way.

In Juanita's case, careful questioning revealed that five months earlier she had been hospitalized with a severe bout of flu that developed into pneumonia. This illness was a major cause of her subsequent hair loss. Another reason was that she often used hair straighteners, strong chemicals that make hair strands brittle. I recommended a gentler treatment plan for her hair. Six months later she phoned to thank me and say that her hair was indeed growing back in, as thick and healthy as ever.

What You Can Do About Hair Loss

Sometimes hair loss proves to be permanent. About 50 million Americans show at least some signs of hair loss.

Most cases result from normal changes in hormonal levels as we get older, coupled with a genetic predisposition. Male pattern hair loss is a common example, in which hair loss happens first at the temples and crown, then gradually widens over the top of the head. Actually, we don't really lose hair; what happens is that terminal hairs are replaced by downy, less visible vellus hairs.

Women may experience a similar problem, called female pattern hair loss, although the female version often takes the form of general thinning, not limited to one area of the scalp. Female pattern hair loss can appear at any age, although it's more commonly noticed in women who've been through menopause. Again, hormonal changes coupled with a genetic predisposition are to blame.

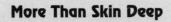

More Than Skin Deep

Alopecia areata is a condition characterized by localized patches of hair loss. The hairless areas are usually round or oval, and located on the head or other hairy parts of the body; aside from hair loss, the skin looks and feels normal. While the cause is unknown, alopecia areata may clear up within six to 12 months without treatment. Shots of cortisone into the bald areas may speed recovery. In rare cases, hair loss can affect the entire scalp or body. If you notice bald spots, consult your doctor.

Men who are balding may not like the idea, but they generally adjust well, thanks in large part to society's tolerance. As one of my male patients remarked to me, "I think of it as mind over matter. If I don't mind, losing my hair doesn't matter!"

Hair loss is more difficult emotionally for women, since our culture is much less supportive of their situation. However, there are steps you can take to make your hair look thicker and reverse hair loss:

Beauty Tips
Hats, scarves, turbans, and broad head-bands can make a flattering fashion statement while hiding hair loss. Browse through the hair accessories section in department stores for ideas.

➤ Consult your hair stylist. A good haircut and style can help disguise thinning hair. Generally, a layered style is best.

➤ Remember that permanents, blow dryers, curling irons, hair dyes, and anything else that could further stress the hair shaft will increase hair breakage. While this does not affect growth from the roots, damaged, brittle hairs will not be as attractive as healthy hair. Be gentle.

➤ Consider a hair weave, a piece of matching hair that's braided into your own hair. A well-done hair weave can look very realistic, though it will need periodic retightening as your hair grows.

➤ Another option: a wig. Before you dismiss the idea, consult a qualified cosmetologist who can demonstrate top-quality hairpieces. They're made with human hair and stay on with two-sided tape that will stick even when wet. Several of my patients wear wigs that are so natural looking I defy anyone to identify them.

➤ Ask your doctor about minoxidil (Rogaine®), a drug that can help some people regrow hair. This topically applied medication slows fallout in the majority of people who use it. A small percentage of men and a larger percentage of women report actual regrowth with minoxidil. However, it must be used indefinitely. When you stop the applications, you lose anything you gained from the drug.

If all else fails, there are some surgical options. A procedure called *scalp reduction* removes bald areas of the scalp and pulls together the remaining (hairy) areas to give the appear-ance of more hair. If your hair is still thick on the sides of your head, this procedure may be a good way to go. It does leave a scar on the top of the scalp, however, where no hair will grow. Scalp reduction is generally more helpful for men than for women, whose hair loss is often more diffuse.

Saving Your Skin
The FDA recently approved a drug, finasteride (Propecia®), for the treatment of male pattern hair loss in men only. Studies in women are not available yet, but because taking finasteride during pregnancy may feminize a male fetus, there are concerns about its use in women.

In another surgical procedure, a hair transplant, hair is removed from a region where it's plentiful, such as the back of your head, and transplanted to bald areas. The trans-planted hair won't spread, but if the transplant is successful, the transplanted hairs will grow normally in their new location. Again, this procedure requires areas of scalp with thick hair growth.

If you decide to have a hair transplant, make sure the transplants are distributed evenly and naturally; otherwise, you could end up with obvious plugs of hair. "Microplugs," which consist of very few hairs per plug, can give you a more natural look.

Finally, let me emphasize again that while most hair loss is normal or temporary and nothing to be alarmed about, in rare cases it can be a sign of a serious underlying condition. I have discussed only the most common hair loss problems here, and this subject alone has filled many books. If you are losing hair, be sure to see your doctor or dermatologist.

Dealing with Dry and Brittle Hair

Like many skin problems in general, we cause many of our own hair troubles.

Is your hair very brittle? Take a good look at how you care for it. Do you frequently subject your tresses to straighteners, hot combs, hot rollers, curling irons, permanents, or hair dyes? Any of these can damage your hair and split hair shafts.

Likewise, dry hair is often caused by overly zealous shampooing and made worse by blow-drying. Washing hair too much strips it of natural protective oils, and exposing it to the hot dry wind of a blow dryer exacerbates the damage.

Occasionally—and I stress occasionally—dry brittle hair can be a sign of poor nutrition, such as a severe vitamin, mineral, or protein deficiency. However, this is rare in developed countries. Most cases of damaged hair are self-inflicted.

Tips for Healthy Hair

When it comes to good hair care, many of the same basic skin care principles discussed in previous chapters still apply:

➤ First and foremost, be gentle! Just like your face, your hair will benefit from the mildest cleanser possible. Even if your hair is very oily, avoid using harsh shampoos. You don't want to turn oily hair into dry brittle hair.

➤ Is your hair too oily? Try washing it every day (but not more than once a day) with a detergent shampoo. Many women automatically follow up with a conditioner, but you might not need one if your hair produces a great deal of natural lubricant. If you regularly use a conditioner, try going without and see if that helps.

➤ Is your hair too dry? As mentioned before, you could inadvertently be making it worse. Cut back

Saving Your Skin
In rare cases, hair loss and dry hair can indicate an underlying health condition, such as hypothyroidism (underactive thyroid gland). Hypothyroidism is most common in women, although it can appear in men, too. If you experience persistent hair problems plus other symptoms—fatigue, weight gain, muscle weakness, dry flaky skin, or deepening voice—consult your doctor. Hypothyroidism is easily treated.

on the rough stuff—chemicals, curling irons, hot combs, and so on. Give your hair a while to recover and it probably will.

➤ If you have dandruff, try a dandruff shampoo that controls scalp flaking. Be aware that some of these cleansers tend to be harsh, so you may need a conditioner afterward.

➤ Go easy on hairstyles that stress your hair: tight buns, ponytails, or braiding. If you have lots of broken strands or pulled-out hairs along the scalp margin, you may be tearing your hair out—literally! Give your hair a rest by alternating tight styles with more relaxed 'dos.

Beauty Tips
How can you learn the pH of your shampoo and conditioner? Order nitrozine paper test strips from a pharmacist. Wet a strip with the shampoo or conditioner and note how it changes color. The change indicates pH level.

➤ Try a shampoo and conditioner with a pH between 4.5 and 5.5.

➤ After shampooing, rinse your hair thoroughly. Soapy residue is drying and can coat your hair, dulling its natural luster. Furthermore, it can flake, making you look like you have dandruff even if you don't.

➤ If you blow-dry, apply conditioner first to put a thin protective film between your hair and the device's dry heat. Use a moderate heat setting and don't dry your hair completely; stop while it is still damp and let it air-dry the rest of the way.

➤ This advice applies to hot rollers and curling irons, too. Remove them before your hair is bone-dry so you don't scorch it.

➤ If your hair tends to be fine and limp, try avoiding body-building shampoos and conditioners. These products contain thickening agents that are supposed to increase the diameter of the hair shaft and boost hair volume. Ironically, they're more apt to deflate your hair because the extra coating weighs your fine hair down. Instead, wash your hair frequently with a mild shampoo to make sure it isn't flattened by excess oil.

➤ Try to let your hair grow out completely between permanents. This will give it a chance to recover from the perm's harsh chemicals.

Perhaps the biggest boost you can give your hair is a good haircut. Instead of fighting your hair's natural tendencies—fine, coarse, straight, curly, whatever—find a hairstyle that makes the most of them.

It's worth investing time and money to find a stylist who can give you a flattering cut that won't require a lot of maintenance. After all, wouldn't you really rather spend less time on your hair, not more?

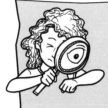

More Than Skin Deep

How do you find a good hair stylist? When you see a haircut you like, ask who did it and set up an interview with the stylist. Collect photos of hairstyles you like and bring them with you so you can discuss them together. Be honest, with yourself and with the stylist, about how much time you want to spend on your hair. If you have straight hair, swim every day and are always on the go, an elaborate curly 'do isn't for you. Choose a hairstyle based not just on how it looks, but also on its suitability for your lifestyle.

What About the Hair You Want to Lose?

Here's an ironic twist: While we worry about losing hair from some parts of the body, we do our best to banish it from others. Let's take a look at how to get rid of hair you don't want.

Shaving

Shaving is the simplest way to remove unwanted hair. It's fast, easy, and, barring accidents, painless. It's also temporary, of course, but you can't have everything.

Do you prefer a safety or electric razor? Safety razors (the traditional type with blades) tend to shave more closely; the downside is that it's easier to cut yourself. If you use a safety razor, always wet the hair first and apply a shaving gel or cream. Personally, I find gels work better. Lathering up with soap also works. Shaving "against the grain" will cut hair shorter. Rinse thoroughly with clean water, and pat with a towel till damp but not dry. If your skin feels abraded, apply moisturizer (except in your armpits, of course).

If you prefer an electric razor, make sure your skin is completely dry; otherwise, the razor will stick and you won't get a close shave. If electrics give you razor burn, try one of the hybrid razors that combine disposable double-edged blades with a battery-driven vibrating head.

Never apply deodorant or antiperspirant right after shaving; the chemicals can make abraded skin sting. And remember to be careful with after-shave lotions; they contain alcohol and can also sting.

Some razors and creams claim to be designed especially for women. If you like them better, fine. But for the most part, there's little difference between supposedly male and female products. My advice is to ignore colors and packaging, and choose what works best for you.

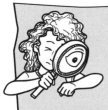

More Than Skin Deep

Some people believe that shaving hair will make it grow back faster and thicker. This is an old wives' tale (or perhaps we should say an old husbands' tale!). Shaving hair, no matter where it is on your body, will not coarsen it or make it grow more rapidly. Hair develops deep inside hair follicles, and how you cut it at the surface does not affect its basic consistency. If you start shaving hair, it may feel more coarse, but only because you are cutting it perpendicular to the skin and leaving a rough tip. The hair's basic structure has not changed.

Since shaving cuts hair at the skin surface, it grows back quickly and soon needs another shave. If you get really tired of having to shave regularly, read on for more options.

Chemical Depilatories

Depilatories are creams, lotions, or powders that can remove hair from slightly below the skin surface. They do this with chemicals that split the chemical bonds in the hair shaft and break it off. Therefore, they're more effective than shaving, and the results last longer.

Skin Smart
Depilatories are creams, lotions, or powders containing chemicals that split the chemical bonds in hair, breaking it off slightly below the skin surface.

Saving Your Skin
Never use depilatories near your eyes; the chemicals they contain are too strong and potentially risky. If you do get any in your eyes, call your doctor immediately.

A depilatory's advantage is also its drawback: Anything that's strong enough to burn off hair can also burn your skin. Many people experience some skin irritation after using depilatories. Try some on a small area first to see how your skin reacts. If it irritates the skin, wash the depilatory off immediately with mild soap and cool water.

You may apply hydrocortisone 1-percent ointment for a few days to decrease the inflammation. Remember, though, that cortisone preparations are not for long-term use. If the irritation persists, discontinue the cortisone and call your doctor. And, if depilatories inflame your skin, consider a different method of hair removal.

Some depilatories are intended for the face; others, for the legs. There are differences between the two types, so follow the package instructions and use them only as directed. They aren't the best choice for underarm hair, since the skin there is especially delicate. Skin in the pubic area is also sensitive; some women can tolerate depilatories there but others can't. If you want to try it, start with a small amount to test how your skin responds. Be sure not to get any on mucous membranes, and be prepared to wash it off promptly if it stings.

Waxing

Just imagine: a soothing film of warm liquid wax is spread over your legs. Slowly, it cools and hardens around your leg hairs. When solid enough, it's stripped off your legs, pulling the hairs with it. Ouch!

If anyone tells you waxing feels good, she's lying. But it can be effective, because it plucks hair from deep beneath the skin surface. It doesn't need to be done as often as shaving or depilatories. On the other hand, you have to let the stubble grow before your next waxing, so it will be long enough to catch in the wax.

You can buy home waxing kits, but I recommend going to a qualified salon professional. It's too easy to irritate your skin and inflame the hair follicles. At the very least, have it done professionally several times and pick up some pointers before trying it yourself.

Bleaching

If the offending hair is fine and downy (like on the upper lip, forearms, or sides of the face), bleaching can be a good alternative. In addition to making the hairs lighter, repeated bleaching can make them so brittle they break off, which also helps to make them less visible. You can buy commercial bleaching products, or have it done professionally at a salon.

Never use bleach on your eyebrows or near your eyes. Needless to say, if the bleach irritates your skin, wash it off immediately with soap and water.

> **Beauty Tips**
> Be aware that bleached hair could become more noticeable if you tan (which, of course, I suggest you never do). The bleach job that hides unwanted hair effectively during winter could actually make it stand out more in the summer.

Electrolysis

Electrolysis destroys hair follicles with the heat generated by an electric current. The electrologist inserts a thin needle into the pore containing the offending hair and zaps it with an electrical impulse. If done properly, electrolysis can remove unwanted hair permanently.

Electrolysis is not something to be undertaken lightly. Depending on the amount of hair to be removed, the procedure may be time-consuming and moderately expensive. The goal of electrolysis is to permanently remove unwanted hair. An individual hair can be destroyed on the first treatment if the needle is inserted accurately and if the intensity and timing of the current are correct. However, it may be difficult to do correctly.

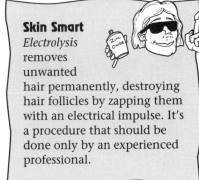

> **Skin Smart**
> *Electrolysis* removes unwanted hair permanently, destroying hair follicles by zapping them with an electrical impulse. It's a procedure that should be done only by an experienced professional.

Even if the procedure is performed perfectly, remember what I said about the hair cycle. Hairs in the resting phase cannot be treated. When they start to grow again, new hairs will seem to appear. They may not represent regrowth, just untreated hairs. Therefore, even in expert hands, more than one treatment will be necessary.

If you want to go this route, choose your electrologist carefully. Good results depend on a skilled operator. The best way to find a good electrologist is to ask your dermatologist. You can also check with the American Electrology Association (or the International Guild of Professional Electrologists. Ask for a licensed or board-certified electrologist. (See Appendix A, "Bountiful Resources for Beautiful Skin," at the end of the book for these and other useful phone numbers.)

Sometimes problems can occur even with experienced electrologists. Follicles can become infected, and damage to the tissue around the follicle can leave scars or colored marks. Electrolysis is even more challenging if you have curly hair or scars.

Yes, you can buy home electrolysis devices, but please, don't even think about it. Electrolysis is challenging even for experienced professionals; doing it yourself will be painful and unproductive. Instead of unwanted hair, you could end up with unwanted infected hair or scars!

Lasers

Some patients ask me about using a laser (a device that produces a concentrated beam of light) to remove hair. There are many kinds of lasers, and more than one kind may be employed to get rid of hair. Each type has its advantages and its drawbacks.

Laser technology is improving all the time. At the present time laser treatments remove hair only temporarily, but there appears to be less hair growth after each treatment. I suspect that in the next few years we'll see laser treatments that can get rid of hair permanently.

Since this field is changing so rapidly, I suggest discussing the most up-to-date technology with your dermatologist to see what's best for you. (For more information on lasers see Chapter 23, "Better Looking with Lasers.")

Tweezing

Well, if all else fails, you can always yank it out by the roots—otherwise known as plucking and tweezing. Tweezing won't make hair grow back coarser, but it could irritate the hair follicle. And of course the hair will grow back again; tweezing isn't permanent. If you decide to go ahead with it, invest in a decent set of tweezers. You could even look into electric tweezers that make the job easier.

Beauty Tips
Eyebrow shape has a big impact on the appearance of your eyes. If you tweeze too much from the inner edge of the eyebrow, it makes your eyes look smaller. Plucking too much from the bottom edge gives you a permanent look of surprise. When in doubt, don't tweeze; natural eyebrows are fashionable, anyway.

Go easy on plucking your eyebrows. Eyebrow hairs have a very brief active phase, which is why they remain short instead of growing as long as the hair on your scalp. Whatever you remove will be very obvious and will take some time to regrow. Proceed slowly, pluck a few hairs at a time, and give yourself several days to assess the look before deciding to tweeze more.

Hiding Your True (Hair) Colors

Like skin, hair gets its color from melanin. Melanin cells at the base of the hair follicles add pigment to the growing shaft; your genetic heritage determines the precise blend of pigments that create your unique hair color.

Until you go gray, that is. For many of us, follicular melanin cells start shutting down when we reach our 30s and 40s. By the time we're in our 70s, only a lucky few still produce enough melanin to enjoy naturally tinted hair.

But don't despair. Hair dyes have come a long way since the platinum-blonde bleach jobs you see in old movies. You can choose from the following:

➤ Temporary rinses that wash out the next time you shampoo

➤ Gradual dyes that alter hair color gradually, over two to three weeks

➤ Semipermanent dyes that wash out after four to six shampoos

➤ Permanent dyes that don't wash out

If you're considering a color change, try a temporary rinse first to see how you like it before committing to the permanent variety. Choose a shade slightly lighter, not darker, than your natural color; too-dark dyes look harsh and unflattering. Another option is to streak or frost your hair. The lighter streaks help camouflage patches of gray.

Unless you want a frankly fake look, take into account your eyebrow color and skin tone. If you have olive skin and black eyebrows, light blonde hair won't be believable. If you're a natural redhead with pale pinkish skin, raven tresses just won't look right.

Here's another option: learn to love your gray. Its softer hue may actually be more flattering to your skin. One of my friends ended up being a lovely, natural ash-blond gray—a color she had spent years trying (and failing) to achieve with dyes. Tinted hair doesn't always look better.

Saving Your Skin
Semipermanent and permanent hair dyes can cause allergic reactions; one frequent offender is the ingredient ammonium persulfate. Test these dyes on a small area of skin behind your ear or inside your elbow before putting them on your hair.

Beauty at Your Finger (and Toe) Tips

As noted previously, nails help us grasp and scratch, and protect the delicate edges of our fingers and toes. The visible portion we call a fingernail is actually the nail plate (see the diagram), which grows outward from specialized cells in the matrix and lunula, the "half-moon" at the base of the nail. Below the nail plate lies the nail bed, a fragile area of skin filled with blood vessels; if you've ever accidentally thunked your thumb with a hammer, you know it doesn't take much to make it bleed.

Fingernails develop from cells in the matrix. Injuring the cuticle, which protects the delicate matrix cells, can damage your nail.

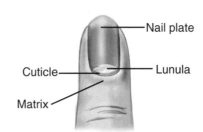

Unlike hair, nails don't cycle through active and resting phases; they grow continuously. It takes roughly 6 months to grow out a fingernail completely, and about 12 to 18 months to grow out a toenail. Serious illnesses can temporarily slow their growth, and nail growth in general slows as you get older.

Nail Care Basics

Since the keratin in the nail plate is dead protein, you can't nourish or feed nails by applying products topically. You can, however, moisturize them and the surrounding tissue. When you rub moisturizer on your hands and feet, be sure to rub it around and on your nails too, including the cuticles.

A word about cuticles: This much-maligned portion of the nail has gotten a bad rap. For some reason, it's considered unsightly, and fashion magazines advise us to cut, trim, or push it into obscurity. But the cuticle plays a crucial role in nail health: It seals out water and impurities from the delicate matrix cells that manufacture the nail. Cutting or removing the cuticle leaves the matrix vulnerable to bacteria and fungi, setting the stage for infection and injury. This, in turn, can weaken nails, deform them, and even make them stop growing temporarily.

Some tips for healthy finger- and toetips:

➤ If you really want to minimize your cuticle, rub it with moisturizer to soften it, then push it back gently with a clean orange stick.

➤ Don't overdo nail polish. Wearing polish all the time dries out the nail plate and makes nails brittle and fragile. The acetone in polish removers makes things worse. Remember, the nail is dead and cannot "recover." Therefore, leave nails unpolished periodically to minimize damage.

➤ Nail polish removers contain acetone, alcohol, and other potential irritants. Look for nail polish removers that also contain moisturizers, such as lanolin and synthetic oils, to counteract the drying effect of the active ingredients.

➤ If your nails break easily, try applying a nail hardener, which contains nylon or rayon fibers, as a base coat under your polish. Check the ingredients list to make sure the hardener doesn't contain formaldehyde, a frequent irritant.

Beauty Tips
To give your nails a rest, try buffing rather than polishing. You can buy an inexpensive buffer at your local drugstore.

➤ Trim toenails after a bath or shower, when they're soft. Trim them straight across, not too short, and don't round off the outside corners too much.

When you have manicures or pedicures, insist that the nail technicians practice good hygiene. They should wash their hands and clean their equipment between customers. Fungal and bacterial infections are contagious; so are viral warts. Dirty hands and nonsterile equipment could transmit these infections to you.

More Than Skin Deep

If the area around your toenails becomes red, sore, and swollen, you could have an ingrown nail. Wash your feet thoroughly with soap and water, and then place a small piece of clean cotton under the nail corner to raise it above the nail bed. Apply an antibiotic cream two or three times daily. If it doesn't get better within a week, or if you notice a discharge, call your doctor. Often ingrown nails result from too-short trims that push the side of the nail into surrounding skin; tight toe-squishing shoes are another factor. Be good to your toenails: Wear comfortable round-toed shoes made of breathable materials like leather.

Taking Your Nails to New Lengths

If you can't get your own nails to behave, you can always try artificial nails instead. You have several options:

➤ Nail tips are artificial extensions glued to the ends of your real nails; nail and tip are then painted with an acrylic solution to smooth out the surface. Although sometimes a bit complicated to apply, they do a good job of making short nails look longer.

➤ Press-on nails are preformed plastic shapes that you glue over real nails. They're probably the easiest artificial nail to work with. One type comes with glue on one side so you just press them on; for the other type, you have to paint your nails with adhesive first, and then apply the nail. Whichever type of press-on product you choose, remember that bacteria, dirt, and humidity can get trapped underneath. Remove them every 48 hours and leave them off for at least one night.

➤ Nail wraps are sheaths made of bendable materials, such as linen, silk, or paper. They're glued to your nails and shaped to resemble nail tips.

➤ Sculptured nails are synthetic polymer pieces custom-fitted to your own fingers. When done well, they look great and very authentic; when done poorly with nonsterile equipment, they can cause infections and damage your real nails.

This industry is not well regulated, so shop carefully for a good nail technician. Qualified professionals can do a great job, but inexperienced operators can leave you with lasting problems.

If you wear any type of artificial nail consistently, you'll find your real nails getting brittle, thin, and dull-looking. Wear them for no more than three months at a time, and then leave them off for a month to let your nails rest.

The Least You Need to Know

➤ Healthy hair goes through cycles of growth, rest, and shedding. Hair loss isn't necessarily permanent.

➤ If your hair is thin, you have a lot of options to choose from: hairpieces, weaves, medications, hair transplants, and scalp reduction.

➤ No matter what your hair's natural tendencies—straight or curly, thin or thick—find a style that makes the most of them. It'll make life easier, and it will also make you less dependent on beauty aids that are so hard on hair.

➤ Many problems with hair and nails result from what we do to them. Overwashing, chemicals, and heat make hair dry and brittle; polish and artificial nails do the same to nails. Be gentle!

➤ Be kind to your cuticles and nails. Avoid trimming and cutting cuticles because they're important for healthy nails. Remove polish and artificial nails periodically to give your real nails a rest.

Part 2
Beauty: It's More Than Skin Deep

Sometimes you can't help noticing the changes in your skin. Every time you glance in the mirror, there they are: freckles and age spots; tiny broken blood vessels; skin color that grows ashy, sallow, or dull; lines that start out faint and slowly deepen over time.

Perhaps you've been telling yourself, "It's only to be expected. I'm getting older, after all." Well, good news! Many of the visible changes we call "aging" are not inevitable. In fact, often they're preventable; they result from our own actions and reflect how we treat our skin through the years.

Coming up in Part 2: taking control of how fast—and how beautifully—your skin ages.

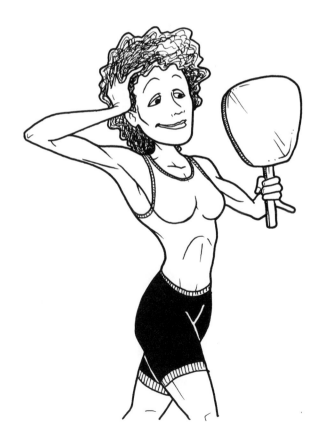

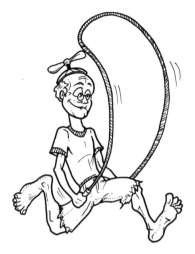

Chapter 8

Keeping That Youthful Look

> **In This Chapter**
>
> ➤ Learn to help your skin age gracefully
>
> ➤ Discover which nutrients help your skin look its best
>
> ➤ Uncover the link between exercise and beautiful skin
>
> ➤ Learn how to choose a great spa
>
> ➤ Enjoy the spa experience at home

When we were in our late 20s, several of my friends and I began to worry about turning 30. In our minds, this particular milestone seemed to mark the beginning of "aging." And, in fact, I was about 30 when I noticed the first fine lines appearing in the folds between my nose and mouth.

Today, I see this sort of self-consciousness about aging in general, and about skin aging in particular, in many of my patients. They grow anxious about any signs of getting older, and they worry that the changes they see aren't normal.

What happens to our skin over time? Which changes can we expect to see, which can be avoided, and what can we do to promote beautiful skin at all ages?

Beautiful Skin: The Long-Term View

Everything in our body changes as we get older, and skin is no exception.

How does it change? While this seems like a simple question, skin aging is actually very complex. It involves a lot of separate but interrelated processes that go on throughout life. Over time, they lead to noticeable differences between the skin of a child and an older adult (see the diagram).

As you get older, skin gets thinner and loses some of its supporting players, like collagen and some small blood vessels, while fat tissue redistributes itself.

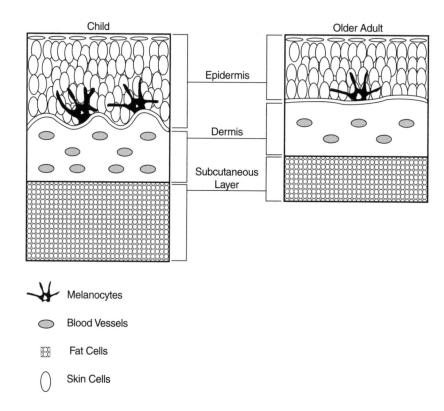

In the adult, collagen and elastin (the proteins that make skin firm and elastic) get a bit weaker. The dermis loses about 20 percent of its volume, and the epidermis grows thinner too. Fat tissue in the subcutaneous layer gradually redistributes itself; for instance, fat that used to plump out the face, neck, and extremities collects in the torso.

Meanwhile, oil and sweat glands get a bit lazy and produce less sebum and perspiration. Some hair follicles decide to retire early, leaving us with less hair. Some blood vessels shut down and our circulation may not work quite as efficiently as it used to, reducing the blood supply that nourishes skin.

Put together, all of these developments can make skin more dry and wrinkled. They also slow down the healing process (ever notice how quickly children's skin recovers from cuts and scrapes?).

In men, these changes take place gradually, over a lifetime. In women, they become most noticeable after menopause, probably because of falling levels of the female hormone estrogen.

"Great," you say. "Now I'm really depressed! Is there anything I can do about all this?" Here's the good news: Yes, there is something you can do. Several things, in fact.

These developments are not inevitable. There's built-in aging (called *intrinsic aging*), and then there's the aging we do to ourselves (called *extrinsic aging*). How you choose to live has a huge impact on your skin; the single most important variable in extrinsic aging is the amount of exposure your skin gets to sunlight.

Throughout this book, I'll discuss ways to prevent and counteract both types of aging. First, in this chapter, let's look at some things that are good for your skin.

> **Skin Smart**
> *Intrinsic aging* refers to the built-in changes that occur over time, as opposed to *extrinsic aging*, the changes we bring on ourselves due to lifestyle factors.

> **More Than Skin Deep**
>
> Some of my female patients ask whether taking estrogen hormones after menopause will help their skin. According to recent studies, estrogen may slow down some age-related changes in skin, including dryness and the tendency to wrinkle. It may limit skin thinning and the loss of collagen, but these results are somewhat controversial. Before you rush out and start taking it, know the pros and cons. Estrogen cuts the risk of heart disease and osteoporosis (brittle bones), but—you knew there'd be a "but"—it may raise the risk of breast cancer and blood clots. This is a decision you should make only after consulting your doctor and weighing your options carefully.

The Skin-Food Connection

Hippocrates, a physician in ancient Greece who's considered the father of modern medicine, once told a patient, "Thy food be thy remedy." Today's doctors still agree with him: A healthy, nutritionally sound diet is crucial to good health.

The Importance of Good Nutrition

Saving Your Skin
As an example of an enriched food, check out the ingredients label on your breakfast cereal. Chances are a long list of nutrients have been added to it.

In many ways your skin is a window into your inner workings; it is a visible reflection of what goes on inside you. If you aren't getting the right nourishment, it will eventually show up in your skin.

How do you know if your diet is nutritious? This is a difficult question; even experts cannot agree on exactly what levels of vitamins and minerals are required for good nutrition. However, the FDA helps you out by setting recommended daily values for many of the nutrients considered important to health. The following table is a partial list of the FDA's recommendations, based on an average diet of 2,000 calories per day.

The FDA's Recommended Daily Values, a Partial List

Nutrient	Daily Value	Nutrient	Daily Value
Fat	65 grams	Folic acid	0.4 milligrams
Cholesterol	300 milligrams	Thiamin	1.5 milligrams
Carbohydrates	300 grams	Riboflavin	1.7 milligrams
Protein	50 grams	Niacin	20 milligrams
Fiber	25 grams	Calcium	1.0 gram
Potassium	3,500 milligrams	Iron	18 milligrams
Sodium	2,400 milligrams	Magnesium	400 milligrams
Vitamin A	5,000 international units	Phosphorus	1.0 gram
Vitamin B_6	2.0 milligrams	Iodine	150 micrograms
Vitamin B_{12}	6 micrograms	Copper	2 milligrams
Vitamin C	60 milligrams	Pantothenic acid	10 milligrams
Vitamin D	400 international units	Zinc	15 milligrams
Vitamin E	30 international units		

Does this list look dauntingly long? Not to worry. In most developed countries, it's easy to obtain these nutrients from foods and beverages. Not only do we have an enormous menu of food choices, but many grocery products have been enriched with extra helpings of these goodies.

Fatty Foods and Skin Cancer

It's rare in this country to suffer from nutritional deficiencies severe enough to affect the skin immediately. Instead, poor nutrition more often exerts a subtle, long-term effect by hurting overall health and contributing to the development of health conditions that gradually sap skin's vitality.

Want an example? Typically, Americans get 40 percent of our calories from saturated fat (this includes fat that comes from animal sources, dairy products, even certain plants). Our high-fat diet has been linked to many health problems, including atherosclerosis (clogged blood vessels) and heart disease. If left untreated, heart disease and atherosclerosis interfere with healthy circulation and reduce blood flow to the skin. Over time, diminished blood flow results in fragile skin, sores, slower wound healing, and unhealthy color.

A high-fat diet may hurt skin in more direct ways too. Recent studies at Baylor College of Medicine in Houston compared the effects of two diets, one with 38 percent of its calories from fat and the other with just 20 percent, on people who had already been treated for skin cancer. During the final eight months of a two-year study, eight people in the first group developed new skin tumors, compared to only one person in the low-fat group. What's more, the higher fat group was also more likely to develop premalignant skin lesions.

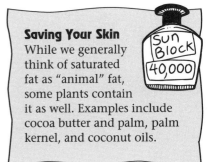

Saving Your Skin
While we generally think of saturated fat as "animal" fat, some plants contain it as well. Examples include cocoa butter and palm, palm kernel, and coconut oils.

Clearly, cutting back on fat can safeguard our skin, perhaps by reinforcing the body's immune system. The good news is that we can benefit from improving our diet no matter what our age. The average age of the Baylor study participants was 51.

What About Supplements?

Unfortunately, most Americans don't take full advantage of the rich bounty available to them. A recent survey shows that more than half of us fail to eat a single daily serving of vegetables or fruit. The FDA recommends eating at least five servings of fruit and vegetables per day, but fewer than 10 percent of Americans achieve this minimum goal.

If your diet is skimpy on fruit and vegetables, my best advice is to make a serious effort to add them to your diet. In my opinion, no supplement is as good as the natural whole food product. A case in point is the controversy over beta-carotene. For years, it has been known that diets rich in beta-carotene are associated with a decreased risk of some cancers, yet vitamin supplements of beta-carotene did not seem to impart the same protective effect. Now it is suspected that another substance found in beta-carotene-rich foods is actually what reduces cancer risk.

However, if you just cannot seem to maintain a balanced diet, you might consider vitamin and mineral supplements. Which vitamins and minerals? All are essential to healthy life, and, consequently, to beautiful skin. Each has a role to play, even the substances of which you need only trace amounts, such as iron and zinc.

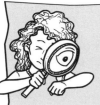

More Than Skin Deep

Vitamin and mineral supplements are so easy to buy, we forget how potent they can be. Large doses can interfere with medications and cause side effects. A few examples: High doses of niacin dilate blood vessels and can cause irregular heartbeats and flushing. Too much vitamin A leads to skin problems, hair loss, and liver and bone damage. Megadoses of vitamin C cause nausea, abdominal cramps, diarrhea, and possibly kidney stones. Always consult your doctor about the supplements and dosages that are best for you.

While all the nutrients are important, some that may be especially crucial for your skin include the following:

➤ Vitamin A (retinol), which helps to regulate cell development and maintain the skin, hair, and mucous membranes. There are two ways to get it from your diet: either as vitamin A itself, or as beta-carotene, a plant-based nutrient that your body converts into vitamin A. Vitamin A and its derivatives have been used to treat acne and some scaly skin disorders, such as psoriasis. (I'll talk more about acne in Chapter 15, "Acne: An Age-Old Problem," and about psoriasis in Chapter 16, "Solving Common Skin Problems.")

➤ B-complex vitamins. Severe B-complex deficiencies, particularly of niacin, can cause *pellagra*, a skin condition characterized by scaly dermatitis and inflamed mucous membranes.

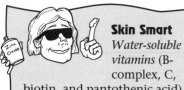

Skin Smart
Water-soluble vitamins (B-complex, C, biotin, and pantothenic acid) are stored in body water. We eliminate them constantly in urine, sweat, and other body fluids, so we need to replenish them daily. *Fat-soluble vitamins* (A, D, E, and K) are stored in fat and stay in our bodies longer. Daily supplements are less important for fat-soluble vitamins, and could even be dangerous if we take too much.

➤ Vitamin C, which helps our bodies synthesize collagen. Vitamin C deficiency causes scurvy. This is one vitamin I do take supplements of, because of its usefulness in collagen synthesis and its antioxidant properties.

➤ Vitamin E (alpha-tocopherol), an antioxidant that helps protect cells from free radicals (high-energy oxygen molecules that destroy body cells). I'll go into more detail about antioxidants in Chapter 13, "Tretinoin and Antioxidants: The Age-Tamers?"

Many vitamins are *water-soluble*, meaning our bodies store and transport them in water. Water-soluble vitamins need to be replaced daily, since we are constantly flushing them out in urine, sweat, and other body fluids. This group includes the B-complex vitamins (thiamin, riboflavin, niacin, pyridoxine, cyanocobalamin, folic acid), vitamin C, biotin, and pantothenic acid.

Other vitamins are *fat-soluble*; they are transported by fats in our bloodstream. Since they are not readily removed from the body in our urine, fat-soluble vitamins last longer. In fact, if you take large doses, you could accumulate toxic levels and literally overdose. Fat-soluble vitamins include A, D, E, and K.

For more advice on nutrition and vitamins, you'll find *The PDR Family Guide to Nutrition and Health* a helpful resource. (See Appendix A, "Bountiful Resources for Beautiful Skin," at the end of the book for more details.)

Should You Drink More Water?

Sometimes patients ask me whether drinking more water will help their appearance. Some beauty magazines recommend this, on the premise that extra water will moisturize and hydrate dry skin.

Certainly, you need to be sure that you get enough water every day. Water is crucial to our health; it's the main ingredient in our cells and accounts for roughly 60 percent of total body weight. Without sufficient water, we can't digest food, absorb nutrients, circulate blood, or eliminate waste products. It keeps mucous membranes moist and transports water-soluble vitamins through our bodies.

How much water do you need? The equivalent of eight 8-ounce glasses per day is a good guideline, but you'll need more if you perspire a lot or feel thirsty. Thirst is your body's way of requesting a drink.

Your water doesn't necessarily have to come in liquid form; many foods and beverages contain H_2O. As long as you meet your daily requirement, there's no point in drinking more water. Your body maintains a fairly constant level and eliminates excess H_2O as urine. Drinking more water will not moisturize your skin. It will, however, make you head for the nearest bathroom!

> **Saving Your Skin**
> Even though beverages containing alcohol and caffeine are fluids, they deplete your body's water supply rather than replenishing it. Why? Because they make you urinate more. If you are thirsty, drink water, not beer or soft drinks.

Exercising Your Skin

Sometimes patients are surprised when I advise them to exercise. "But you're a skin doctor!" they protest. "What does exercise have to do with skin?" My response: Just like good nutrition, regular physical activity is crucial to your overall health, and thus to the health of your skin.

Regular exercise helps in a lot of different ways. It perks up your metabolism and keeps your blood pumping healthfully to your skin (and everywhere else, for that matter). Regular exercise also helps counteract the changes that occur with age. Between ages 30 and 65, muscle mass shrinks by an average of 10 to 12 percent. This depletes the muscle tissue that helps to anchor and support skin.

Less muscle also makes it easier to gain weight (every pound of muscle on your body burns over 30 calories a day, so losing muscle leaves more calories to turn into excess pounds). Staying active will help you burn calories more efficiently and maintain a healthy amount of muscle tissue. This keeps your skin firm and helps you hold those unwanted pounds at bay.

Ready, Set, Go!

If you already exercise regularly, more power to you. Keep it up! You're already enjoying the benefits of exercise.

Many of us aren't in that category, though, and we need a bit of help getting started on a regular exercise program. Just remember you don't have to be an athlete, or even athletically inclined, to enjoy and benefit from exercise.

Here are some tips as you get underway:

➤ Always consult your doctor before starting a new exercise or activity. This is particularly important if you have a health condition of any kind.

➤ Start slowly and ease into your new exercise gradually. Don't overdo, or you could end up sore and discouraged, sapping your resolution to continue.

➤ Probably the easiest way to start is by walking. Wear supportive shoes and (if you'll be walking near a road) bright-colored or reflective clothing. If you're new at this, start by walking 10 to 15 minutes, nonstop, every other day. Gradually increase the duration of your walks.

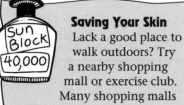

Saving Your Skin
Lack a good place to walk outdoors? Try a nearby shopping mall or exercise club. Many shopping malls open early so walkers can exercise before they get crowded.

➤ Forget the phrase "No pain, no gain." Exercise doesn't have to be painful to be good for you. In fact, unless you are a body builder, it shouldn't hurt. If you feel any discomfort, stop and consult your doctor.

Furthermore, exercise doesn't have to be strenuous or formal. If the thought of an organized exercise program leaves you cold, just think in terms of incorporating more activity into your everyday life. For instance, I don't like formal workouts either, but I run my errands on foot and walk home from my office when I can.

Here are some other possibilities to consider:

➤ Instead of cruising for the closest parking spot, park farther away and walk.

➤ Take the stairs, not the elevator.

➤ Get off the bus or train one stop early and walk the rest of the way.

➤ Stand up and walk around while you're talking on the phone or dictating a report.

➤ Reserve at least part of your lunch hour, a few days a week, for exercise. Take a walk or work out in a nearby health club. If your employer has a gym, take advantage of it.

Exercise can open new opportunities for networking. Organize a regular walking or exercise club with co-workers.

Beauty Tips
Some exercise teachers will make "house calls" to company facilities, especially if the company can guarantee a certain number of participants. Talk to your human resources department about setting up an exercise program.

Can Facial Exercises Help?

Patients sometimes ask if they should do facial exercises. Some fashion magazines recommend them, the idea being that if exercise helps other muscles in your body, it'll benefit facial muscles as well.

I don't recommend facial exercises. The muscles in your face get a constant workout from your expressions. Every frown, smile, laugh, even blink, calls on them to stretch and contract. Over time, some of the lines in our faces (the so-called expression lines) deepen from the frequent exercise of facial muscles, so working them still more isn't likely to help.

Many of us could benefit, in fact, from exercising our facial muscles a little less. If you frown a lot, you will develop lines between your eyebrows. Tightening your lips encourages wrinkles around the mouth; squinting creates crows' feet around eyes (especially when combined with sun exposure); raised brows leave lines on your forehead—you get the idea.

This is not to say that you shouldn't be expressive; life is meant to be enjoyed, and a deadpan expression isn't attractive either. Chances are, however, you give your facial muscles a good workout now, and doing exercises will just place more stress on facial skin that's already stretching and contracting daily.

Going to a Spa . . . Ahhhh

One skin treatment that's getting steadily more popular is a visit to a spa. Once the exclusive province of the wealthy, spas have become much more democratic in recent years. Today there are wonderful facilities all over the world, ranging from reasonably priced to fabulously expensive.

If you decide to try a spa, you have a lot of options to choose from. Many facilities specialize in certain types of experiences. Some focus on exercise, others on nutrition. You can choose from spas that offer Japanese mud baths, holistic therapies, New Age philosophy, martial arts, massages, training in coping with chronic medical conditions—the list is endless.

Before committing to a big-bucks adventure out of town, you might sample spa life at a day spa. These facilities, available in your community, offer many of the same services and perks without the expense of an overnight stay.

Another option is a department store spa. Several companies, such as Estee Lauder, Lancome, and Clarins, have opened in-store spas in a few cities. An in-store Estee Lauder spa typically includes at least four facial treatment rooms, two body treatment rooms, and three or more manicure stations. Lancome's in-store facilities offer massages, pedicures, facials, and free makeup demonstrations. Ask company representatives in your area whether spas are available.

More Than Skin Deep

Some spas offer "oxygen bars" that administer pure oxygen, which is supposedly purifying. The truth is that oxygen does nothing to cleanse your body and it could be dangerous, especially if you have a lung condition. We breathe because our brains signal us to take in oxygen and expel carbon dioxide, a waste product of cell metabolism. People with certain severe lung conditions can lose the ability to respond to these signals; given pure oxygen, they could theoretically stop inhaling. Even if you don't have lung problems, breathing pure oxygen for extended periods is thought to be damaging to the lungs. While short exposures—under half an hour—may not hurt, I don't recommend them.

Choosing a Spa

Here are some tips for choosing a good spa and getting the most from it:

➤ Check the staff's credentials and training. It's not enough for them to look good; they should also be knowledgeable. If the spa offers exercise classes, is there an exercise physiologist on staff? If it offers massages, what type of training do the massage therapists have?

➤ If you have a health condition, look for a facility with a health care professional on staff, such as a doctor, nurse, or physical therapist. The staff should be responsive to your needs and knowledgeable about ways to tailor their program to your condition.

➤ Some elements of your spa stay, such as physical exams, physical therapy, or stress reduction exercises, might qualify for health insurance coverage. Consult your doctor about the possibility of at least partial coverage.

➤ Schedule "detoxification" and exfoliation treatments (salt rubs, mud baths, seaweed wraps, loofah rubs) early in your stay, preferably in the mornings. This will prepare your skin for all the treatments, exercises, and activities you'll enjoy the rest of the time.

➤ If you plan to try new exercises and activities, plan ahead for massage appointments. Since it can take 24 hours for muscles to reach maximal soreness, book a massage about 24 hours after every strenuous workout. A massage is a nice way to finish off the day; try to schedule it as your day's last activity.

➤ Schedule other relaxing treatments (aromatherapy, hydrotherapy, reflexology, herbal wraps, facials) for late afternoons when you're winding down. After all, you won't want to gear up for a six-mile hike later.

➤ Book beauty sessions (hair care, cosmetics demonstrations, manicures and pedicures) for your last day, and don't schedule any strenuous activities afterward. This will give you visible benefits to bring home and keep you from chipping those carefully pedicured toenails in your hiking boots.

Facials are another popular treatment at spas. Be sure that the facial is gentle: no pulling on the skin. If you have sensitive or allergy-prone skin, beware of fragranced lotions used in some facials. And, if you're acne prone, remember to ask for oil-free, noncomedogenic products.

Saving Your Skin
If you go to a spa, don't overdo. You can't compensate for five years of sedentary living with five days of strenuous exercise and dieting. Abrupt changes in nutrition and activity level could lead to constipation, pulled tendons, torn muscles, and worse.

Beauty Tips
If your spa is located in the mountains, remember to bring sunscreen and a hat. Higher elevations mean less atmosphere to screen the sun's UV rays, so you'll burn faster than you would at sea level.

Bringing the Spa Experience Home

The most economical way to enjoy a spa is to create one in your own home. Stock up ahead of time with the basics: candles, body brushes, essential oils, jars of facial mud, moisturizers, large soft towels. That way, you'll be prepared to indulge when you get a free evening or weekend.

Here are some ideas to try. (For other soothing suggestions, check out the books by Stephanie Tourles and Kathi Keville and Mindy Green listed in Appendix A, "Bountiful Resources for Beautiful Skin.") You can enjoy these indulgences by yourself, but they'll be even more fun with a partner:

Saving Your Skin
Some people experience allergic reactions to essential oils. Before using an oil on your face, test by rubbing it into a small area on the soft underside of your wrist, and then leaving it for 24 hours. If any reaction occurs, wash it off immediately with soap and water.

Saving Your Skin
Plan ahead to avoid jarring interruptions during your home spa treatments. Pick a quiet time of day, then unplug the phone or turn on your answering machine.

➤ Give yourself a relaxing facial massage (better still, sit back and let your partner do it!). Mix one ounce of a base oil (jojoba, macadamia, or hazelnut) with five drops of an essential oil (chamomile or rosemary for dry skin; basil, ylang-ylang, or lemongrass for oily skin; rose, geranium, or neroli for normal skin). Spread the oil over your face, rubbing gently in circles; do not rub hard or pull at your skin. Rinse your face by splashing gently with tepid water. (Remember to avoid oils, though, if you have acne-prone skin.)

➤ To exfoliate skin cells, try a salt scrub. Place one-half cup of table salt in a bowl near the shower, and pour one cup of quick-cooking oats into a fine-textured muslin bag and close it tightly with a rubber band. Combine one quart of hot water in a large bowl with two drops of scented essential oil, and then soak the oatmeal bag in this solution and place next to the salt bowl.

Wet yourself thoroughly in the shower. Rub the salt over your body (not your face), using your hands, a loofah, or a washcloth. Rub in gentle circles (not hard) moving from your extremities toward your torso. Rinse the salt off thoroughly, and then rub your body gently with the oatmeal pouch and rinse again. Blot yourself dry with a clean towel and apply moisturizer.

➤ Ready for a foot scrub? Combine one-fourth cup of ground oatmeal, one-fourth cup of cornmeal, and one tablespoon of salt (sea or table). Add enough warm water to create a smooth paste, and then mix in six drops of essential oil, such as lemon or peppermint.

Massage your feet with the paste, paying particular attention to calluses and roughened areas. This can get a bit messy, so do it over the bathtub or a basin. Rinse thoroughly, pat feet dry with a warm towel, and apply moisturizer.

➤ Do your feet ache? Try a foot bath and do-it-yourself massage. Find a foot tub, pour in enough marbles to cover the bottom, and then fill with cool water (if your feet feel hot and tired) or warm water (if you're more in the mood for a relaxing soak). Mix in one-half cup salt and five to ten drops of essential oil (peppermint and lavender are particular favorites). Place the tub in front of your favorite chair and soak your feet for 15 minutes. Rub your soles across the marbles. With your toes, pick up and release marbles to stretch and exercise your tendons. Blot feet dry and rub them with moisturizer.

And finally, how about an herb wrap? This one is definitely easier with a partner.

Set a waterproof plastic lounge chair on a hard floor (I don't recommend doing this on a carpeted or wood floor; it'll get too wet). Cover the chair with a heavy blanket, and then spread a drop cloth over that.

Bring two gallons of water to a boil; remove from heat, add four cups of dried herbs, cover, and steep for at least 20 minutes. (You can use any herbal combination that appeals to you; many people swear by rose petals, chamomile, elder flowers, peppermint, yarrow, and lavender). While the herb soup is steeping, take a warm bath or shower. After 20 minutes, strain out the herbs, close the drain on your sink, and pour the scented water into the sink.

Take one flat twin-size bedsheet and fold it till small enough to fit in the sink. Soak the sheet, and then wring it out till it's wet and warm but not dripping. Have your partner unfold the sheet and wrap it around you, loosely enough that you can pull your arms out if necessary. Have your partner wrap the drop cloth, then the blanket, around you. Close your eyes and relax on the lounge chair for 15 minutes or so.

For even deeper relaxation, have your partner place a washcloth soaked in cool water on your forehead. Ahhhhh!

Treating yourself, and your skin, well is important at any age. There are plenty of things you can do to promote healthy, beautiful skin. These activities don't have to hurt; in fact, as you can see, they can feel wonderful. Try them, and your skin will thank you!

Saving Your Skin
If you have an herb wrap, or indeed any spa treatment that makes you sweat profusely, remember to replace the water you're losing so you don't become dehydrated. Keep a glass of water nearby and take periodic sips. Don't drink alcohol or coffee, because they will dehydrate you even more.

The Least You Need to Know

➤ While some skin changes occur with age, others depend on lifestyle. How you treat your skin has a lot to do with how well it ages.

➤ Good nutrition benefits your skin in lots of ways, both directly and indirectly. A low-fat diet appears to lower your risk of certain skin cancers and premalignant lesions.

➤ Like good nutrition, a good exercise program is one of your skin's best friends. However, facial exercises are unnecessary and may even contribute to facial lines.

➤ Spas are a great way to relax and pamper your skin. Choose one with a qualified staff and programs suited to your interests and abilities.

➤ With a little planning, you can enjoy spa-style treatments in the privacy of your home. Your stress level (and wallet) will appreciate it!

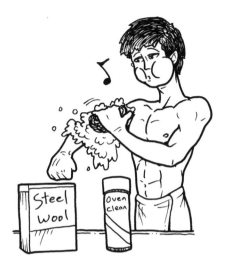

Skin No-Nos

Recently my friend Marti had a terrible day. A busy pediatrician, she saw patients all day long, and then rushed to pick up her kids from daycare and get home in time to fix dinner. The baby was crying, the older kids were fighting, and in the midst of it all, her husband called to say he would be late and ask if she could please take their eldest daughter to softball practice. Marti drove her daughter to practice, rushed to the grocery store, picked up her daughter, drove home, and worked on a report till 1 a.m. Then she got up five hours later and did it all again.

The next day was just as busy, and so was the day after that. By week's end, Marti noticed small red bumps breaking out on her arms. Soon the bumps spread into patches of red, inflamed skin that drove her crazy with itching.

After three days of torture, Marti had enough. She made an emergency appointment with me.

"Look at this!" she gasped, showing me her arms. "Where on earth did this come from?" "Those are hives," I said. "Are you allergic to anything?" "No," she said wryly. "Except maybe my own life!"

Stress and Your Skin

Marti's self-diagnosis was more accurate than she realized. Intense stress had given her a bad case of hives. Indeed, you could say she had become allergic to her life.

Marti's case is not unique. Many of us suffer from stress, which can show its ugly self in a lot of unexpected places, including our skin. Why does stress affect us this way? The answer lies deep in our history.

Fight, Flight, and Flesh

Thousands of years ago, our ancestors faced danger every minute of the day. When a wild beast attacked, they had to spring into action immediately; they grabbed a spear and fought back, or they ran for their lives. The ones who could respond quickly were the ones who lived to brag about it.

From them, we have inherited the same physiological responses to stress. When we feel threatened, hormones flood into our bloodstream and jump-start our metabolism. Our pupils widen to admit more light. Our hearts beat faster to pump blood more efficiently to our muscles. Blood pressure rises, muscles tense, and the liver speeds up its conversion of molecules to sugars to provide energy. For obvious reasons, this response is called "fight or flight."

The fight-or-flight response came in handy when we needed to outrun a woolly mammoth, and our ancestors burned up all that extra energy just to stay alive. It's less helpful when the challenge is to outrun tomorrow's deadline or that co-worker who's competing with you for promotion. Today we still face danger, although it takes other forms; office politics, family problems, and financial worries are wild beasts of a different breed. Your supervisors may have the personality of a woolly mammoth, but challenging them with a spear is no longer socially acceptable.

Saving Your Skin
Hives are caused by reactions to medications, foods, insect bites, exposure to heat or cold, and even exercise more often than they are caused by stress.

Today we can't fight and we can't flee, but we must remain ready to meet all challenges, personal and professional. Meanwhile, our bodies are still flooded with all those energizing hormones. No wonder stress is linked to so many health conditions, including high blood pressure, heart disease, and digestive problems. And, of course, to many skin problems, including—but not limited to—hives.

Recognizing Stress

A certain amount of stress is necessary, even healthy. Without it, we couldn't rise to the ordinary challenges of everyday life, let alone the extraordinary demands of emergencies. If it becomes a constant in your life, however, it leads to problems.

How do you know if the stress in your life has reached an unhealthy level? Check out the following list of danger signals. Do you often . . .

➤ Feel nervous, irritable, or depressed?

➤ Have trouble controlling your moods?

➤ Have trouble sleeping?

➤ Find it hard to make decisions?

➤ Find it difficult to think clearly and learn new information?

➤ Suffer from headaches, backaches, or chest pain?

➤ Notice your heart pounding?

➤ Suffer from shortness of breath, diarrhea, or indigestion?

Obviously, stress affects a lot of body systems, and it can certainly do a number on your skin. One nasty side effect may be hives; just ask Marti. Hives are actually an allergic reaction in which cells release chemicals that cause itching and also cause fluid to leak from blood vessels into the skin. Voilà—red, itchy, raised areas.

Saving Your Skin
One unexpected effect of stress: it can play tricks with your memory. Stressed-out folks have more trouble remembering things, even recent events.

Beauty Tips
What else can stress do to your skin? Well, it can turn your nose red. No, I'm not kidding. Surging stress hormones can dilate blood vessels and make your skin appear flushed. In some people, this effect really shows up in the nose and cheeks. So the next time your friends say you look like Rudolph, take a good look at your stress level.

Another unpopular result: pimples. Many factors cause acne, and certainly many calm people suffer with this condition. However, stress does seem to aggravate acne in predisposed individuals. (For more on treating acne, see Chapter 15, "Acne: An Age-Old Problem.")

Just to make things more fun, stress pushes sweat glands into overdrive, leaving you with cold clammy palms and armpits. It's also associated with dandruff flakes in some people. Those irritating white flakes can result from a skin condition called *seborrheic dermatitis* and, less often, from other skin disorders such as psoriasis or other types of dermatitis. All may be exacerbated by stress. (See Chapter 16, "Solving Common Skin Problems," for more on these disorders.)

As we saw in Chapter 7, "Beautiful Hair and Nails," an acute episode of severe stress can influence your hair growth cycle, causing a lot of hairs to enter the resting phase simultaneously. Subsequently these hairs all shed simultaneously in preparation for a new active phase. Usually this does not mean permanent hair loss, but nonetheless, it can be terrifying. I've had to reassure many worried patients who brought me handfuls of hair from their shower drains.

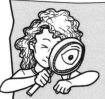

More Than Skin Deep

Legends tell of people whose hair turned white after enduring some terrible event. This reaction is seen in people who already had a fair amount of gray or white hair and is thought to be due to a preferential retention of nonpigmented hairs. That is, in some people the pigmented hairs may be more likely to enter the resting phase and then be shed than their nonpigmented neighbors.

Saying No to Stress

So what, you ask, can I do about it? While you can't get rid of stress entirely, you can do a lot to minimize its negative effects.

When you feel an anxiety attack coming on, try the following techniques:

➤ Take several deep breaths. This is not just a feel-good maneuver; it may temporarily enhance circulation, allowing you to relax tight muscles and think more clearly.

➤ Pay attention to how stress tenses your facial muscles. Consciously relax them. Blink your eyes; rub your forehead; work the corners of your mouth to relax the muscles. Tight worried expressions etch lines in your face, so don't let them become a habit.

➤ Move around. Stretch your arms, shrug your shoulders, go for a walk if you can. Exercise releases hormones into your bloodstream that act as natural tranquilizers. Furthermore, as we've seen, regular exercise is a great beautifier for body and skin.

➤ Take a good look at what causes the stress in your life. Job? In-laws? Personal relationships? Try to analyze what upsets you and what you can do about it.

➤ Many of us feel stressed out because we find it so difficult to say no. If you feel overextended, it's time to prioritize activities and weed out the ones that are less important to you.

➤ Talk about what's bothering you. You'll feel better if you share your troubles with someone else, perhaps a friend or trained counselor. Another option is a self-help group whose members can empathize with your situation and suggest practical courses of action. Groups have been organized to help people deal with a wide variety of medical and lifestyle concerns. No matter what bothers you, there's a support group available.

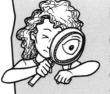

More Than Skin Deep

Once dismissed as unscientific, stress-reduction techniques are now recognized as valid treatments for stress and related health conditions. Case in point: The National Institutes of Health recommends meditation, not medications, as the treatment of choice for mild high blood pressure. Meditation doesn't have to be formal or complicated. Just take 15 to 20 minutes to sit quietly, close your eyes, breathe slowly, and relax. Clear your mind and focus on the rhythm of your breathing. Then rouse yourself gradually, stretch, and ease back into the day's activities.

Smoking and Skin: What a Lot of People Don't Know

Recently I checked a medical book for data about smoking. It contained multiple pages of information on how smoking affects various parts of the body: lungs, heart, blood vessels, and so forth. But guess what? Comprehensive though this book was, it said nothing about how smoking hurts your skin.

More Reasons to Quit

Smoking is so bad in so many ways that it's easy to overlook one more. But here's a great reason to quit smoking: It makes you look older. Since the mid-nineteenth century, doctors have noticed that chronic smokers' skin tends to be yellowish, thick, and wrinkled. In this century, scientific studies show that heavy smokers are 4.7 times more likely than nonsmokers to develop premature facial wrinkles.

Why the link between smoking and wrinkles? Smoking actually alters the cellular structure of skin. Over time, elastin fibers become thicker and more fragmented. Cells in the horny layer lose some of their normal water content, becoming dehydrated and rough.

In addition to the effects that some of these chemicals have on the skin, I'm convinced that another reason for the extra wrinkles is the way you hold your mouth when you smoke. Next time you light up, glance in a mirror. Note the lines as you purse your lips around the cigarette, and then blow out the smoke. Another contributing factor: frowning and squinting from the smoke.

Saving Your Skin

Every time you inhale tobacco smoke, more than 4,000 chemicals enter your body. They include such appetizing substances as carbon monoxide, ammonia, formaldehyde, vinyl chloride, and hydrogen cyanide. The Surgeon General warns that nicotine, the habit-forming ingredient in cigarettes, is as addictive as heroin. Is it any wonder that exposing your face to this chemical soup can be damaging to the skin?

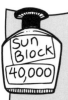

Saving Your Skin
Smokers are not the only ones hurt by smoke. Family members, co-workers, and anyone else within "nose shot" are also affected by the chemicals. Secondhand smoke is responsible for 5 to 10 percent of all cases of lung cancer. It also irritates bystanders' eyes, mucous membranes, and throats. Children of smokers are more likely to suffer from asthma and ear problems.

Need more reasons to quit? A study at the University Hospital of Wales, United Kingdom, revealed a link between smoking and psoriasis, a chronic skin condition characterized by thickened patches of inflamed red and scaly skin. In the study, 55 percent of patients with psoriasis smoked before they developed the condition, compared with only 32 percent in the control group. What's more, the more they smoked, the greater their risk.

Smoking narrows blood vessels and raises carbon monoxide levels in the bloodstream, restricting healthful circulation to the skin. Not surprisingly, smokers' skin takes longer to heal from all types of injuries, including surgical incisions, and surgical skin grafts in smokers have a much higher failure rate.

You may know that tobacco increases your risk of lung cancer (by up to 24 times), but did you know that it also raises your chance of skin malignancies? If you smoke, you more than double your odds of lip and mouth cancer.

Kicking the Habit

"Okay," you say. "So cut the lecture and tell me how to quit!"

You'll be glad to know that your skin, and your body in general, will start to repair itself the minute you stop smoking. As the chemical level in your blood goes down, its oxygen content increases. Blood vessels widen, heart rate slows down to normal, and your lungs begin a grand spring house cleaning.

To kick the habit, try these strategies:

➤ Write down all the reasons you want to stop smoking and review the list every day. Look at it every time you're tempted to resume.

➤ Set a date with yourself to quit. Some of my patients choose a date of personal importance, like a birthday or holiday. Others prefer to wait till after holidays because they tend to be high-stress occasions. Don't set a date two weeks before a big report at work is due.

➤ Announce ahead of time to family and friends that you're going to quit. Ask for their support.

➤ After you quit, particularly during the crucial early weeks, spend as much time as possible with nonsmokers in smoke-free premises. Most relapses occur within the first few months, so avoid temptation.

➤ Stock up on healthy snacks: fruit, sugarless gum, popcorn (hot-air popped), carrots and celery, seltzer, herbal tea. When you get the urge to smoke, munch and sip to keep mouth and hands busy.

Exercise can help when you're having a craving. Remember those stress-relieving hormones that are released into the bloodstream when you exercise? They can help you get past an acute craving. When you want a cigarette, get up and take a walk around the block.

As you are breaking the habit, you will have periods when you crave a cigarette as strongly as ever. Know that these episodes will occur less frequently as time passes. Just knowing that they will pass may give you the strength to resist.

Take another look at the stress-reduction techniques mentioned earlier in this chapter and the home spa procedures in Chapter 8, "Keeping That Youthful Look." When a craving becomes great, these techniques can help you through.

Most doctors recommend quitting cold turkey. If you prefer a more gradual approach, ask your doctor about nicotine patches or gum. These medications deliver small doses of nicotine to gradually wean you off cigarettes. Remember, they're supposed to help you quit smoking, not become a new habit. Follow the package directions. You should cut back on, then stop, these aids within a set period of time.

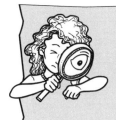

More Than Skin Deep

If you use nicotine patches, dispose of used patches properly in a covered container inaccessible to kids and pets. They could be poisoned by the nicotine that still remains on the patches. And be sure not to smoke while using the patch. You could overdose.

The Perils of Weight Gain (and Weight Loss)

Beth's primary care physician referred her to me because she was worried about persistent stretch marks and sagging skin on her face, arms, and neck. "It's so ugly!" she complained to me. "How do I get rid of it?"

Beth was very pretty but overweight—standing five feet two inches, she weighed 220 pounds. As we discussed her medical history, she revealed that she had gone on several crash diets over the past five years. Each time she lost about a hundred pounds, only to gain it back in several months. "This is the reason for your stretch marks and skin folds," I told her gently. "When you gain weight, your skin stretches. Then when you lose weight, it takes time for the skin to shrink back down to match. And, I'm sorry to say, it is possible that some never will."

"But what can I do about it?" she wailed. "I want to lose weight for good, and I want to lose that skin too!"

Why It's Bad

Like Beth, many of us want to know how to lose weight and keep it off. Almost one-third of Americans, roughly 34 million of us, are over our ideal weight. Over the past decade, our average weight has risen by 10 pounds apiece.

How much should you weigh? This chart summarizes weight ranges according to height. Note that there is no one ideal weight for your height; if you are anywhere within the healthy range, good for you! Muscle and bone weigh more than fat tissue, so if you are muscular or big-boned you'll be at the high end of the healthy range.

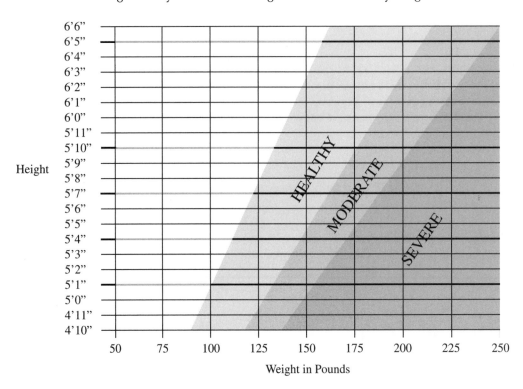

Are you a healthy weight for your height? (Adapted by permission of the U.S. Department of Agriculture.)

If this chart shows you to be heavier than you'd like, it's time to take charge of your weight. Like smoking and stress, excess weight affects your skin both directly and indirectly. Among the results are the following:

➤ Stretch marks and sagging folds

➤ Varicose veins

➤ Increased risk of high blood pressure, certain types of cancer, arthritis, heart disease, and diabetes—conditions that impair your circulation, energy level, and general appearance

As your weight rises, so does your risk. People who are *obese* (more than 20 percent above their healthy weight) have dramatically higher rates of health problems.

Losing Weight for Good

So how can you lose weight and, even more important, keep it off? Here's a tip: don't diet.

Sound strange? Not really. When you cut back drastically on food, your body's metabolism slows way down. Just like the fight-or-flight response, this is something we have inherited from our ancestors. In the good old days, humans were in more danger of dying from too little food than too much, so our bodies developed this efficient technique for conserving calories.

From your body's point of view, a crash diet is a period of famine. This is why dieters complain they can't lose weight no matter how little they eat; their bodies are trying to help by hoarding calories. Eventually, tired of deprivation, they return to old eating habits. When they do, those pounds are waiting. It's estimated that 90 percent of crash dieters regain the weight they lost, just like Beth.

Rather than starving yourself, think in terms of developing healthy eating habits. Aim for a gradual loss of one-half to one pound per week. Fill up on stuff that's good for you, like fruit, vegetables, and whole grains. Cut back on empty calories—candy, desserts, soft drinks, alcohol. You don't need to give them up entirely, but make them special treats rather than everyday staples.

Some other tips:

➤ Substitute. Instead of whole milk, drink skim (non-fat) or one-percent. Instead of ice cream or potato chips, try low-fat frozen yogurt and pretzels. Enjoy low-fat equivalents of your favorite foods.

Saving Your Skin
Being extremely overweight may even be bad for your immune system. A Japanese study measured levels of T lymphocytes (crucial defender cells in the body) in a group of obese people enrolled in a weight loss program. After losing an average of 50 pounds, their T lymphocyte activity doubled.

Skin Smart
In medical terminology, *obese* doesn't just mean overweight; it means being 20 percent or more over your healthy weight.

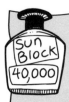

Saving Your Skin
Emotional support is crucial to successful weight loss. If you have trouble losing weight on your own, ask a friend or family member to keep you company, or join a support group like Weight Watchers or Overeaters Anonymous.

Beauty Tips
There are reports that tretinoin cream may diminish stretch marks. Talk to your dermatologist for more information.

➤ Cut back on red meat. Smother your pasta with mushroom or tomato sauce, and make burgers with ground turkey. When you do eat beef, buy lean cuts and trim off visible fat. Red meat is high in saturated fat, which is loaded with calories and clogs arteries. But don't remove protein entirely. It's necessary for good nutrition.

➤ Cut the late-night snacks. Your metabolism is highest during your first 12 waking hours, so consume most of your calories then. If you really get the evening munchies, stick to low-calorie eatables like fruit, carrots, celery, and popcorn (hold the butter).

➤ Take the focus off food. If you know you've eaten enough but you still have the munchies, try focusing on something else. Take a walk, go to the movies, or pick up a good book.

➤ Above all, exercise! Regular physical activity speeds up your metabolism and burns calories. It's crucial to keeping the weight off over the long haul.

If, like Beth, you're bothered by stretch marks and excess skin, consider plastic surgery or laser treatments. Don't be fooled by cosmetics that promise to tighten skin: Surgery is the only effective way to remove it. For more information, and the latest on lasers and tretinoin in treating stretch marks, see Chapter 13, "Tretinoin and Antioxidants: The Age-Tamers?," Chapter 23, "Better Looking with Lasers," and Chapters 24 and 25, "Should You Try Plastic Surgery?" and "Popular Choices in Plastic Surgery."

Please, Be Gentle

Many patients come to see me because their skin is inflamed or irritated. Sad to say, often they are suffering from their own actions. Picking and squeezing pimples, sudsing with strong soaps, overusing toners, scrubbing with harsh exfoliants, rubbing with abrasive loofahs and washcloths—these are just a few of the abuses people inflict on their skin.

Talk about stress! Over time, these habits take their toll. As I've said before, if you wouldn't do it to a baby's face, please don't do it to your own. Always use the gentlest products that are effective on your skin, and apply them gently too.

What else can you do to protect your skin? Lots of things. The biggest skin no-no of all is sun exposure. In the next chapter, you'll learn how ultraviolet radiation ages your skin.

The Least You Need to Know

➤ Stress saps your energy and the health and vitality of your skin. Over time, frowns and tense expressions turn into permanent lines. Learning to relax will make you look and feel better.

➤ You've heard how bad smoking is for your heart and lungs. Turns out it's bad for your skin, too. Over time, smoking turns skin yellow, leathery, and wrinkled. Quitting is a great way to add years to your life while taking them off your appearance.

➤ A healthy program of regular exercise benefits your entire body, including your skin, and helps you stay slender.

➤ Gaining weight stretches your skin, and is one of many factors that may impair skin-nourishing circulation. Cycles of weight gain and weight loss leave skin sagging and wrinkled.

➤ Sometimes we are our own worst enemies. Many cases of dry, irritated, and inflamed skin result from our own rough handling.

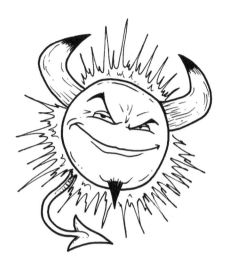

Chapter 10

The Sun Is No Fun

In This Chapter

➤ Discover what really happens when you sunburn

➤ Learn why there's no such thing as a healthy tan

➤ Find out why tanning beds should be illegal

➤ Learn what longtime sun exposure does to skin (here's a hint: It's not pretty!)

➤ Discover the only safe way to "tan"

The daughter of one of my friends, blonde blue-eyed Brittany, is an athletic high school student who spends a lot of time outdoors. Last July she came to see me because of a mild case of acne. After I prescribed medication, we chatted for a few minutes.

I noticed she had a very dark suntan. "Do you use sunscreens?" I asked her.

"Nope," she replied. "They just sweat off anyway. Besides, I hate my light skin. I love getting a tan because it looks sexy! In the winter I look like a ghost. A lot of my friends go to tanning salons during the winter so they can stay dark all year. I'd like to go too, but my mom won't let me."

Too Much Sun: Public Enemy Number One

Let's hear it for Brittany's mother! If more people said no to tanning beds and dark suntans, I'd see a lot less wrinkling and skin cancer in my practice.

In Chapter 8, "Keeping That Youthful Look," you looked at how skin changes over time. Some of these changes are built-in and will happen anyway with the passage of time. However, research shows that much of what we call "aging" is self-inflicted; it has nothing to do with getting older and a lot to do with how we treat our skin. In Chapter 9, "Skin No-Nos," you looked at some of the things that age skin prematurely.

In this chapter, I discuss the single most important enemy to beautiful skin: the sun.

The ABCs of UV

Sunlight comes in a variety of wavelengths, only some of them dangerous to skin. The wavelengths we're concerned about in this chapter are *ultraviolet (UV) rays*, which account for only 2 or 3 percent of solar radiation. As shown in the drawing, ultraviolet rays are intermediate-length waves that fall on the spectrum between longer-wavelength visible light and short, invisible x-rays. (They're called "ultraviolet" because they lie just beyond the violet rays of visible light.)

In the spectrum, the three types of ultraviolet rays fall between visible light and invisible gamma rays and x-rays.

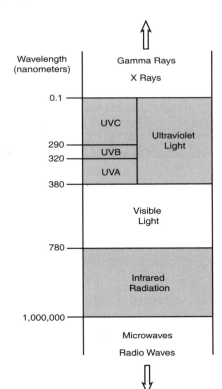

There are three wavelengths of ultraviolet light: A, B, and C. Most of the light that reaches the earth is *UVA*, the wavelength largely responsible for suntans; chronic exposure to UVA damages skin and plays a role in aging and skin cancer. Sunlight contains a smaller amount of *UVB*, which makes us sunburn. The third type, *UVC*, certainly has the potential to injure skin; fortunately, it doesn't get the chance because it's absorbed above the earth by the ozone layer.

What Happens When You Sunburn?

A small amount of sunlight, but not much, is necessary for your skin to produce vitamin D. The minimal exposure you get every day from going to work and running errands is enough. Beyond that, there's no health-related reason to sunbathe your skin.

What happens if you do sunbathe? After you've been in the sun for a while, your skin becomes a little red. This effect signals an inflammatory response as your skin works to protect you against UV damage. The longer your sun exposure, the more serious the UV bombardment becomes. UV rays injure and then kill skin cells in the epidermis and damage the tiny blood vessels underneath that nourish the skin.

Skin Smart
Ultraviolet rays are medium-wavelength light rays that get their name from being located next to violet light on the spectrum. *UVB* rays are responsible for sunburn; *UVA* rays tan skin and play a role in long-term skin aging. *UVC* rays don't reach the earth because they are absorbed by the ozone layer.

Skin Smart
A *sunburn* is an inflammation of the skin caused by overexposure to the sun's UVB rays.

Generally, this slight flush fades within half an hour after you go inside. The real *sunburn* appears many hours later when your sun-exposed skin turns pink and tender. If you really overdid it, forget pink and tender; your skin will be red, painful, and blistered. After several days, your skin peels as it sheds the layer of dead cells.

If You're Fair, Beware

As we saw in Chapter 2, "Your Skin: Don't Leave Home Without It," melanin has the job of protecting you against UV radiation. Sun exposure signals your melanin-making cells, called melanocytes, to step up production. How does this signal work? Recent research shows that within minutes, sunlight starts to damage the DNA in skin cells. When the skin senses light-injured DNA particles, it issues a call for more melanin.

Melanin production rises slowly and results in a suntan. The bronzed tan we admire so much is actually a sign of skin damage from too much UV.

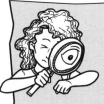

More Than Skin Deep

The image of suntans as sexy is relatively new. Before 1900, a suntan was frowned upon because it meant you had to work outdoors. Members of the upper class were proud of their light, non–sun-exposed skin. Women wore broad-brimmed hats and carried parasols to preserve their pale complexions. Today, when so many of us labor in offices, the ability to spend time outdoors has become a perk, not a punishment. We consider suntans attractive because they are associated with the luxury of leisure time.

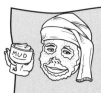

Beauty Tips

Sometimes we're told that tanning slowly, over several days to weeks, is safer than tanning rapidly. This is a myth. While gradual tanning may reduce your risk of a sunburn, any tan, whether acquired slowly or quickly, indicates skin damage from sun exposure.

The lighter your skin, the less melanin it can marshal to protect you. Not surprisingly, skin cancer is much more common in Caucasians than in Asians or African Americans. If you have extremely light skin, especially if you're a redhead or blonde, you may not make enough melanin to tan, period. Even a mere 20 minutes outdoors can leave you looking like a boiled lobster. (You might feel like one too!)

But remember: Even if you do tan, no tan is safe. No matter how readily your melanin cells rush to your aid, you are still exposing your skin to harmful UV—and the damage, unfortunately, accumulates over time.

I realize that we all love being outside, and it's unrealistic to advise avoiding the sun entirely. Life is too short to spend all your time indoors. Fortunately, you can still enjoy sunlight while minimizing its harmful effects; we'll talk more about that in Chapter 11, "Fighting Back Against Photoaging."

Do After-Sun Products Help Your Tan?

Some companies sell creams and lotions that supposedly make your tan stick around longer. These "after-sun products" are really nothing more than moisturizers. While a good moisturizer can slow down the skin's natural peeling process, making tanned skin cells stay in place longer, eventually they will slough off. In fact, if they remain on your skin too long, they could make it dull, dry and flaky, giving your tan a patchy look.

I don't recommend spending extra money on an after-sun moisturizer. Your regular moisturizer will do just as good a job and is probably cheaper.

Ouch! Soothing a Sunburn

So what can you do if, despite all your good intentions, your skin gets that ominous pink tinge? Here are some tips for soothing sunburn:

➤ Go inside immediately. If that's not possible, move to the shade or cover the sunburned area with clothing.

➤ As soon as you can, apply cool compresses. Do this for 20 minutes, two times a day, for the first several days.

➤ Apply a soothing moisturizer several times a day, either your regular brand or a sunburn cream with a mild topical anesthetic.

➤ If you notice any blisters, call your doctor. Blisters are pools of fluid that accumulate within the epidermis; if they rupture, they open your skin to microorganisms and infection. Your doctor may prescribe medications to head off any trouble.

➤ If the sunburn is severe, your doctor may prescribe corticosteroids. These medications suppress skin inflammation and moderate some of the pain.

➤ Protect your burned skin from the sun until it has completely healed.

Ask your doctor about taking over-the-counter painkillers, such as aspirin or ibuprofen; they will help you feel a little better. Another option is to apply aloe vera gel, a time-honored home remedy for irritated skin.

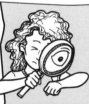

More Than Skin Deep

As far is your skin is concerned, a sunburn is like any other burn in many ways. Doctors classify burns according to how much of the body is affected and how deep the damage goes. A mild sunburn is comparable to a first-degree burn, with damage confined to the superficial layers of the epidermis. If you blister, you have a second-degree sunburn, which destroys superficial and deep cells in the epidermis down to the junction with the dermis.

No Tanning Beds, Please

Remember when Brittany said her friends visit tanning salons during the winter and she wants to go too? Like all dermatologists, I am dead-set against the use of tanning beds and home sun lamps for tanning.

Tanning beds (also known as *tanning booths* or *beaches-in-a-box*) emit concentrated bursts of UVA rays. Tanning salon owners insist they're safe because they don't produce UVB. Supposedly, this lets you tan safely without having to worry about sunburn.

There's just one problem: This isn't true. While UVA rays generally do not cause visible sunburn, they are responsible for many of the long-term changes that age skin. UVA actually penetrates more deeply into the skin than UVB; it reaches the dermis, where it damages collagen and elastin fibers. You might not get sunburn from a tanning bed, but you will get wrinkles, tiny spider veins, bumpy skin, and all the other hallmarks of premature skin aging.

You can also get skin cancer. A study in Sweden showed that people who use tanning beds more than 10 times a year have a seven times greater risk of melanoma, the most deadly type of skin cancer.

Saving Your Skin

Visits to tanning beds are not just bad for your skin. They can also cause burns to the cornea (the transparent outer layer of the eyeball) and retina (the tissue inside the eye), eventually leading to cataracts.

Another scary fact about tanning beds: The industry is poorly regulated. A typical sun lamp emits two to three times more UVA radiation than does natural sunlight. Some lamps put out even higher doses, and there's no way to know how much you're getting. In terms of UVA exposure, the average salon visit is equivalent to a full day at the beach. (Incidentally, while sun lamps are not supposed to contain UVB, some do. The proportion of UVB may actually be higher than that found in sunlight.)

"But surely I can ask the tanning salon owners," you may protest. "Can't they tell me how safe their lamps are?" Probably not. A recent survey of 31 tanning salon proprietors found that most were woefully ignorant of their products and the associated risks. For example, 71 percent insisted that tanning beds were safer than tanning outdoors, and only 7 percent knew they could cause cancer. The folks at your local salon may not be any better informed.

Ordinarily, your risk of sun-related skin damage is highest during summer, when the sun is brightest. Thanks to the miracle of sun lamp technology, we can now experience this risk year-round, even in winter. Every day, one million Americans visit tanning salons; at least two thirds are young women, average age 26. One to two million of them are devoted fans who broil themselves 100 times a year or more. Unfortunately, the people fondest of tanning beds are often the fair-skinned types who have the most to lose.

The bottom line: Don't use tanning beds, and don't let your kids use them either.

What the Sun Does to Skin

When it comes to skin, a lot of what we call "aging" is actually *photoaging*—deterioration caused by exposure to sunlight. (*Photo* means "pertaining to light.") I've seen youthful people in their 70s with very few wrinkles, and others, ardent sunbathers in their 30s, who look 15 years older than the age on their drivers' licenses. While your genetic heritage certainly influences your skin's durability, the single biggest factor is the amount of time you have spent in the sun.

Photoaging begins at the level of the tiniest skin cell. Cells in the horny layer that used to interlock neatly become rough and thickened. Melanocytes distribute their melanin unevenly, elastin fibers clump together, collagen structure changes, and the connective tissue that keeps skin smooth and firm slowly breaks down. Eventually, all these changes combine to produce the pebbled, leathery texture of photoaged skin.

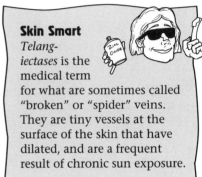

Skin Smart
Photoaging refers to skin deterioration caused by exposure to sunlight.

The all-too-common signs include the following:

➤ Wrinkles. Many scientists believe that wrinkles have less to do with chronological aging and more to do with sun exposure.

➤ Dull complexion. Caucasian and Asian skin may take on a yellowish sallow tinge; African-American skin looks ashy.

➤ Leathery, rough texture.

➤ Age spots. These patches of pigmented skin, variously called freckles, liver spots, or age spots, grow darker with time and sun exposure. Depending on your skin color, they may be pale beige, almost black, or somewhere in between. (Incidentally, liver spots, despite the name, have nothing to do with the liver.)

Skin Smart
Telangiectases is the medical term for what are sometimes called "broken" or "spider" veins. They are tiny vessels at the surface of the skin that have dilated, and are a frequent result of chronic sun exposure.

➤ Tendency to bruise easily. Over time, sun exposure injures tiny blood vessels and supporting connective tissue. These tiny vessels break and bleed more readily than they used to.

➤ *Telangiectases*, also called spider veins. These are tiny blood vessels in the skin that have dilated or stretched out. They are seen in increased numbers in many conditions, including chronic sun damage. If enough telangiectases are present, they may impart a reddened appearance to the skin. While telangiectases are sometimes called "broken" veins, the blood vessels are dilated rather than broken. The most common places you can see them are the nose and cheeks.

➤ Various types of bumps and lumps. Some are flesh-colored, others dark or reddish. Occasionally they are precancerous, although most simply indicate sun damage. (I'll go into more detail about how to tell the difference in Chapters 18, "Benign Bumps," and 19, "Skin Cancer: The Dark Side of the Sun.")

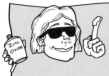

Skin Smart
Dihydroxyac-etone (*DHA*) is the active ingredient in artificial tanning products. It interacts with the proteins in superficial skin layers to darken your skin temporarily.

Saving Your Skin
Have you seen ads for artificial tanning pills? The active ingredient is usually *canthaxanthin*, a distant relative of vitamin A. This coloring agent deposits in subcutaneous tissues and turns your skin orange. Canthaxanthin is risky as well as unattractive; it's been pulled off the U.S. market because of adverse reactions. You can still mail-order it from catalogs, but please don't.

Is your skin photoaged? Here's a simple test: Compare skin that hasn't seen a lot of sun, like your buttocks or inner arm, with your face and forearms. If you detect a noticeable difference, don't be discouraged, but do take steps to protect yourself. I'll tell you how in the next chapter.

Artificial Tans: Tanning from a Tube

Like Brittany, you might think you just plain look better with a tan. "So what am I supposed to do?" you ask. "Is there any good way to get a suntan?" Yes, there is. The only safe way to tan is with an artificial tanner, a product that stains your skin to give it that just-spent-all-day-at-the-beach look.

Artificial tanners contain *dihydroxyacetone* (*DHA*), a colorless substance that interacts with proteins in the outer epidermal layers to create a brownish compound that dyes your skin temporarily. DHA is the only substance approved by the FDA for this purpose.

Artificial tans may look like a "real" tan, but be aware that they are completely different. Unlike a sun-induced tan, they have no effect on your melanocytes, so they offer no protection against ultraviolet rays. You are just as liable to sunburn with an artificial tan as you are without it. In fact, you may be even more vulnerable because the dye will mask the pinkness that warns you to go indoors. I've had patients who used artificial tanners, then ended up in my office with incredibly painful sunburns.

Applying a Beautiful Tan

Artificial tanners come in a variety of forms: creams, lotions, sprays, and gels. Choose the type that goes on the smoothest because, when getting your tan from a tube, that's the real challenge.

Follow these steps:

➤ Before smearing the stuff all over your body, try a small test patch on the underside of your arm. Wait 24 hours and make sure you like the color (and you don't have an allergic reaction) before committing yourself.

➤ If you decide to go ahead, exfoliate first; the smoother your skin, the better your tan will look. Rub your face gently with a cosmetic scrubbing cream, or apply alpha hydroxy acids the night before (see Chapter 12, "Help from Hydroxy Acids"). If you plan to apply tanner on areas of thicker skin, like elbows, knees, or the soles of your feet, rub them gently with a pumice stone or loofah.

➤ Just before applying the tanner, bathe or take a shower, shave, then blot skin lightly with a towel. The tanner will go on more easily if your skin is a little damp.

➤ Apply a very thin layer of the product; if in doubt, use less than you think you will need. It's easier to rub on a small amount smoothly and evenly. You can always apply more later if you want to go darker.

➤ Be very careful when rubbing tanner on calluses and rough areas like elbows and knees. The extra layers of thick skin will absorb more of it. Rather than looking like you spent the day at the beach, you'll look like you played in the dirt and forgot to wash up.

➤ Wash your hands carefully afterward, and clean fingernails and cuticles with a nail brush, or they may develop a tanned color too.

➤ Give yourself a good 30 minutes to dry. Stay away from clothing, bed linens, and all other fabrics because the tanner will stain them.

➤ If you're not dry after 30 minutes, you probably applied too much. Next time, go a little lighter.

An artificial tan lasts only a few days. As your skin sheds the dyed cells, your color will gradually fade to your normal complexion. If you want to stay dark, you'll have to reapply the product every few days.

Some people have good luck with artificial tanners, but others find them frustrating. It's all too easy to end up with streaks and dark spots, and some people find the color too orange. Another problem is that your tan may start to look patchy after you shave or take a shower.

The percentage of DHA in these products varies, although it's relatively low (you'll notice it's often listed near the end of the ingredients). If you consistently get streaks and blotches, you may be using one of the higher-formulation products. Try one with less DHA and a lighter texture.

> **Beauty Tips**
> If you acquire a tan, whether artificial or natural, remember to adjust your makeup accordingly. Choose a slightly darker foundation and blush. Stay away from orange and coral hues; many artificial tanners have an orange undertone that orange-toned makeup will exaggerate. As your tan fades, lighten your makeup to suit.

A Message About Tan Accelerators

Tan accelerators (also called "amplifiers" or "activators") are topically applied products that supposedly expedite the skin's ability to produce melanin. Generally they contain *tyrosine*, an amino acid found in melanin. The manufacturers claim they make the tanning process more efficient so you tan faster with the same amount of sun exposure.

Fact is, tan accelerators really don't help you tan. Several companies have been censured by the FDA for making misleading statements on their packaging. In any case, I question anything that encourages you to spend more time in the sun. So, the message on tan accelerators is "Don't bother."

You'll learn more about the adverse effects of too much sun in Chapter 19, where I tell you how to protect yourself against skin cancer. Meanwhile, in the next chapter, I'll show you how to safeguard your beautiful skin against those damaging ultraviolet rays.

The Least You Need to Know

➤ Much of what we call "aging" is actually skin damage from sun exposure. If you want to look younger when you're older, cut your sun exposure now.

➤ There's no such thing as a healthy suntan. Both suntans and sunburns signal cell damage from ultraviolet radiation.

➤ Stay away from tanning beds, which emit high doses of UVA rays that age skin even when they don't cause visible sunburn. The industry is poorly regulated and filled with misleading claims about the safety of their products.

➤ The safest way to tan is with an artificial tanner. Exfoliate your skin first, and apply the tanner lightly to damp skin. But remember, artificial tans do not offer any protection against the sun; you will sunburn just as though you had no tan at all.

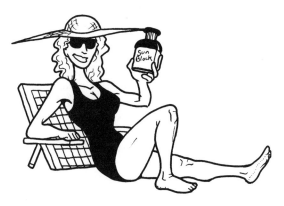

Chapter 11

Fighting Back Against Photoaging

In This Chapter

➤ Find out why sunscreens are so important

➤ Discover what SPF does and doesn't tell you

➤ Go beyond SPF and learn more about sunscreens

➤ See how photosensitive reactions sneak up on you

➤ Learn why "mad dogs and Englishmen stay out of the noonday sun"

The other day I went shopping for a sunscreen. "Which do you recommend?" I asked the sales representative. "This is our top seller," she said confidently, displaying a small (and expensive) bottle. "But this is only SPF 8," I pointed out. "I really would like something stronger."

"Oh, don't worry, this is as strong as you'll ever need," she assured me. "SPF 8 is high enough to protect you against the UV rays that burn you, but it still lets through the safe UV rays that give you a tan. I've seen lots of studies that say the ideal sun protection is to combine a natural tan with an SPF 8 sunscreen."

Hmmmm...

Sunscreen: Your Skin's Best Friend

Here's a quiz: Of all the products on the market that promise to keep you looking young, which comes closest to keeping that promise? The answer: sunscreens, one of the most promising cosmetic developments in years.

A *sunscreen* is an oil, lotion, or cream containing compounds that filter out UV rays. A good sunscreen can do more to prevent wrinkles than the best-hyped wrinkle cream or the most expensive moisturizer. When it comes to fighting photoaging, an effective sunscreen is your skin's best friend. Short of avoiding the sun entirely, it's the best way to preserve the beautiful skin you were born with.

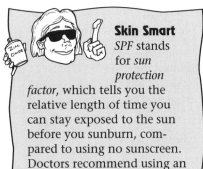

Skin Smart

A *sunscreen* is an oil, lotion, or cream that contains compounds to filter out UV rays. It's an important weapon in the fight against photoaging.

But not just any sunscreen. As my conversation with the salesperson shows, there's a lot of false information out there about sunscreens. Her advice certainly conflicts with anything I (or any other doctor) would tell you. Who knows how many customers have bought this sunscreen based on her well-meaning, but misinformed, recommendation?

A Consumer's Guide to Sunscreens

All sunscreens are not created equal. Some ingredients protect against UVB rays only, others shield against UVA, and a few offer protection against both. How can you know what you're buying? Fortunately, the FDA makes your decision easier by mandating that companies label their products with an SPF number.

SPF and Your Skin

SPF stands for *sun protection factor*, which tells you the relative length of time you can stay in the sun before you sunburn, compared to using no sunscreen at all. To compute your sun protection factor, multiply the SPF number by the number of minutes you can typically spend in the sun without getting burned.

Skin Smart

SPF stands for *sun protection factor*, which tells you the relative length of time you can stay exposed to the sun before you sunburn, compared to using no sunscreen. Doctors recommend using an SPF of 15 or higher.

For example, suppose that without sunscreen, you ordinarily turn pink after 10 minutes. An SPF of 4 would extend that to 40 minutes, an SPF of 8 to 80 minutes, an SPF of 15 to 150 minutes (see the following diagram). Clearly, the higher the SPF, the better.

SPF does not tell you the whole story, however. It primarily measures your protection against UVB rays, the ones responsible for sunburn. It does not gauge a product's effectiveness against UVA very well, and UVA, as we saw in

Chapter 10, "The Sun Is No Fun," may be even more dangerous than UVB for long-term skin aging. A sunscreen may do a great job of blocking UVB but let longer-wavelength UVA rays pass through to harm your skin with no burn to warn you to take cover.

Skin Type	Time to Burn			
	Using No Sunscreen	Using Sun Protection Factor		
		4	8	15
FAIR	10 minutes	40 minutes	80 minutes	2 1/2 hours
MEDIUM	30 minutes	2 hours	4 hours	7 1/2 hours
DARK	1 hour	4 hours	8 hours	All day

The higher the SPF, the longer you can stay outdoors without burning.

Understanding Sunscreen Ingredients

To get the broadest range of protection possible, take a look at the active ingredients listed on the product label. Sunscreens work by absorbing or blocking sunlight. All the ingredients in the following list absorb sunlight except for titanium dioxide and zinc oxide, which block it.

These are the most common sunscreen ingredients:

➤ *Anthranilates*: Moderately effective at screening out both UVA and UVB.

➤ *Benzophenes (oxybenzone and methoxybenzone, sulisobenzone)*: Have coverage that extends into the UVA range.

➤ *Cinnamates*: Block mainly UVB.

➤ *PABA (para-amino-benzoic acid; related compounds are glyceryl, padimate 0, and padimate A)*: Very effective at screening UVB, but does not stop UVA.

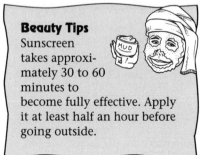

Beauty Tips
Sunscreen takes approximately 30 to 60 minutes to become fully effective. Apply it at least half an hour before going outside.

➤ *Parasol 1789*: Effective for UVA.

➤ *Titanium dioxide, zinc oxide*: "Physical" sun blocks that screen out both UVA and UVB by forming a layer that stops them from reaching the skin.

The cosmetics industry refers to titanium dioxide and zinc oxide as "non-chemical" sunscreens because they physically reflect ultraviolet light, as opposed to chemical sunscreens that absorb UV. Titanium dioxide and zinc oxide seem to cause fewer allergic reactions than some chemical sunscreens. That, coupled with their broad range of protection in the UVB and UVA wavelengths, make them excellent sunscreens.

Getting the Most from Your Sunscreen

Beauty Tips
Although an effective sunscreen, zinc oxide has rarely been used in cosmetics because it tends to be opaque. (Maybe you've seen lifeguards wearing zinc oxide paste on their noses.) New zinc oxide preparations are nearly transparent, however, and worth checking out.

Saving Your Skin
Even "waterproof" sunscreens aren't really waterproof. To be labeled waterproof, FDA guidelines say that a sunscreen must maintain its SPF for 80 minutes underwater; a "water-resistant" sunscreen must maintain its SPF for only 40 minutes. If you spend more time than that in the water, keep putting on more sunscreen.

Many of my patients ask for advice on selecting and using sunscreens. Here's what I tell them:

➤ Always choose a sunscreen with an SPF of at least 15. It's estimated that this screens approximately 94 percent of UVB radiation. Lower numbers simply don't offer enough protection. If you're fair-skinned or spend a lot of time outdoors, look for an even higher SPF.

➤ Make your first choice a sunscreen with titanium dioxide or zinc oxide as the active ingredient. This "non-chemical" block does a better job than most chemical sunscreens of protecting your skin against both UVA and UVB. The downside is that some of these products are greasy and leave a whitish film on the skin.

➤ If you can't find a titanium dioxide or zinc oxide sunscreen you like, select one that combines UVA and UVB blockers from the previous list. Look for "broad-spectrum" on the label.

➤ Be good to yourself and use plenty. Most people need at least one ounce of sunscreen to cover their entire body. If you use less, you're not getting the full SPF benefit.

➤ Price is immaterial; an expensive sunscreen is no better than a drugstore brand. Both contain the same basic ingredients. The inexpensive product may actually be better because you'll be less tempted to economize when slathering it on.

➤ Sunscreens do wear off, especially if you perspire or spend any time in water. Look for one labeled "waterproof" or "water-resistant." Reapply it frequently throughout the day.

➤ Remember, geographic location makes a difference. The closer you are to the equator, the stronger the UV rays. An hour on the beach in the Bahamas is more intense than an hour on the beach near Boston.

➤ Wear sunscreen year-round. While the sun's rays are less intense during the winter, they're still not good for your skin.

➤ More and more cosmetics companies are including sunscreen in their products. If you can find a good SPF 15 moisturizer or foundation that you like, great. But please don't sacrifice SPF power for the convenience of an all-in-one product. A foundation with an SPF lower than 15 simply doesn't offer enough protection for daily wear. Apply an SPF 15 sunscreen first, and then smooth your foundation over it.

➤ Most sunscreens sting if they get in your eyes. One solution: Apply an SPF 15 sun block for the lips around your eyes. It's more waxy than sunscreen lotions and won't sweat into your eyes. Another solution is to try the "sports" brands meant for people who perspire a lot.

Water, snow, sand, and pavement reflect UV rays. If you're skiing on the slopes or lounging next to a swimming pool, take this into account and put on extra sun block.

Beauty Tips
Many cosmetics contain titanium dioxide as a coloring agent, but this ingredient does not make them sunscreens. Make sure titanium dioxide is cited as an active ingredient, not in the list of other ingredients, and that an SPF number is listed.

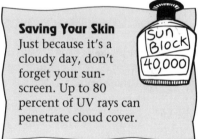

Saving Your Skin
Just because it's a cloudy day, don't forget your sunscreen. Up to 80 percent of UV rays can penetrate cloud cover.

Making Up for Lost Time

At what age should you start wearing sunscreen? As young as possible. Research shows that people who begin before age 18 lower their lifetime risk of skin cancer by a whopping 78 percent. Indeed, most of the sun damage to our skin occurs before we reach our 20s. Those freckles that look so cute on kids are really a signal of too much sun exposure. Many doctors recommend starting kids on sunscreen as early as six months, so make it a routine part of their morning, just like brushing their teeth.

"But hold on," you may be thinking. "What if we didn't have sunscreens when we were teenagers? Do we have to just give up and get wrinkles?"

Not at all. When it comes to sunscreens, the old adage "better late than never" certainly applies. Experiments with lab animals show that even sun-damaged skin can repair itself to some degree with regular applications of SPF 15 sunscreen. And, of course, it also prevents further UV damage.

Fielding Photosensitive Reactions

Bob, a friend of mine, came down with a bad case of flu, and his doctor prescribed an antibiotic to get him over the worst of it. One evening, I got a worried phone call from him. "I'm sunburned!" he said.

"What do you mean, you're sunburned?" I asked. "Haven't you been staying home in bed?" "Yeah," he said, "but it's the weirdest thing. This morning I walked to the drugstore to pick up some decongestants and tissues. I noticed right away that my skin felt a little tingly and hot. Tonight my face is red and so are my hands. And they feel kind of tender. I swear it's just like a sunburn!"

"What medications have you been taking?" I asked. He mentioned a commonly prescribed antibiotic and a well-known over-the-counter pain reliever. "There's your answer," I said. "You've become photosensitive from the medication. That little bit of sunlight from your walk this morning was enough to make you sunburned."

There was a long pause. "I've become photo *what*?" he asked.

What Causes Photosensitivity?

Photosensitivity is an unusual reaction to sunlight. Often, it takes the form of a skin rash that occurs as a reaction to the effects of light on the skin. As Bob found out, it can look a lot like sunburn.

What causes photosensitive reactions? In Bob's case, it was the antibiotics. Many commonly prescribed drugs, not to mention many over-the-counter brands you can buy in any drugstore, can have this effect.

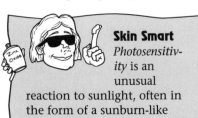

Skin Smart
Photosensitivity is an unusual reaction to sunlight, often in the form of a sunburn-like skin rash. Medications, dyes, perfumes, soaps, and plants can all cause photosensitive reactions.

Table 11.1 lists common photosensitizing drugs. It is not by any means an exhaustive list. More than 150 medications can be photosensitizing, including tetracycline antibiotics, sulfonamides ("sulfa drugs"), and some pain relievers.

The culprit doesn't have to be a medication, though; handling certain foods (celery, parsnips, limes, and many more) can cause photosensitization. So can some substances you put on your skin, including ingredients in cosmetics (musk ambrette, sandalwood oil, bergamot oil); deodorants; and some antibacterial soaps (although this is rare now, as most photosensitizers have been removed in the United

States). Fluorescent brightening agents, used to treat nylon, wool, and cellulose fibers, can photosensitize if they come into contact with your skin.

Exfoliants can also make your skin more vulnerable to UV because they strip its outer protective layer of cells. They include alpha hydroxy acids, beta hydroxy acids, cosmetic scrub creams, and chemical peels. They expose underlying cells, which ordinarily are protected by an intact horny layer.

> **Beauty Tips**
> You can even get a photosensitive reaction from a tattoo! Cadmium sulfide, a chemical injected into the skin during the tattooing process, is a notorious photosensitizer.

Table 11.1 Common Photosensitizing Drugs

Advil™	Cordarone™	Motrin™	Tetracyclines
Aleve™	Crystodigin™	Nuprin™	Thiazides
Azulfidine™	Diabinese™	Orinase™	Tolinase™
Bactrim™	Duraquin™	Phenergan™	Vibramycin™
Ciprofloxacin	Feldene™	Sinequan™	

When you take a photosensitizing substance, it reacts with your skin to increase your sensitivity to both natural sunlight and artificial UV rays from tanning beds and sun lamps.

Sometimes the chemical absorbs energy from UV rays and releases the energy into your skin, injuring or killing skin cells, and sometimes UV light changes the drug or chemical into one that you are allergic to. The reaction may take anywhere from a few minutes to several hours before it appears. In rare cases, people have continued to suffer skin eruptions up to 20 years later.

While photosensitive reactions usually resemble sunburn and fade within a few days, sometimes they are more serious. They can cause rashes, swelling, blisters, itching, scaling, or even eye burns. Long term, they may damage small, superficial blood vessels, cause cataracts and skin cancer, and age your skin prematurely.

Fending Off Photosensitivity

Many photosensitive reactions go unreported. People assume it's sunburn or allergies, and often they don't associate sunlight with the development of their symptoms.

There's really no way to predict who will be photosensitive. While fair-skinned folks seem to have more problems, dark-skinned people suffer them too. Some reactions follow a mysterious logic that only the body understands. One study reported on 17 people, all allergic to the antiseptic thimerosol (used in some contact lens preparations), who became suddenly photosensitive to the painkiller Feldene™.

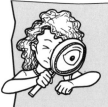

More Than Skin Deep

While some substances make you more vulnerable to the sun, others may protect you. In one experiment, Australian scientists exposed two groups of lab mice to UV rays; one group had been fed black tea, and the others water. The tea-drinkers developed 50 percent fewer skin cancers than the water-drinkers. The scientists believe that chemicals in black tea may counteract some of the cell damage caused by sunlight.

How can you protect yourself from a photosensitive reaction?

➤ Always wear sunscreen, and follow the tips in this chapter to protect yourself from the sun. As mentioned earlier, look for a broad-spectrum sunscreen. Most reactions are activated by UVA rays, so a UVB-blocking sunscreen might not protect you.

➤ Read the inserts that come packaged with every medication you take, both prescription and over-the-counter. (This is a good habit to get into anyway.) Drugs that are known photosensitizers will say so in their literature.

➤ If you get a sunburn that seems out of proportion to the time you spent outdoors, get out of the sun and limit further exposure until you know what's going on. Follow the advice in Chapter 10, "The Sun Is No Fun," for soothing a sunburn.

➤ If any skin reaction lasts more than two days, call your doctor. Tell your doctor about all the medications you take, and try to remember if you've been exposed to any of the photosensitizers mentioned in this chapter. Incidentally, don't forget to mention herbal preparations. Some herbal remedies contain natural equivalents of standard medicines and could interact with or exaggerate their effects.

Saving Your Skin

In rare cases, photosensitivity can signal a health condition, such as lupus erythematosus or certain types of porphyria. If you experience a photosensitive reaction for no apparent reason, consult your doctor.

A word about sunscreens: Ironically, some contain ingredients that cause photosensitive reactions. Occasionally, people report trouble with sunscreens containing bergamot oil, sandalwood oil, benzophenones, PABA, or cinnamates. Titanium dioxide seems to be the least troublesome sun block ingredient.

Avoid That "Mid-Day Sun"

Years ago, British author Noel Coward penned a song about "mad dogs and Englishmen" who "go out in the mid-day sun." Coward was shaking his head over the sunburned

Britons who insisted on braving the hot sun of India and other tropical climates. Today, he would probably shake his head about us Americans!

Coward had a point: It's sensible to stay out of the sun during the hottest part of the day. Sunburning UV rays are most intense between 10 a.m. and 2 p.m. UVB strength peaks during this time because the sun is directly overhead and its shorter wavelengths can reach the earth's surface more easily. This is when the sun is hardest on your skin. If you have yard chores to do or outdoor errands to run, save them for early morning or late afternoon, when UVB is less intense.

In addition to wearing sunscreen and taking Coward's advice, follow these steps to fight photoaging:

> ➤ Clothing can be a good sunscreen. Instead of baking bare limbs, don a long-sleeved white shirt; opt for pants instead of shorts. Avoid loose-weave and see-through fabrics; if you can see through them, so can the sun.

> ➤ Wear sunglasses. Choose dark polarized lenses (gray offers the best color resolution) large enough to cover your eyes. Be sure they have UV filters. A good pair of UV protective sunglasses shades the delicate skin around your eyes to help prevent crow's feet.

> ➤ Wear a hat, preferably made of tightly woven straw or light-colored cloth. Baseball caps are better than nothing, but they don't protect the side of your face. Instead, I recommend a hat with a brim of at least three inches.

Saving Your Skin
Many cities across the United States now include an ultraviolet radiation index (1 to 15) in their weather forecasts. An index of 8 or above indicates high levels of UV in your area. On days like this, it's especially important to guard your skin.

The bigger your hat, the better. One study found that a four-inch hat brim blocks more than 80 percent of sunlight from your face. And there's a bonus: In addition to protecting your face, hats help keep you cooler.

More Than Skin Deep

Some of my patients look at me like I'm crazy when I suggest covering up against the sun. "But I want to wear shorts and tank tops! Otherwise, I'll get too hot!" they protest. The truth is you'll feel a lot cooler if you block the sun's rays from your skin. We could learn a lot from the cultures of the Near East, where traditionally they have coped with torrid temperatures by wearing voluminous white robes and flowing headdresses. This protects them from both the burning rays of direct sunlight and reflected UV from sand and pavement.

The Least You Need to Know

➤ Wearing sunscreen is one of the most important things you can do to beautify your skin. It wards off wrinkles better than any "wrinkle cream" could possibly do.

➤ Look for a sunscreen with an SPF of at least 15. Those that contain titanium dioxide and zinc oxide are very effective. If you can't find a titanium dioxide or zinc oxide product you like, choose a sunscreen that combines UVA- and UVB-blocking ingredients.

➤ A lot of chemicals found in medications, foods, exfoliants, and cosmetics can make you photosensitive and give you a bad case of instant sunburn. Always read the warning labels on prescription and over-the-counter drugs. After you exfoliate your skin, be sure to wear sunscreen.

➤ Don't neglect commonsense precautions. Wear loose-fitting, light-colored clothing, a hat, and UV-filtering sunglasses. Limit your outdoor activities to early morning or late afternoon, when the sun's rays are less intense.

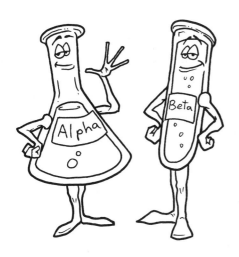

Chapter 12

Help from Hydroxy Acids

In This Chapter

➤ Learn why there's so much excitement about alpha and beta hydroxy acids

➤ Find out how to know what you're buying

➤ Discover the importance of pH and percentage

➤ Learn about the difference between alpha and beta hydroxy acids

➤ See how to get the biggest benefit from hydroxy acids

"Wow! Did you see this?" said Maria. She handed me a magazine opened to an article. The headline blared: "Finally—the miracle we've all been waiting for! Scientific studies prove alpha hydroxy acids erase wrinkles!" Below was an article announcing a wonderful new cream that could make you look 20 years younger.

Several other friends came over to look at the article. "I've heard about alpha hydroxy acids," said Teresa. "They're supposed to be great. What do you think, Marsha?"

"Oh, don't ask her," said Maria good-naturedly. "She'll just tell us it's all hype. She knows too much!"

"Certainly this article is a lot of hype," I responded, "but alpha hydroxy acids themselves may be valid. I'm not saying to believe everything you read about them, but they may be useful."

"In that case, I repeat my earlier comment: Wow!" said Maria. "This is a historic occasion. We may have found a cosmetic that Marsha likes!"

Alpha and Beta Hydroxy Acids: The Facts Behind the Fiction

All kidding aside, my friends (and my patients) know that I take product advertising claims with a great deal of salt. In this chapter, I'm glad to say, we will look at a category of nonprescription skin-care products that may really be able to help you. Of course, I will still advise you to be skeptical of publicity claims. (After all, I have a reputation with my friends to maintain!)

No, alpha and beta hydroxy acids do not work miracles, but they may be worth looking into. In this chapter, you will see why.

Alpha Hydroxy Acids and Ancient History

Alpha hydroxy acids (*AHAs*) are acids that are derived from various plants; the acid extracts act as mild exfoliants. Often, although not always, they're derived from fruit, which is why they're sometimes called "fruit acids." Other natural sources include ginger, wine, sugar cane, tomato juice, and milk. These days, AHAs can be produced in a laboratory too.

From all the excitement, you'd think that alpha hydroxy acids are something new and innovative. In fact, they have been with us for a long time.

In ancient times, Queen Cleopatra of Egypt bathed in sour milk and skimmed dirt and oil from her royal body with a specially designed scraper. Upon occasion, she would also wash her face with red wine, a habit she may have picked up from beauties in old Rome who dredged up sludge from the bottom of wine barrels and applied it as a facial mask.

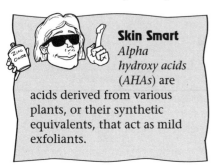

Skin Smart
Alpha hydroxy acids (AHAs) are acids derived from various plants, or their synthetic equivalents, that act as mild exfoliants.

Several centuries later, a Spanish noblewoman, the Duchess of Alba, applied facial masks of orange pulp, which she left in place for 20 minutes. In the nineteenth century, Queen Elizabeth of Hungary also went in for washing her face with wine, in this case with herbs added. The queen was also known to bathe in water from a mineral-rich Hungarian spring that had been infused with lemons, roses, violets, and peppermint leaves.

Recognizing Alpha Hydroxy Acids on Labels

In a modern-day list of alpha hydroxy acids, you will recognize some of the ingredients just mentioned. AHAs you will encounter on product labels include the following:

➤ Glycolic acid, derived from sugar cane juice, sugar beets, and unripe grapes (also known as hydroxyacetic acid, alpha hydroxyacetic acid, hydroxyethanoic acid, ammonium alpha hydroxyethanoate, ammonium glycolate)

➤ Lactic acid, from tomato juice and sour milk (other names include 2-hydroxypropanoic acid and ammonium lactate)

➤ Malic acid, from apples

➤ Tartaric acid, found in grapes and wine

➤ Citric acid, occurring in citrus fruits and pineapples

The best-known are glycolic and lactic acid, on which research began more than 15 years ago. Some cosmetic chemists consider them superior to the others because they may be better at penetrating skin's outer layers. Research on other AHAs is far more recent and, therefore, less conclusive.

For this reason, I recommend looking for products that contain glycolic or lactic acid as the active ingredient. Lactic acid may be a better moisturizer.

Saving Your Skin
No matter which alpha hydroxy acid you choose, be careful. Some people find glycolic acid, as well as the other alpha hydroxy acids, to be irritating. If you experience any skin reactions, you might try a product with a different active ingredient.

And Now, a Few Ingredients That Are Not AHAs

Since AHAs have become so popular, some companies have been known to imply that their products contain AHAs even when they don't. Non-AHA compounds that are sometimes mistakenly identified as AHAs include the following:

➤ Acetic acid

➤ Benzoic acid

➤ Formic acid

➤ Fruit extracts

➤ Oxalic acid

➤ Monochloroactic acid

➤ Retinyl palmitate

➤ Sodium hyaluronate

➤ Sugar cane extract

➤ Trichloroactic acid

While these ingredients may be useful in a product, they are not alpha hydroxy acids.

Saving Your Skin
In addition to watching for misleading ingredients, be alert for misleading brand names. You might think a name including "fruit," "alpha," or "beta" would have to include hydroxy acids, right? Not necessarily. When it comes to naming products, companies have a lot of leeway. Don't assume something contains hydroxy acids unless you see them in the ingredients list.

How Do Alpha Hydroxy Acids Work?

Why all the excitement about substances that have been around since Cleopatra?

As you might guess from their name, alpha hydroxy acids are naturally derived (although gentle) acids. When you apply an alpha hydroxy acid preparation topically, it penetrates the superficial horny layer of your skin and breaks apart the bonds that hold skin cells together. This makes it easier for your skin to shed those dead cells and make way for the newer ones underneath.

Sound familiar? Essentially, alpha hydroxy acids act like mild exfoliants, similar to the ones we looked at in Chapter 4, "Clean Living: The Best Way to Clean Your Skin." The difference is that exfoliants physically scrub the skin cells off, while alpha hydroxy acids are chemicals that act on the connecting bonds between cells.

You could say these mild acids literally burn away the bonds between skin cells. The speed with which they do this depends on the concentration of alpha hydroxy acids in the product. This is why you may notice your skin tingling and getting a little pink after you apply an AHA. The redness and tingling should subside within 20 minutes. If it does not, or if your skin becomes red and inflamed, discontinue the product until your skin has had a chance to recover and then switch to a product with a lower concentration (see "How to Know What You're Buying," below).

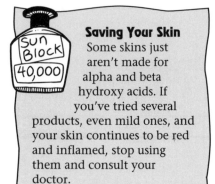

Saving Your Skin
Some skins just aren't made for alpha and beta hydroxy acids. If you've tried several products, even mild ones, and your skin continues to be red and inflamed, stop using them and consult your doctor.

Your skin may get a little flaky and dry at first. These flakes are the cells being shed from the horny layer. Your skin should become smoother within a few weeks. Again, if it does not improve, or if it becomes extremely dry and irritated, try a different product.

Even if you've already been using AHAs, your skin may change when you switch to another brand. The new one may make you tingle more, and you may start flaking all over again, which indicates a different active ingredient, a different concentration, a different moisturizer in the base, or a different delivery system. Even alpha hydroxy acids in identical concentrations can have very different effects on your skin, depending on the nature of the preparation they are in.

What Research Tells Us

Despite the popularity of AHAs, there's still a lot we don't know about them. Some experts feel they are effective mainly because they're good moisturizers, while others praise their ability to exfoliate. Doctors disagree over whether exfoliation makes you look better just because it exposes fresh new cells, or whether it can actually stimulate new cell growth and new collagen deposition.

Scientific research into alpha hydroxy acids is beginning to accumulate. Dermatologists at Ohio State University studied the effects of a 12 percent AHA lotion on 21 volunteers who applied it twice a day to one side of their faces. After eight weeks, the researchers reported that the treated skin felt a bit softer and smoother in 18 of the volunteers, and 15 seemed to have fewer wrinkles on that side. (Perhaps the most telling comment is that after the study ended, 17 of the 21 decided to keep using the lotion!)

In another study, researchers at Massachusetts General Hospital examined whether low concentrations of alpha hydroxy acids can really be beneficial. They concluded that a moisturizer containing 8 percent glycolic or lactic acid was slightly, but noticeably, better at improving skin's appearance than the same moisturizer without the acid. The AHA cream smoothed subjects' skin slightly and made freckles and sun-induced brown marks a little less noticeable.

While these studies say more about alpha hydroxy acids' effect on photoaging, the acids can also aid acne. Blemishes often result from dead skin cells collecting in pores and blocking them. By encouraging your skin to shed cells, AHAs help to clean out your pores.

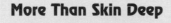

More Than Skin Deep

You've heard of cosmetics, and you've heard of pharmaceuticals. Some experts believe alpha hydroxy acids are a hybrid of the two, sometimes referred to as "cosmeceuticals." This classification puts them in a regulatory no-man's-land. Officials at the FDA are increasingly uncomfortable with all the fuss over cosmeceuticals. After all, they reason, if AHAs really can cause changes in the skin, they should be reclassified as drugs and regulated accordingly. The idea makes cosmetics companies nervous, since many products already on the market would have to undergo testing. The FDA is continuing to investigate some of the more extravagant AHA marketing claims.

What Alpha Hydroxy Acids Can't Do

Notice that the summaries of the previous studies used words like "slightly," "a little," and "a bit" to describe their results. This terminology sums it up. I would love to promise you a dramatic change from using alpha hydroxy acids, but in all honesty, I cannot.

After several weeks, you may notice a slight improvement in the appearance of your skin. It might seem a little smoother, and blotchy pigment irregularities may start to fade. Moisturizers might become more effective because your skin absorbs them more easily. If you have dark skin, you may notice your color becoming a little less ashy.

What alpha hydroxy acids won't do: They won't banish wrinkles forever, close pores, eliminate acne completely, or make you look 20 years younger. You won't look like a different person, but you may look like the same person with slightly better skin. Considering that all this treatment requires is the regular application of an over-the-counter cream, that's not bad.

Beta Hydroxy Acids: "New" Kids on the Block

Now that alpha hydroxy acids have been on the market for a while, companies are searching for fresh marketing ploys. Beta hydroxy acids are poised to become the new darling of the skin care industry.

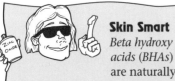

Skin Smart
Beta hydroxy acids (*BHAs*) are naturally occurring acids derived from plant sources such as willow bark, or their laboratory-produced equivalents. Common BHAs include salicylic, benzoic, and buteric acids.

Like AHAs, *beta hydroxy acids* (*BHAs*) are naturally occurring acids from plant sources or their laboratory-synthesized equivalents. The beta hydroxy acid most commonly used in cosmetics is salicylic acid, derived from willow bark. Other BHAs include benzoic and buteric acids.

Although they have a slightly different chemical structure from AHAs, beta hydroxy acids also serve as mild exfoliants. Makers of BHA products claim that beta hydroxy acids are more gentle than their alpha cousins. However, this claim is controversial at best. What's more, the effectiveness of BHAs (salicylic acid in particular) at improving the skin's appearance is less clear than that of AHAs. New research in this area is underway, and the final word is just not available to us yet.

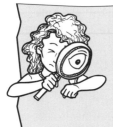

More Than Skin Deep

If you have ever applied a liquid to zap a stubborn corn or callus, you have already used a beta hydroxy acid. Salicylic acid has long been the active ingredient in corn and callus removers. Liquid solutions are 12 to 18 percent salicylic acid. On medicated disks, pads, and plasters, its concentration can go as high as 40 percent.

Is Exfoliation a Good Thing?

Is exfoliation a good thing? To be honest, we really don't know. Constant exfoliation might sound like a good idea; however, its long-term effects are unknown. Some dermatologists fear that alpha and beta hydroxy acids could leave skin in a state of perpetual irritation.

Another concern: By constantly removing the protective outer layer of dead cells, exfoliants leave you vulnerable to UV. Unless you compensate by wearing sunscreen and cutting back on sun exposure, you could actually be harming your skin in the long run.

Until we know more about the long-term effects of alpha and beta hydroxy acids, be prudent. Choose products carefully and use them in moderation. Read on for more information on how to keep your skin safe as well as beautiful.

How to Know What You're Buying

When shopping for alpha and beta hydroxy acids, you need to consider two factors: the percentage of active ingredients and the acidity level (pH) of the whole product.

Most AHA cosmetics range from 1 percent or less alpha hydroxy acids up to about 15 percent. Generally, 4 percent is the minimum for effective exfoliation. Less than 4 percent, and the acids are so diluted you won't notice any effect. It may be a good moisturizer, but that's about it.

Between 4 to 7 percent AHAs, the product is an extremely mild exfoliant. If it contains 8 percent to 15 percent, it becomes more effective at shedding cells. At the same time, it also becomes more effective at irritating skin.

How can you tell the hydroxy acid percentage of a product? It's not always easy to do. This information isn't necessarily given on the label, and some salespeople are not well informed. If you can, avoid the unknown and choose well-labeled products.

Here are some other tips for choosing a good alpha hydroxy acid product:

➤ The most effective pH is between 3 to 5. Lower than that, and the product is acidic and irritating. Higher than that, and it doesn't exfoliate well. If you thought you had trouble finding out the percentage of AHAs, just wait until you ask about pH! Even the most helpful salesperson will probably not be able to answer this one. You might try calling the company's headquarters (see Appendix A, "Bountiful Resources for Beautiful Skin," for information on contacting cosmetic firms). Or, test the item yourself with nitrozine test strips, which you can get at your local pharmacy.

➤ Check the ingredients list. If the AHA is listed near the end, chances are the brand does not contain enough to be effective; if it comes first, it

Saving Your Skin
Chemical face peels use higher alpha hydroxy acid concentrations than what's available over the counter, usually 30 to 70 percent. These are strong solutions with potential for burns and skin reactions. Peels are performed by cosmetologists and dermatologists. While there are many competent cosmetologists, it may be safer to be under a doctor's supervision during this procedure. See Chapter 20, "Make Your Skin More A-Peeling," for more information.

may be too strong. Look for one with the AHA listed second to midway through the ingredient list.

➤ If the item contains both alpha and beta hydroxy acids, make sure it does not contain a lot of both. One should be near the beginning of the ingredients list, the other near the end.

➤ As noted earlier, lactic and glycolic acid have undergone more testing than other alpha hydroxy acids, and salicylic acid is the best-known beta hydroxy acid. This makes them the active ingredients of choice. Other acids may perform just as well, but we simply don't know that for sure.

➤ Since hydroxy acids can be rough on your skin, note the other ingredients, too. Avoid anything that also contains too much alcohol or other known irritants. They will exaggerate the already irritating effect of the acids. Look for ingredients that make good moisturizers (see Chapter 5, "Choosing the Right Toner and Moisturizer") to counteract the drying effect of AHAs and BHAs.

➤ Try a small size first, so you don't invest a lot of money in an unknown. Ask for a sample; it's surprising how many companies will provide them on request. If no samples are available, create your own by bringing a small clean container and asking the sales rep for a few days' supply from a tester.

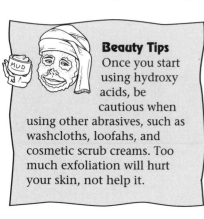

Beauty Tips
Once you start using hydroxy acids, be cautious when using other abrasives, such as washcloths, loofahs, and cosmetic scrub creams. Too much exfoliation will hurt your skin, not help it.

➤ Before committing your face, rub a small amount on the underside of your forearm. Do this several days in a row and note the results. If your skin looks extremely red or irritated, forget about putting it on your face. Try another brand.

Ultimately, it comes down to trial and error. No one can tell you for sure how your skin will react to a given pH or AHA/BHA percentage. You may have to try several brands before finding one you really like.

How you use a hydroxy acid product can make a big difference in its effectiveness, so next you'll see how to make it work well for you.

Getting the Biggest Benefit from Hydroxy Acids

Hydroxy acids come in a lot of different forms, including creams, gels, and lotions. If you have dry skin, I recommend using a cream because it will be more moisturizing. If your skin is oily, try an oil-free lotion or gel.

Unless your skin is extremely sensitive, a 7 to 8 percent alpha hydroxy concentration is a good starting point. This is a moderate concentration that will let you see how your skin reacts. Stay at this level for at least four to six weeks before considering something stronger.

When using any hydroxy acid, follow these guidelines:

➤ First, wash and rinse your face thoroughly. Be sure to rinse off all traces of cleanser, because many leave a residue that will counteract the mild acidity of AHAs and BHAs.

➤ Wait 15 minutes after washing to apply hydroxy acids as applying to moist skin seems to increase the likelihood of irritation.

➤ Apply a small (pea-sized) amount of the hydroxy acid product to your face. Smooth it on gently with clean fingers. Be careful not to tug or pull at your skin. Don't worry about rubbing it in; just let it dry naturally.

➤ Start by using hydroxy acids once a day, at bedtime. Note how your skin reacts. If your skin gets persistently dry, flaky, pink, or sore, cut back to once every other day. If problems continue, switch to a lower concentration.

➤ After four to six weeks, if you don't notice any results and haven't had any problems with irritation, you might increase applications to twice a day, or try a stronger product.

➤ Always wear a sunscreen with an SPF of at least 15, either as part of your foundation or applied separately. (See Chapter 11, "Fighting Back Against Photoaging," for tips on choosing sunscreens.) As mentioned earlier, alpha and beta hydroxy acids make your skin more vulnerable to UV. There's no point in making your skin smoother now only to give yourself wrinkles later!

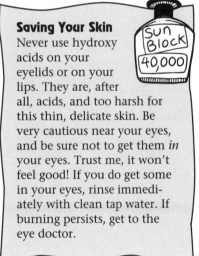

Beauty Tips
Some companies will try to sell you a different hydroxy acid product for every part of your body: eye area, neck, throat, thighs, feet, nails. This is unnecessary and expensive. Generally speaking, only two products are usually necessary: a higher-concentration AHA product for the body and a milder product for the face.

Saving Your Skin
Never use hydroxy acids on your eyelids or on your lips. They are, after all, acids, and too harsh for this thin, delicate skin. Be very cautious near your eyes, and be sure not to get them *in* your eyes. Trust me, it won't feel good! If you do get some in your eyes, rinse immediately with clean tap water. If burning persists, get to the eye doctor.

After you find a hydroxy acid product you like, I recommend using it consistently, once or twice a day, for six months to a year, or until you stop seeing continued improvement. Then try cutting your usage in half to see if that is enough to maintain your results; for example, you could switch to one application every other day.

By the way, hydroxy acids have become so popular they're turning up everywhere: shampoos, cleansers, facial masks, toners, you name it. Alpha hydroxy acid cleansers and toners may be very helpful, especially if your skin is oily.

Some people feel that if a little is good, a lot must be better. This is not necessarily true. As a general rule, I don't recommend using two or more hydroxy acid products together because their combined effect could inflame and irritate your skin. Let your skin be your guide: If it reacts negatively (to hydroxy acids or indeed anything else), cut back or try another product.

The Least You Need to Know

➤ Alpha and beta hydroxy acids are naturally occurring acid extracts from plants that act as mild exfoliants.

➤ The two factors to look for in a product are pH and the percentage of hydroxy acids. Look for a pH of 3 to 5 and a concentration of at least 4 percent alpha hydroxy acids. Four to 7 percent AHA is a mild exfoliant; 8 to 15 percent is more effective but also more irritating.

➤ Hydroxy acids will not work miracles. They won't erase wrinkles or take years off your face. With consistent use, however, you may see your skin become a little smoother and fresher, and your color a little more even.

➤ Use hydroxy acids consistently for six months to a year, or until you are no longer seeing continued improvement. Then cut your usage by 50 percent.

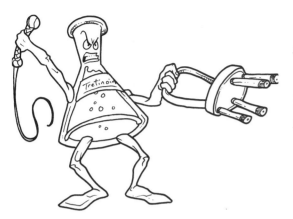

Tretinoin and Antioxidants: The Age-Tamers?

One rainy afternoon, Sally made an appointment with me. "Congratulate me!" she said. "Today I'm 50." "Congratulations," I responded. "While I'm certainly glad to see you, what on earth are you doing here? Why aren't you out celebrating and having fun?"

"But this is fun," she said cheerfully. "Today I'm going to do something I've wanted to do for a long time. It's time I did something to make myself look better. I want to get a prescription for Renova®!"

What Is Tretinoin?

Like Sally, many people who consult me are interested in trying *tretinoin*, a long-time acne drug that is becoming popular as a treatment for photoaging. Often it's referred to by its brand names: Retin-A®, Renova®, or Avita®.

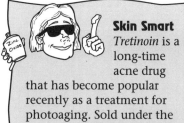

Skin Smart

Tretinoin is a long-time acne drug that has become popular recently as a treatment for photoaging. Sold under the brand names Renova®, Retin-A®, and Avita®, it is classified as a *keratolytic drug*, which loosens and removes cells in the skin's horny layer.

A synthetic derivative of vitamin A, tretinoin is classified as a *keratolytic drug*, which loosens and removes the keratin-rich horny layer of the skin. (Other keratolytic drugs include sulfur preparations and salicylic acid, the beta hydroxy acid we discussed in the previous chapter.)

From Acne to Wrinkles

For more than a quarter-century, doctors have prescribed tretinoin to treat acne. Like alpha and beta hydroxy acids, it is a mild acid that, when applied topically, helps dissolve the bonds connecting skin cells in the horny layer. The skin sheds cells more easily, which unplugs pores, increases cell turnover rate, and counteracts the formation of pimples.

Among the acne patients who benefited from tretinoin were a number of women in their 30s and 40s. They reported that in addition to minimizing pimples, tretinoin also seemed to make their skin smoother and less wrinkled. This result piqued the interest of researchers, who began to explore the use of tretinoin to treat photoaging.

Can tretinoin really make you look better? Several studies have tried to answer this question. While results vary widely from person to person, many dermatologists believe it can make a positive difference in the appearance of your skin. "Before" and "after" photos, magnified hundreds of times through a microscope, reveal that after six months of tretinoin skin cells become larger, more regular, and more evenly distributed. The horny layer becomes thinner and smoother.

While tretinoin thins the horny layer, it makes the epidermis thicker. It evens out the distribution of melanin and may stimulate the production of collagen. Another interesting result: It encourages the development of new blood vessels. Over time, chronic sun exposure injures and destroys some of the tiny blood vessels that nourish facial skin; months of tretinoin treatment can cause new vessels to form.

Does Tretinoin Make You Look Younger?

Apparently, tretinoin changes skin at the cellular level. Do these changes translate into noticeable improvements in appearance?

Good question. Unfortunately, there's no easy answer. According to Ortho Pharmaceuticals, the company that markets Renova®, 64 percent of people who used Renova® in clinical trials experienced at least minimal improvement in wrinkling, 65 percent experienced at least some improvement in freckling and pigment irregularities, and 41 percent developed smoother skin. However, 35 percent of the subjects experienced no improvement in fine wrinkling or freckling, and 49 percent had no change in skin texture.

More Than Skin Deep

How do scientists measure improvements in wrinkling? One method is *optical profilometry*, a tool originally developed by NASA to evaluate craters on the moon's surface. To evaluate wrinkles, researchers take a soft cast of the subject's skin, shine a fiber-optic illuminator on it, and then feed information about shadows and light into an image analyzer. The computer translates this data into a picture from which they can calculate irregularities in surface texture and depth of wrinkles.

This diversity is reflected in my patients' histories. Some of them swear by tretinoin. Sally, for example, has been very pleased. As she told me the other day, "I can definitely see a difference. It's not just the lines, either; I feel like my skin has a new glow!" (Some dermatologists attribute this "new glow" to renewed circulation.)

But then there's Helen, another patient who has tried tretinoin with less success. "I can't really say that it helped me," she admits ruefully. "It made my face red and blotchy, and my skin felt irritated all the time. I just can't see what the fuss is all about."

Based on my experience, I'd say that tretinoin is most effective in evening out color irregularities—freckles, liver spots, and the mottled hyperpigmentation that comes from sun damage—and minimizing very fine wrinkles. This effect may be due to increased collagen production, although this is not certain. We do know that tretinoin improves wound healing, perhaps because it stimulates the formation of new small blood vessels. This is why many doctors like to prescribe it before and after certain procedures, such as facial peels, laser resurfacing, and dermabrasion.

I must tell you, though: Tretinoin is not a face lift. It only helps signs of photoaging, as opposed to the changes that occur with chronological aging. It will not tighten your skin, erase deep wrinkles, or rebuild elastin tissue, and it will not make you look dramatically different.

Will Tretinoin Help You?

So, should you try tretinoin? And if you do, will you be a Sally or a Helen?

Tretinoin seems to be most effective at reversing photoaging early in the process, before there is a great deal of sagging skin or deep wrinkles. Deep furrows will not respond to it, and only plastic surgery or possibly laser work can tighten excess folds of hanging skin.

If your skin shows any of the following characteristics, you could be a good candidate for tretinoin:

➤ Fine wrinkles

➤ Some brown marks, such as persistent freckles or "liver spots"

➤ Rough, leathery skin texture

It also helps if your skin isn't hypersensitive, since many people experience skin irritation when they first start using the drug. Fair-skinned people are most likely to suffer from this.

Another plus: patience. Often it takes at least six months of steady use to notice any improvement.

More Than Skin Deep

A few studies indicate tretinoin may help prevent the squamous cell type of skin cancer. In some cases, it eliminated precancerous skin growths (actinic keratoses). Some researchers believe that topical applications of retinoids (tretinoin's chemical family) are beneficial not because they kill precancerous cells, but because they promote the cells' development into normal cells. While promising, this does not make tretinoin a home remedy for skin cancer. Always consult your doctor about any marks that look suspicious. See Chapter 19, "Skin Cancer: The Dark Side of the Sun," for more information.

Getting the Most from Tretinoin Treatment

Remember, tretinoin is a prescription drug, not a cosmetic. Always follow your doctor's guidelines for using it because this will make it safer and more effective.

Here are some tips for getting the biggest benefit from tretinoin treatment:

➤ Apply the cream only once per day, at bedtime. People with sensitive skin may need to start with every-other-night applications. Don't use more than the recommended amount. Using more will not help your skin, but it may leave it sore, inflamed, and peeling.

➤ Wash your face gently with a mild soap or water-soluble cleanser, then blot dry with a clean towel. Make sure all makeup has been removed.

➤ Wait 20 to 30 minutes before applying tretinoin. Apply a pea-sized amount of cream to cover your entire face. Smooth it over the skin gently—don't rub it in vigorously. Wash your hands with soap afterward.

➤ You may notice a feeling of warmth or slight stinging; it should go away in a few minutes.

➤ Do not apply tretinoin too close to your eyes or on your eyelids, mouth, nostrils, or ears—it can cause severe reactions. Theoretically, you could put it anywhere else on your body (except mucous membranes), and it has been used on the neck, chest, back, forearms, and hands. However it may be a bit less effective in these areas.

➤ Many people experience some type of skin reaction when they first start using the drug, including itching, dry skin, stinging, burning, redness, and skin peeling. Moisturizers can help; ask your doctor about the best way to use a moisturizer with your tretinoin therapy. Some people may notice acne getting worse initially. All these reactions should improve within two months.

➤ Several forms and concentrations of tretinoin are available. Gels and liquids are usually stronger; creams are milder. As a general rule, I recommend gels and liquids only for people with extremely oily skin and persistent acne; photoaged skin is better off with a cream. If your skin gets irritated easily, consider starting with a lower-strength cream until your face gets used to the idea. Then, if irritation is not a problem, you can switch to a stronger formulation.

➤ Tretinoin is likely to make your skin photosensitive. Please take this warning seriously. After you start using it, stay out of direct sunlight as much as possible; avoid sun lamps and tanning salons entirely. When you are outdoors, wear protective clothing and a hat, and always apply a sunscreen with an SPF of 15 or higher. (Remember, if you are using tretinoin in an attempt to reverse the signs of photoaging, getting more sun just doesn't make sense.)

➤ Tretinoin can also make your skin more sensitive to wind and cold. Avoid them when possible.

> **Beauty Tips**
> If you are already taking a medication that makes you photosensitive, tretinoin may make it worse. Before starting tretinoin, tell your doctor about everything you take, including prescription, over-the-counter, and herbal remedies.

> **Saving Your Skin**
> Skin reactions to tretinoin tend to be worse during the cold windy days of winter. Consider starting therapy in the spring when the weather is easier on your skin. However, be sure to wear sunscreen!

According to Ortho, most visible improvements occur during the first six months of therapy. Generally, subsequent use simply maintains these initial changes. If you use tretinoin faithfully, following all directions, for more than six months without noticing any improvement, you may be one of those people it doesn't help. (Don't give up yet, though; you have many other options. See Chapters 20 to 25 for more ideas.)

If you do notice an improvement, congratulations! Do be aware that you will have to continue using tretinoin on a regular basis, although your doctor may recommend a less frequent schedule. If you discontinue the drug, your skin will gradually go back to its old ways.

Available Only by Prescription

As this book goes to press, the only brand of tretinoin that has been approved by the FDA for treating photoaging is Renova®. The FDA still views Retin-A® and Avita® as acne medications. All three are available only by prescription.

Some cosmetics companies try to capitalize on tretinoin's fame by implying that their products contain it. Don't be fooled. You can't buy it over the counter; you have to consult your doctor first.

You may see some of the following ingredients on cosmetics labels:

➤ Vitamin A

➤ Retinol

➤ Retinyl palmitate

➤ Palmitic acid

Some salespeople may insist these goodies are Renova® or Retin-A® in disguise. Not true! While chemically related to vitamin A, tretinoin has specific effects on skin that vitamin A and other derivatives do not have. These ingredients may make a good skin-care product, but they aren't tretinoin.

More Than Skin Deep

Once you start using tretinoin, stop using anything else that could irritate or dry your skin—including alpha and beta hydroxy acids, cosmetic scrubs, loofahs, and washcloths. Alpha hydroxy acids may be cautiously and slowly added back to your regimen after your skin has acclimated to the tretinoin. Ortho also recommends staying away from medicated shampoos and soaps, hair depilatories, hair waxes, permanent wave solutions, astringents, and any products containing alcohol, spices, or lime.

Can Antioxidants Keep You Young?

During another appointment, Sally asked me, "Doctor, what's your opinion of antioxidant moisturizers? Do you think they're better than regular moisturizers without antioxidants?" Good question. Like tretinoin, antioxidants have come in for heavy marketing hype. Let's see what they can really do for you.

Antioxidants Versus Free Radicals: A Fight for Life?

Antioxidants are chemicals that absorb or quench harmful molecules called free radicals. Oxygen-centered free radicals develop in our body as a byproduct of normal metabolism. They are also formed by certain known carcinogens, such as cigarette smoke and sunlight.

Free radicals are unstable, high-energy molecules that damage components of the cells in our bodies, such as proteins, fats, and DNA. As they interact and damage essential cellular molecules, they start long chain-reactions that produce more free radicals, which in turn cause more damage.

One theory suggests that this damage is cumulative and leads to the physical deterioration we call aging. A diet rich in antioxidants may interrupt these chain reactions. Certainly, evidence is mounting that a nutritious diet reduces your risk of cancer, heart disease, and many other health problems. (For more on nutrition and vitamins, see Chapter 8, "Keeping That Youthful Look.")

Important antioxidants include the mineral selenium and vitamins A, C, and E. Antioxidants aren't new; they have long been a staple in the food industry. For example, when vitamin E is added as a preservative, it slows down deterioration and keeps food fresh longer. Now some scientists believe that antioxidants can keep people "fresh" longer too!

Cosmetic companies have jumped on the bandwagon by adding antioxidants to almost everything they make. Makeup, cleansers, moisturizers, body lotions, shampoos, toners, sunscreens, exfoliants—everywhere you look, product labels advertise the presence of vitamins C, E, and A.

Skin Smart
Antioxidants (like selenium and vitamins A, C, and E) are chemicals that prevent or slow down the destructive effects of free radicals. Some researchers believe *free radicals*, unstable, high-energy molecules that damage body cells, play a big role in the aging process.

Saving Your Skin
Here's another reason to stay out of the sun: It robs your skin of natural antioxidants. When researchers at the University of California-Berkeley exposed lab mice to ultraviolet rays, the animals' skin lost a significant amount of vitamins C and E. It may be that sun exposure creates free radicals, even as it weakens skin's antioxidant protection.

Vitamins C and E

While I encourage you to include lots of antioxidants in your diet, research is still under-way as to whether applying them topically will help your skin. As you know from reading Chapter 2, "Your Skin: Don't Leave Home Without It," skin has multiple layers, and the top one (the horny layer) consists of dead cells. Generally, rubbing vitamins on these surface cells will not nourish your skin or enhance its underlying structure. In fact, most products wear off and never penetrate to deeper layers anyway.

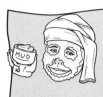

Beauty Tips
Vitamin C creams appear to reduce the skin's inflammatory response to UV radiation. Some researchers believe these preparations also encourage the synthesis of collagen. These experiments are promising, but still preliminary.

That being said, some dermatologists do think topical applications of C and E are beneficial. Some forms of vitamin C can penetrate through many skin layers. Vitamin C may inhibit free radicals, and some researchers believe vitamin C and E creams may offer some protection against ultraviolet rays. They caution, however, that this research is still in experimental stages. Antioxidants are not a substitute for sunscreen.

Vitamin A

As we've seen, vitamin A is related chemically to tretinoin. Some of my patients ask whether they can skip the prescription and simply take vitamin A supplements instead.

Some people with certain skin conditions do report good results to their skin from taking vitamin A. However, I do not believe that you can reverse photoaging by taking safe doses of vitamin A supplements. Remember, you must be very careful when taking supplements. As you saw in Chapter 8, vitamin A is a fat-soluble vitamin readily stored in the body's fat tissue. That means it stays with you for a long time. If you continue to take supplements, body levels will build until it's possible to overdose. Too much vitamin A causes headache, nausea, bone pain, muscle weakness, blurred vision, and dry, peeling skin. It can also make your hair fall out. Extremely large amounts can even be fatal.

Sometimes patients ask whether they should apply vitamin A oil or other products containing vitamin A directly to their skin. If you're pestered by dryness, vitamin A oil is a good emollient, but not significantly better than any other moisturizer. Even the most optimistic reports imply that topical vitamin A gives only a fraction of the benefit derived from tretinoin, and even this is controversial.

My advice: Get a healthy dose of vitamin A from your diet (good sources include carrots, sweet potatoes, spinach, and tomatoes). Then, if you still have the urge to apply retinoids to your skin, talk to your doctor about a prescription for tretinoin.

The Least You Need to Know

➤ Tretinoin (brand names Renova®, Retin-A®, and Avita®) is a synthetic derivative of vitamin A that helps your skin shed cells from the horny layer.

➤ Research shows that tretinoin can have a positive effect at the cellular level: thinning the horny layer, thickening the epidermis, normalizing skin cells, distributing melanin more evenly, improving circulation, and possibly stimulating the formation of collagen.

➤ In terms of overall appearance, the drug may lighten pigmented areas, smooth very fine wrinkles, and promote wound healing. While it can improve the appearance of your skin, it is not a face lift, and it doesn't work for everyone.

➤ Benefits often take six months or more to become visible, and you have to continue using the drug on a regular basis to maintain them.

➤ Antioxidants (such as selenium and vitamins A, C, and E) are substances that absorb harmful free radicals. While antioxidants are important in your diet, we aren't sure how much benefit rubbing them on your skin provides. Vitamin C may inhibit free radicals, and vitamins C and E might help protect skin against ultraviolet rays.

Part 3
Staying Healthy

Good health is the best beautifier of all. But sometimes, through no fault of your own, skin problems occur. In Part 3, you'll learn how to protect your exterior against the challenges life hands you.

A few of these challenges you're born with, like moles and birthmarks. Others, such as acne, first plague you during adolescence. Some are exciting (pregnancy), others less so (cold sores, warts, poison ivy). Some, like skin cancer, require medical treatment.

I cover a wide range of situations in the next six chapters. The common theme: They all affect your skin somehow. You'll learn about practical ways to prevent them, treat them, and restore your skin to radiant health.

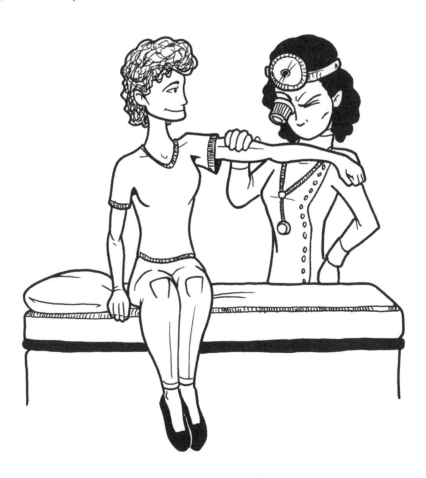

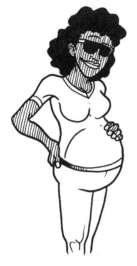

Chapter 14

Baby and You: Your Skin During Pregnancy

In This Chapter

➤ Find out what to expect from your skin when you're pregnant

➤ Discover why you get dark patches, and what you can do about them

➤ Learn to cope with that mysterious itch

➤ Get the bottom line on hemorrhoids

➤ Learn the bad news, and the good news, about your hair

An attractive 30-year-old, Jan ordinarily had a smooth olive complexion. Skin complaints were the furthest thing from her mind.

Until she became pregnant, that is. She came in to see me recently, very pregnant and very uncomfortable. "What's wrong with me?" she asked, looking worried. "My cheeks, chin, and forehead keep getting darker, and I have an incredibly itchy rash on my belly! I expected the weight gain and the morning sickness, but I didn't expect my skin to act so weird. What's going on?"

"Nothing dangerous," I reassured her. "Your body is going through a lot of changes right now, and that means your skin is, too. I'm glad you came to see me, though, because there are things we can do to make pregnancy a little easier on your skin."

Said Jan: "Great. I'm ready!"

Pregnancy: A Special Time for You—and Your Skin

Congratulations! You're pregnant, and you're excited. You may even be a little nervous. This is natural because there are a lot of changes and new developments ahead of you.

If you haven't already seen a doctor, I urge you to do so immediately. Find a health professional you trust and make regular visits a habit because good prenatal care is vital to the health of both you and your baby. Many doctors recommend office visits once a month during the first seven months of pregnancy, every two weeks during month number eight, and once a week during your final month.

Saving Your Skin

If you are taking Accutane® (isotretinoin), a drug used to treat acne, you should stop taking it at least a month before you try to conceive. Accutane® can cause severe birth defects, including heart disease, central nervous system problems, and abnormal development of the baby's face and ears. Consult your doctor for advice.

Be sure to tell your doctor about any health conditions you have and any that seem to run in the family—both yours and your partner's. Also mention all medications you take (this includes prescription drugs, over-the-counter medications, and herbal remedies). Unless drugs are important for controlling a health problem, your doctor will recommend as few as possible, since most things that enter your bloodstream will end up in your baby's too.

Some drugs like Accutane® (isotretinoin) and Propecia® (finasteride) are absolutely contraindicated in pregnancy. (Propecia® is not approved for women at all as this book goes to press.) Accutane® must be stopped at least one month before you conceive. If you are pregnant and think you may have been exposed to one of these drugs, tell your doctor immediately. If you are on Accutane® and would like to become pregnant, stop taking it at least one month before trying to conceive. Discuss your medications and the timing of conception in detail with your doctor.

Other tips for radiant prenatal health:

➤ If you smoke, stop. Tobacco reduces the amount of oxygen that reaches your baby, and mothers who smoke more than a pack a day bear smaller, weaker infants than do nonsmokers. They are also more likely to suffer miscarriages. As we saw in Chapter 9, "Skin No-Nos," smoking is bad for you as well as your child; it ages your skin prematurely and gives you wrinkles. This is a great time to quit.

➤ Cut back on alcohol, or stop drinking entirely while you're pregnant. Alcohol is a potent drug that has the potential to injure your child. Up to 33 percent of babies born to mothers who drink heavily, especially six or more drinks per day, have some type of birth defect, compared to fewer than 5 percent of those born to women who abstained during pregnancy.

Needless to say, it's crucial to eat right and exercise regularly, with the guidance of your doctor, of course. In addition to benefiting your overall health, exercise can help with some of the skin problems we'll discuss in this chapter, like varicose veins and water retention.

"Doctor, What's Wrong with My Skin?"

Like Jan, up to 90 percent of pregnant women notice their skin getting darker in certain areas. This is probably due to heightened levels of estrogen and other hormones, which stimulate melanocytes.

Dark-skinned people seem especially prone to this effect. The dusky patches may be most noticeable in the armpits and around nipples and genitals. Moles and freckles can become darker, and some mothers-to-be develop a dark vertical line (called the "linea nigra") between belly button and pubic hair.

Jan noticed more pigmentation in her cheeks, forehead, and chin especially. This is known, appropriately enough, as the *mask of pregnancy* (the medical term is *melasma* or *chloasma*). You don't have to be pregnant to develop this mask, although it helps; between 50 to 70 percent of expectant mothers notice some facial darkening. It's probably related to estrogen levels coupled with exposure to sunlight, and can also appear in women taking oral contraceptives.

> **Skin Smart**
> Between 50 to 70 percent of expectant mothers develop the *mask of pregnancy* (the medical term is *melasma* or *chloasma*)—increased facial pigmentation, especially in the cheeks, forehead, and chin.

Sun exposure makes the mask of pregnancy worse. Always wear sunscreen, stay out of the sun as much as possible, and avoid tanning salons and sunlamps. (See Chapter 11, "Fighting Back Against Photoaging," for advice on choosing a good sunscreen.)

Dark patches usually fade within a year after delivery. If not, you may be able to reverse them with a prescription for hydroquinone, an FDA-approved skin-lightening drug. Some doctors recommend using tretinoin as well, since tretinoin helps even out irregular skin tone. (Neither should be used if you are pregnant or nursing.) Truly stubborn melasma may respond to a chemical peel (see Chapter 20, "Make Your Skin More A-Peeling") or to treatment with lasers (see Chapter 23, "Better Looking with Lasers").

Gaining the Right Kind of Weight

Being pregnant, of course, means gaining weight. How much? Most obstetricians recommend 20 to 30 pounds. Too little, and your baby may not be getting the nutrition it needs. Too much, and you increase the risk of complications for both you and your child.

What does that extra weight consist of? See Table 14.1, which summarizes the distribution of an average weight gain.

Table 14.1 Average Weight Gain During Pregnancy

Where Does It All Go?	
Baby	38 percent
Blood and fluid	22 percent
Uterus, breasts, buttocks, legs	20 percent
Amniotic fluid	11 percent
Placenta	9 percent

In addition to healthy weight gain, you will probably notice some swelling. Many of my patients report swollen faces, ankles, feet, and hands, especially during later months. Often you feel most puffy in the mornings and better as the day goes on. If you have a heart or kidney condition, this will make the swelling worse.

If you notice swelling, please consult your doctor to rule out any underlying problems. Generally, however, the swelling simply indicates that you're retaining water. Here are some tips for combating water retention:

➤ Cut back on salt, which makes water retention worse. To reduce your salt intake, read product labels carefully. In addition to checking for sodium and sodium chloride (table salt), avoid monosodium glutamate (MSG), a related compound often added to seasonings and Chinese dishes. Even if the label says "no salt added," this doesn't mean it's not salty; the food could have been loaded with the stuff to begin with.

Saving Your Skin
According to the FDA, "sodium-free" on a product label means less than 5 milligrams per serving; "very low sodium" means 35 milligrams or less; "low-sodium," 140 milligrams or less; and "lightly salted" means the item contains at least 50 percent less sodium per serving than its regular counterpart.

➤ Exercise regularly (remember, this should be done under the guidance of your doctor). This stimulates circulation, which helps keep fluids from pooling in your ankles and feet. As a bonus, it will tighten abdominal muscles, boost your stamina, and make labor easier.

➤ Not sure how to get started with exercise? Many YMCAs, schools, and health clubs offer exercise classes geared to the special needs of pregnant women. (Consult your doctor before beginning any exercise program.) This is not the time to embark on a strenuous new sport; go for low-impact activities like swimming, water aerobics, walking, cycling, and slow jogging. Let your body be your guide. If you start feeling tired or sore, cut back or try a different activity.

➤ Do not take diuretics ("water pills"). While diuretics help you get rid of excess water through urination, they can be dangerous for your baby.

➤ Rest assured, this swelling is annoying but temporary. It will disappear after your baby is born.

More Than Skin Deep

Exercise is great for you and baby, but remember your body has unique requirements during this special time. Changing hormone levels make your joints looser. While this will come in handy during delivery, it increases the risk of injury because your joints are less stable. Also, as you get larger, your center of gravity shifts, so it's easy to lose your balance. Avoid deep bending, intense stretches, downhill skiing, and high-impact aerobics that could strain your joints. This is not the time for tennis, racquetball, basketball, or other sports that call for abrupt changes in direction.

Coping with Stretch Marks

When you gain weight, your skin stretches, and many women retain souvenirs of pregnancy in the form of *stretch marks* (*striae*). Stretch marks generally first appear during the sixth or seventh month as raised lines, pink to violet in color. Eventually they turn purple, then flatten and fade to become flesh-colored shiny streaks.

Most common in Caucasians (up to 90 percent of pregnant white women get them), stretch marks show up on the abdomen, breasts, upper arms, and buttocks.

Unfortunately, you can't prevent stretch marks, although keeping your weight gain within reasonable limits helps minimize them. Usually they fade and become less visible several months after delivery, but they never really go away on their own.

If the lines bother you after delivery, ask your doctor about trying a tretinoin preparation, such as Retin-A® or Renova®. Some reports suggest that topical applications of tretinoin cream can improve the appearance of patients' stretch marks. (But remember, tretinoin should be avoided if you are nursing.) Laser treatments may also help (see Chapter 23 for more information).

Skin Smart
Stretch marks (*striae*) are raised pink or violet lines that appear as the skin stretches. Eventually they flatten and fade to become shiny flesh-colored streaks.

"Doctor, I Itch Like Crazy!"

Like Jan, many expectant mothers complain of mysterious rashes and itches. Perhaps the most common example is a condition with the impressive name of *pruritic urticarial papules and plaques of pregnancy*. Don't bother memorizing this mouthful; most doctors just call it *PUPPP*.

PUPPP appears during the third trimester, usually in women who are giving birth to their first child. Often it starts near abdominal stretch marks and spreads to thighs, hips, and arms. The stretch marks become red and raised and itch intensely. Treatment is complicated by the need to avoid internal medications during pregnancy, and many of the usual topical anti-itch remedies don't seem to help.

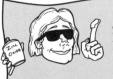

Skin Smart

Many pregnant women are plagued by *PUPPP* (*pruritic urticarial papules and plaques of pregnancy*). This itchy rash appears during the third trimester, usually of the first pregnancy, and usually near stretch marks. It may spread from this point, but it disappears harmlessly after delivery.

PUPPP can be incredibly annoying, but you'll feel better if you just keep reminding yourself that it's harmless. The rash should go away within a few weeks after you give birth, and it won't hurt your baby. And here's more good news: It generally does not recur with later pregnancies.

When it gets to you, try an oatmeal or a cornstarch compress to soothe the itching temporarily. Another option: emollients. Keeping the skin well lubricated can help. If you are really miserable, ask your doctor about antihistamines. Some antihistamines seem to be safer than others during pregnancy, but these decisions are complex and must be discussed with a physician who is carefully watching your pregnancy.

One study found that mothers plagued by PUPPP tended to gain a lot of weight and had a higher-than-average rate of twin pregnancies. This leads some researchers to speculate it's caused by excessive skin stretching.

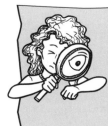

More Than Skin Deep

Always consult your doctor if you develop any skin rash or persistent itching. While PUPPP is the most common itchy rash of pregnancy, occasionally these symptoms indicate an infection, liver condition, or other health problem. Seek treatment immediately to make sure it doesn't affect your child.

How Your Blood Vessels Change

During pregnancy your estrogen levels soar, which dilates blood vessels. This dilation, plus the pressure of your swollen abdomen and general weight gain, can make your blood vessels do strange things.

For instance? Many expectant mothers develop reddish palms. This is normal and usually disappears within two weeks after the baby is born. Many pregnant women find their legs bruise easily, especially in the later months as pressure on leg veins builds. If this becomes a problem, or if you bruise easily in other parts of the body too, consult your doctor.

Up to 40 percent of pregnant women develop *varicose veins*—swollen, twisted veins just beneath the skin surface. They most often show up in the calves, thighs, vagina, and anus. Varicose veins won't win any beauty prizes, and they can sometimes be painful. They may improve after you deliver and lose weight, but unlike your pink palms, they won't go away completely. However, medical science is constantly developing new treatments to get rid of them. Since varicose and spider vessels are a concern for many people, not just expectant mothers, I devote Chapter 22, "Zapping Varicose and Spider Veins," to discussing ways to prevent and treat them.

Getting the Low-Down on Hemorrhoids

When varicose veins develop in the lining of the anus, they're called *hemorrhoids*. They may be near the beginning of the anal canal (in which case they're called *internal hemorrhoids*) or at the opening to the anus (*external hemorrhoids*).

You don't have to be pregnant to get hemorrhoids; according to the National Institutes of Health, about half of all Americans over age 50 have them, the result of too much pressure on anal veins. Contributing factors include constipation (straining during bowel movements distends the veins), obesity, and liver conditions.

And, of course, pregnancy. Your baby's weight puts pressure on these veins and makes them swell. If you also become constipated (as some pregnant women do), this makes matters worse.

Hemorrhoids may be symptomless; you may not even know you have them. If you do experience symptoms, common signs to watch for include:

➤ Pain, itching, or tenderness in the anal area, especially during bowel movements.

➤ Blood on toilet paper, surface of the stool, or in toilet bowl. Hemorrhoids are the most common cause of anal bleeding, especially if the blood is bright red; dark red may indicate bleeding from higher in the colon. A brown-black "coffee grounds" appearance means blood originating even higher in the gastrointestinal tract.

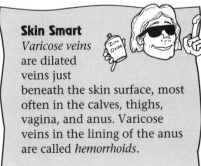

Skin Smart
Varicose veins are dilated veins just beneath the skin surface, most often in the calves, thighs, vagina, and anus. Varicose veins in the lining of the anus are called *hemorrhoids*.

➤ Occasionally, internal hemorrhoids protrude through the anal opening, sometimes producing a mucous discharge. You may be able to feel a bit of soft tissue, and it will be visible when your doctor does a physical exam.

Saving Your Skin
Yes, hemorrhoids are the most frequent cause of anal bleeding, but always consult your doctor if you see any blood. It may also be a sign of ulcerations, benign growths, or colon cancer. Don't just describe your symptoms; have a thorough physical exam to rule out all other possibilities besides hemorrhoids.

If you do develop hemorrhoids, should you get them removed? If you have no symptoms, or if you can tolerate the symptoms you have, most doctors advise against it. Generally hemorrhoids aren't serious, and they do not turn into cancer. They will probably improve after you deliver and return to your normal weight. In the meantime, there are several things you can do to minimize discomfort and stop them from getting worse:

➤ Eat more fiber. Many doctors blame hemorrhoids on constipation, and they blame constipation on the typical North American diet of highly refined foods. Added fiber creates soft bulky stools that are easier to eliminate without straining. See Table 14.2 for good dietary sources of fiber.

Table 14.2 Looking for Fiber in All the Right Places

Food	Dietary Fiber (Grams)
Kidney beans, $^1/_2$ cup	7.3
Navy beans, $^1/_2$ cup	6.0
Bran cereal, $^3/_4$ cup	4.0
Lentils, $^1/_2$ cup	3.7
Green peas, $^1/_2$ cup	3.6
Apple, 1 medium	3.5
Wheat germ, $^1/_4$ cup	3.4
Strawberries, 1 cup	3.0
Prunes, dried, 3	3.0
Orange, 1 medium	2.6
Potato, with skin, 1 medium	2.5
Bran muffin, 1 medium	2.5
Banana, 1 medium	2.4
Oatmeal, cooked, $^3/_4$ cup	1.6

➤ If you find yourself straining on the toilet, stop; continued straining puts more pressure on the veins. Instead, leave the bathroom. Eat a nutritious snack (digestion stimulates colon contractions). Drink lots of fluids, take a walk, and try again later when you feel the urge.

➤ Many hemorrhoid sufferers make things worse with over-zealous cleaning. Avoid frequent rubbing, harsh soaps, and abrasive washcloths.

➤ If dry toilet tissue is irritating, try cleansing gently with a moist baby wipe after a bowel movement. You don't have to invest in expensive brand-name wipes; buy generic towelettes from a drugstore or supermarket.

➤ Try a sitz bath—soak your rump in a hip bath filled with clean warm water or saline solution, which can soothe sore swollen tissues. (Please okay this first with your doctor, as many doctors will not recommend baths late in pregnancy.)

If you really are miserable, hemorrhoids can be surgically removed. But if at all possible, I recommend waiting until after delivery.

Spider Angiomas

During pregnancy, roughly 70 percent of white women and 10 percent of African-American women develop *spider angiomas*, small red dots surrounded by tiny radiating branches. (They are different from spider veins, which we'll discuss with varicose veins in Chapter 22.) Spider angiomas are most common on the arms, face, and neck, and usually appear toward the end of the first trimester.

Spider angiomas are painless and usually nothing to worry about; they do not signal a problem with your circulation. (Rarely, when many appear all at once, they can indicate a liver problem.) Sometimes they fade after delivery. If they persist, your doctor can get rid of them with a procedure called *electrocautery* (electrodesiccation), the use of electric current to seal blood vessels by heat. The current is applied through a slender needle. Complications are uncommon, although in rare cases electrocautery can leave a scar. If electrocautery fails, lasers are another option.

Saving Your Skin
Don't increase the amount of fiber you eat all at once; even if you weren't constipated before, this will do it to you! Instead, alter your diet gradually, and be sure to drink plenty of fluids and exercise regularly.

Skin Smart
Spider angiomas are small red dots surrounded by tiny radiating branches. A common development toward the end of the first trimester, they may fade after delivery. If not, *electrocautery* (electrodesiccation), the use of electric current to seal blood vessels by heat, can get rid of them.

Beauty Tips
After delivery, some of my patients lose almost 50 percent of their scalp hair, and it may take over a year to grow back fully. Don't panic, because this is not dangerous. You may find you feel better wearing a wig for a while. Refer to Chapter 7, "Beautiful Hair and Nails," for other tips on coping with temporary hair loss.

"What's Happening to My Hair?"

You may not be crazy about some of the changes we've discussed in this chapter, but here's one I think you'll like: Your hair will probably get thicker during your pregnancy. Again, this effect is caused by hormones, which propel large numbers of hair follicles into the active phase.

Many of my patients are delighted with their lush new tresses. Unfortunately, this situation is not permanent. Two to three months after delivery, many women begin to shed as hairs in the active phase move to the resting phase and then fall out. Sometimes this shedding is quite dramatic. Again, this situation is not permanent. In another two to three months, the shedding subsides, new hairs begin to grow in, and the entire process begins to shift back to your prepregnancy state.

The Least You Need to Know

➤ Just like everything else, your skin will change during pregnancy. Many women notice dark areas, especially on the face ("mask of pregnancy") and belly, around nipples and genitals, and in armpits. Always wear sunscreen, avoid tanning salons and sunlamps, and stay out of the sun as much as possible.

➤ You can't prevent stretch marks entirely, and generally they fade partially after delivery. If they don't, some doctors recommend topical applications of tretinoin. (Tretinoin should be avoided if you are nursing, however.) Laser treatments are another option.

➤ Some mothers-to-be develop itchy skin rashes. Often this is caused by PUPPP, a harmless (though extremely annoying) rash that starts near stretch marks, generally during the third trimester of the first pregnancy. While you should ask your doctor about any rash, PUPPP will not hurt your baby and should vanish after delivery.

➤ Varicose veins and hemorrhoids are common during pregnancy because of increased strain on blood vessels. To soothe hemorrhoids, eat plenty of fiber to prevent constipation, clean the area gently with moist towelettes, and soak in a warm sitz bath if okayed by your doctor.

➤ Scalp hair will probably grow thicker during pregnancy, but you may notice increased shedding two to three months after delivery. Don't panic about this hair loss; in time your hair should return to its prepregnancy thickness.

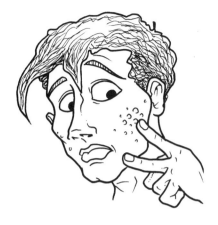

Chapter 15

Acne: An Age-Old Problem

In This Chapter

➤ Learn why acne starts during adolescence, just when you need it least

➤ Find the acne treatment that works best for you

➤ See why you can eat chocolate without guilt—about pimples, anyway

➤ Get the facts about Accutane®: very effective, serious medicine

➤ Discover the skin condition that looks like acne but isn't

Sixteen-year-old Josh, the son of one of my friends, looked absolutely miserable. "Who would want to go out with me?" he said. "There's this girl I want to ask to the prom, but I know she's just going to laugh in my face! That is," he added gloomily, "if she can even stand to look at my face."

Josh did have special reason to be concerned. He had a severe case of acne that covered his face, neck, chest, and shoulders, and the condition was beginning to affect his self-esteem. "He's starting to avoid all his friends," his mother confided to me. "They ask him to do things, but he just says no and stays home."

Josh and his parents were frustrated because nothing seemed to help. "He really watches what he eats," continued his mother. "He's cut out chocolate and fried foods completely. He scrubs his face four or five times a day with really strong soap and an abrasive pad, but it doesn't seem to be working. Is there any way to get rid of acne?"

"Yes indeed," I reassured both her and Josh. "There are a number of treatments we can try. Furthermore, some of the things you're doing now may actually be making it worse—the strong soap and all that scrubbing, for instance, may be irritating the skin unnecessarily. And doctors no longer think that chocolate causes acne."

For the first time during the appointment, Josh smiled. "Awesome," he said. "Less soap and more chocolate!"

What Is This Stuff?

To understand acne, let's return for a minute to Chapter 2, "Your Skin: Don't Leave Home Without It," where we discussed pores and sebum. As we saw, sebum is a waxy, oily substance that serves as a built-in moisturizer. Produced by oil glands in the skin's lower layers, it travels via pores to the skin surface.

Ideally, sebum travels smoothly, but sometimes it mixes with sticky skin cells that block the pores. This blockage is the first step in the formation of acne. The affected pore looks enlarged and dark. We call it a "blackhead" (*comedo* is the medical term). The dark material in a blackhead is not dirt, however; it is dried oil and shed skin cells that block the pore opening.

Skin Smart
Acne is a skin condition characterized by inflammation of the pores and surrounding skin. It can take many forms, including *blackheads* (enlarged dark pores), *papules* (red bumps), *pustules* (pus bumps), or *cysts* (larger swellings beneath the skin surface). Severe cases are referred to as *cystic acne*.

If sebum continues to pour into this blocked pore, it has no exit to the surface. The pore swells and may eventually rupture, releasing the oil and debris (as well as any bacteria trapped inside the pore) into the surrounding skin. The skin near the affected pore becomes red and inflamed. While the characteristic signs of acne are popularly known as "pimples," doctors have specific names to describe the different types. A red acne bump is called a *papule*. If the inflammation is severe enough, a pus bump (called a *pustule*) forms. And when the inflammation is severe and occurs below the surface of the skin, the resulting lump is called a *cyst*. Severe cases of acne, like Josh's, with many cysts, are called *cystic acne*.

Acne: Not Just for Teenagers

Many of us first encounter acne during our teenage years. Why? During adolescence, levels of certain hormones called *androgens* rise. While androgens are referred to as "male" hormones because they spur the development of male characteristics like facial hair and bulky muscles, women have them too. Surging androgen levels enlarge oil glands and stimulate the secretion of sebum. Many of these glands are located in the face, chest, and upper back; it's no coincidence that this is where the majority of blemishes appear.

Acne may be most widespread during adolescence, but it can hit at many different ages. At least 85 percent of us will have acne at some point in our lives. I've seen it in newborn babies (as a result of maternal hormones still circulating in the baby's bloodstream) and in adults in their 20s, 30s, 40s, and beyond. Some women report breaking out in regular patterns that correspond to their menstrual cycle. If your blemishes appear or get worse at certain times of the month, mention this to your doctor. It may be a normal part of your cycle, but it might also signal a correctable hormonal problem.

Thankfully, acne becomes more rare after age 50. But no matter when it appears, it's important to treat it properly. Inflamed lesions can lead to permanent scarring. This is especially true of cysts, although even pustules and papules may scar. But don't despair. As we will see, a lot of different treatments are available, both over the counter and by prescription.

Some of what's diagnosed as "acne" in adults may actually be a condition called *rosacea*, which resembles acne. We'll discuss rosacea later in this chapter.

> **Beauty Tips**
>
> If you get an occasional pimple, don't worry; most of us go through times when our skin acts up. Apply an oil-free foundation or tinted moisturizer, and relax. The pimple should heal on its own in a few days if it isn't disturbed. Chances are it's less noticeable than you think.

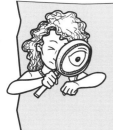

> **More Than Skin Deep**
>
> Stubborn acne may occasionally be a sign of an underlying hormonal abnormality, especially if it is seen in a person who has other signs of a hormonal problem such as irregular periods, excessive facial hair, or scalp hair thinning. If this sounds like it could be you, please have a hormonal work-up by your doctor.

What Else Causes Acne?

In addition to androgenic hormones, what else can cause acne? Here are some possibilities:

➤ **Oral contraceptives:** Some pills contain androgen-like substances that cause acne or make it worse. However, other birth control pills are known to improve acne. If you start seeing pimples after you begin taking oral contraceptives, ask your doctor about the pills' ingredients. Switching to another formulation could help.

➤ **Medications:** Some drugs can give you pimples. These include corticosteroids (used for a wide variety of inflammatory conditions) and lithium (used to treat bipolar disease, a psychiatric disorder). Anabolic steroids (used by body builders to increase muscle bulk) may also make you break out. If acne suddenly appears or worsens within a few months after starting a new medication, consult your doctor.

➤ **Ingredients in cosmetics and skin care products:** Many cosmetic ingredients can cause acne. Oil and petroleum products are common offenders. If your pimples sprout mainly around your mouth and chin, think about what you put on your lips. Do you wear a greasy petroleum-based lubricant for chapped lips? It could be spreading onto the surrounding skin, or you might be sensitive to an ingredient in your toothpaste or mouthwash. Bumps around the hairline may be caused by an oily conditioner or other oily hair preparations. It can take months to clog pores (and months to unclog them), so don't rule anything out, even if you've used it for a while. Experiment with different products or ask the advice of your dermatologist to determine which ones are best for you.

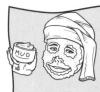

Beauty Tips
Sleeping with makeup on, or not removing it completely, can bring on blemishes. Remove all cosmetics and leave them off overnight. Try the fingernail test: Gently scratch your cheek after washing. If you still get makeup under your nails, either wash again, try a different makeup remover, or follow up with a toner, especially if you have oily skin.

➤ **Chemicals:** Soldiers exposed to Agent Orange (dioxin, a chlorinated hydrocarbon) during the Vietnam War developed severe cystic acne called "chloracne." Some tar derivatives cause similar reactions.

➤ **Oil and grease:** Some people have problems with mineral oil and petroleum jelly. I've also seen restaurant employees react to cooking oil in their kitchens.

➤ **Heat and humidity:** If you break out more during the summer, it may be because hot sticky weather and increased perspiration are clogging your pores.

➤ **Genetics:** The tendency toward acne runs in families. If your siblings and parents had trouble with it, you may too.

What Doesn't Cause Acne?

And now, let's debunk a few myths. Those pimples that drive you crazy are *not* caused by the following:

Saving Your Skin
I don't recommend facials when your skin is broken out. Rubbing and massaging can irritate your skin further, especially if the operator uses oil-containing lotions or helpfully tries to squeeze blemishes for you.

➤ **Chocolate, fried foods, or anything else you eat:** Unless you are sensitive to a particular food or beverage, diet is not responsible for acne. Eating oily foods will not increase the oil on your face (although it could increase your waistline and cholesterol level!).

➤ **Dirt:** Some acne sufferers believe that if only they get their faces really clean, their blemishes will fade forever. Unfortunately, acne has little to do with external dirt.

The mechanisms that produce blemishes start below the surface, deep inside pores and hair follicles, and scrubbing the skin surface has little effect.

➤ **Sexual activity:** This long-standing myth probably reflects the association between acne and surging adolescent hormones. Fact is, your sexual behavior does not influence your pimples.

By its nature, acne tends to flare up and calm down. It's tempting to blame these cycles on one of the factors listed here. However, blemishes seem to be largely independent of chocolate consumption, personal hygiene, and social life.

Getting Rid of It

When your face breaks out, it's tempting to scrub as hard as you can—but please don't. Even the most oily, acne-plagued skin should be treated gently.

Above all, avoid picking and squeezing blemishes. Scratching and pinching them will hurt your skin, not help it. It will increase the inflammation, making the area even more red and swollen. Also, it's easy to damage the inflamed skin around the pimple, and permanent scarring could result. The only person who should open your pimples or remove blackheads is your dermatologist. Here are some more tips:

➤ Wash your hair regularly, especially if it's oily. As mentioned earlier, if you tend to break out around the hairline, try a different shampoo, conditioner, hair spray, gel, or pomade.

➤ Elsewhere in this book, I've noted that often we cause our own skin problems, and this can be true for acne too. Use the mildest products you find effective, and avoid irritating, scrubbing, or drying out your skin. Refer to Chapters 4, "Clean Living: The Best Way to Clean Your Skin," 5, "Choosing the Right Toner and Moisturizer," and 6, "At the Cosmetics Counter," for tips on choosing skin care products. Many women automatically apply moisturizer, but if your skin is oily, you might not need to. If you're acne prone and feel you need a moisturizer, be sure it's oil free.

➤ Men with acne can try both electric and safety razors to see which works better. If you choose an electric razor, make sure your face is completely dry or the razor will catch on your skin. If you prefer a safety, always use a sharp blade and soften your whiskers with warm water and soap before applying shaving gel. I'm sure I don't have to warn you to shave lightly around pimples!

Beauty Tips

If you're bothered by oily shine through the day, try carrying a purse-size package of blotting papers. They come in handy for quick touch-ups.

Should you use alcohol on your skin? Doctors disagree about this. Some feel its drying effect can be beneficial for oily skin; others find it too irritating. Drying out surface skin won't necessarily help your pimples. Since many topical acne medications tend to dry the skin, I usually avoid alcohol in favor of these more effective products. And, fortunately, there are a lot of effective products to choose from these days. Read on for information about the latest acne treatments.

Saving Your Skin

If you have acne that is leaving scars, do not bother to buy hydroxy acids or benzoyl peroxide. You should go to your dermatologist as soon as possible to prevent further scarring.

Hydroxy Acids

Some people benefit from using mild exfoliants, like alpha or beta hydroxy acids, on their acne. This is a good place to start. By helping your skin shed surface cells, hydroxy acids open blocked pores and keep sebum moving smoothly onto the skin surface like it's supposed to.

Refer to Chapter 12, "Help from Hydroxy Acids," where I discuss effective ways to select and use these over-the-counter products. Try them for two months and see if they help.

Benzoyl Peroxide

If hydroxy acids don't make a dent in your acne, another option is *benzoyl peroxide*, a drying agent with antibacterial properties that's available both by prescription and over the counter.

Some tips for using benzoyl peroxide:

➤ Wash your face (and other acne-prone areas) with warm water and a cleanser twice a day. Try a cleanser that contains a beta hydroxy acid (such as salicylic acid), an alpha hydroxy acid (such as glycolic or lactic acid), benzoyl peroxide, or an antibacterial agent. Don't wash more than twice a day. Remember, dirt is not the problem, and since many of the medications used for acne are drying, you don't want to overdry the surface of your skin.

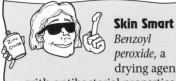

Skin Smart

Benzoyl peroxide, a drying agent with antibacterial properties for treating acne, is available in both prescription and over-the-counter preparations.

➤ After washing and gently blotting your skin dry, apply a benzoyl peroxide product. You can buy it in a lot of different forms, including lotions, gels, and creams.

➤ Benzoyl peroxide comes in several concentrations; my advice is to start with a low over-the-counter concentration and see how that works. If it doesn't seem effective, move to a higher strength.

➤ Some companies market different concentrations of benzoyl peroxide for different areas of your skin.

Instead of buying several products, find one you like that doesn't irritate your skin, and use it anywhere you feel you need it. On tougher areas, like the back, you may apply it twice a day, while more sensitive areas may only be able to tolerate once-a-day applications.

Benzoyl peroxide can dry your skin and make it somewhat red and flaky. If this gets too annoying, try applying it only once a day. Another option is to try a lower strength formulation or a different brand that's more moisturizing. A small percentage of people are allergic to benzoyl peroxide. If your skin becomes itchy, very red, or inflamed after using a benzoyl peroxide product, discontinue it and consult your doctor.

Try benzoyl peroxide for two months. If the routine described in this section hasn't helped your skin by then, it's time for stronger measures available only by prescription.

Retin-A®

In Chapter 13, "Tretinoin and Antioxidants: The Age-Tamers?" I discussed using tretinoin to combat photoaging. Before doctors used tretinoin on wrinkles, we used it on pimples, in the form of Retin-A®.

Saving Your Skin
Keep benzoyl peroxide away from hair, clothing, and towels. It's a bleach, so it could lighten your hair and fade fabrics.

Beauty Tips
If you have oily skin, you may want to try a mud facial mask. Mud masks contain clay, which helps absorb oil. Apply the mask to a clean face, and be careful with topical acne treatments afterward. Since the mask is exfoliating, topical medications could be more irritating than usual.

Many of the points covered in Chapter 13 apply here as well. Some additional tips to keep in mind:

➤ Don't apply benzoyl peroxide and tretinoin at the same time because peroxide may inactivate tretinoin. If you want to use both, try benzoyl peroxide in the morning and Retin-A® at night.

➤ Be very cautious when using hydroxy acids with either tretinoin or benzoyl peroxide. This is a potentially irritating combination.

➤ Some doctors recommend high percentages of Retin-A® for patients with oily skin. If this works for you, great. However, many people find Retin-A® irritating at first, and this is even more likely with stronger formulations. Consider starting with a lower strength, as recommended in Chapter 13, and graduating to stronger products as necessary. Many people find they must start by using tretinoin every other night, increasing to nightly applications once their skin has acclimated.

➤ If you experience severe chapping, burning, or irritation, ask your doctor about switching to a cream form, which will be less drying than the gel or solution.

➤ If you use Retin-A® faithfully for two months with little improvement, your doctor may want to increase the strength or change to a different medication.

In Chapter 13, I noted that you have to continue using Retin-A® permanently to continue enjoying its benefits for photoaging. The same is true for acne. If it helps, your doctor may suggest a maintenance dose of two or three times a week until you "outgrow" the acne.

Topical Antibiotics

If your acne is mild to moderate but shows signs of inflammation, your doctor may prescribe a topical antibiotic that you apply to your skin. These drugs come in a variety of forms, including lotions, creams, roll-ons, and pads. Sometimes you use them with Retin-A; sometimes you don't.

Topical antibiotics you may encounter include:

➤ Clindamycin

➤ Erythromycin

➤ Tetracycline

Your doctor will probably suggest applying them once or twice a day. All these drugs work about equally well, which means they don't work miracles. If you see roughly half of your blemishes disappear, this is considered a good result. Clindamycin and erythromycin are the most commonly prescribed. Some doctors think clindamycin may be slightly more effective.

Oral Antibiotics

For moderate to severe acne, your doctor may want you to take antibiotics by mouth, in addition to applying topical medications. The idea is to start antibiotics to decrease the inflammatory lesions while waiting for the topicals to begin working. Sometimes patients can be weaned off oral antibiotics and maintained on topicals alone. If this is not possible, oral antibiotics may be taken for more extended periods.

Oral antibiotics include the following:

➤ Tetracycline, which is moderately effective and inexpensive. It used to be the mainstay for oral acne therapy. (As you will see in a moment, doctors now often prefer tetracycline derivatives.) Usually, you take it twice daily until the acne has improved, and then slowly cut back on your dose. Many people stay on it for at least three months, or longer if needed. You should take tetracycline on an empty stomach. Don't eat or drink any dairy products or other calcium-containing foods or supplements within two hours before or after because they will inactivate the drug.

In rare cases, tetracycline can cause liver problems, so your doctor may order periodic blood tests.

Tetracyclines (and its derivatives) may make you more sensitive to the sun, so be sure to protect yourself. Very rarely, they can also cause allergic reactions.

➤ Minocycline and doxycycline, which are tetracycline derivatives. They are more expensive than tetracycline, but also tend to be more effective. Each has its own rare side effects. For example, doxycycline may cause nausea in some people, and minocycline can cause headaches and a dizzy feeling if the dose is high. If you experience any of these symptoms, stop the pills immediately and call your doctor.

➤ Erythromycin is another option, especially if you can't tolerate medications in the tetracycline family. You start by taking it twice a day and then cut back as your complexion improves. Many people find that erythromycin upsets their stomachs; taking it with food may help, although doing so could make the drug less effective. Some of the newer erythromycin derivatives are effective and easier on the stomach, but they are considerably more expensive than erythromycin.

➤ Clindamycin, usually a last resort, is sometimes helpful for treating acne that has resisted more commonly used antibiotics. Doctors prescribe it with caution because, in rare cases, it can cause a severe and dangerous form of diarrhea. Call your doctor promptly if you experience any problems.

Saving Your Skin
Some women who take oral antibiotics get vaginal yeast infections. If you develop vaginal itching or a whitish discharge, call your doctor immediately. There are many effective treatments for these yeast infections. If they keep recurring, switching to another antibiotic could help. Sometimes antibiotics have to be stopped altogether if the yeast infections are particularly difficult to control.

Saving Your Skin
If you experience any unusual or questionable reactions to any antibiotic, including tetracycline, stop taking the drug. Contact your doctor immediately.

More Than Skin Deep

There is a controversy among doctors about whether oral antibiotics make birth control pills less effective. One report says yes, another says no. If you have breakthrough bleeding, consider this a danger sign. Even if you don't, the controversy still exists. Please discuss this with your doctor. To be on the safe side, consider a backup form of birth control until you finish antibiotic therapy.

Hormones

Hormonal irregularities are occasionally responsible for outbreaks of acne. These conditions are usually not dangerous, just troublesome. If a patient does not respond to conventional treatment or if I have reason to suspect a hormonal problem (such as excessive facial hair, thinning scalp hair, irregular periods, or obesity) I will suggest a checkup by an endocrinologist or gynecologist. In cases like these, oral contraceptives and/or other medications that suppress androgens can make a world of difference.

Accutane®

If you have severe cystic acne, or acne that scars, and nothing else has worked, your doctor may prescribe the drug Accutane® (isotretinoin). A derivative of vitamin A, Accutane® is taken orally. It's a powerful drug that cuts oil glands' production of sebum, temporarily shrinks the glands, and causes permanent changes in the skin that may cure most cases of acne permanently.

Saving Your Skin
If you wear contact lenses, Accutane® could make it harder to tolerate them due to dry eyes. I always recommend a visit to the eye doctor for contact lens wearers who complain of dryness.

Saving Your Skin
Sometimes, people who take Accutane® develop permanent changes to the skeleton called *hyperostosis*, an outgrowth of bone. At the doses taken for acne, these changes are minimal and have no symptoms. As far as we know now, these changes have no associated long-term problems.

Sound wonderful? Sometimes patients beg me to go ahead and prescribe Accutane®. I tell them what I'm telling you now: Remarkably effective though this drug is, it has potentially serious side effects you should discuss with your doctor before deciding to use it. Be sure you know which symptoms to watch for, and call your doctor immediately if you experience any problems.

Some of the possible side effects of Accutane® include the following:

➤ **Very dry skin and mucous membranes:** Your lips and skin will become dry and possibly chapped. Your skin might start to itch from dryness, and your eyes may feel dry and scratchy. Your dermatologist can help alleviate the dry skin and lips with prescription and over-the-counter remedies; for help with eye problems, consult your ophthalmologist.

➤ **Sore muscles and joints:** Many people complain of musculoskeletal aches and pains while on Accutane®. Often they have to cut back on physical activity. Sometimes lowering the dose of Accutane® will help; in rare cases the drug may have to be discontinued.

➤ **Rising levels of cholesterol and other blood fats:** Most people don't stay on Accutane® long enough for this to be a problem, but it may be a concern if your levels rise dramatically or if they are already high. Your doctor should take blood tests regularly to monitor these levels.

➤ **Liver problems:** In rare cases, Accutane® can cause reversible elevations of liver enzymes. Your doctor will take blood tests regularly to monitor liver enzyme levels.

➤ **Eye problems:** In addition to dry eyes, some people report a decrease in their night vision.

➤ **Headaches:** Some people report headaches while taking Accutane®. Headaches in association with nausea, vomiting, and/or visual disturbances might indicate a serious side effect called *pseudotumor cerebri*. It is treatable if caught early, but stop the Accutane® and contact your doctor at once.

One of the worst side effects of Accutane® is serious birth defects in babies whose mothers take it at any point during pregnancy. You should have a negative pregnancy test immediately before starting this drug. Also, use two reliable forms of birth control the entire time you take it, and for one month before you start and another month after you quit. After finishing Accutane® therapy, you must wait at least one month to become pregnant because the drug will still be in your body.

Your doctor will probably prescribe Accutane® for a period of four to five months. In some cases a second course of treatment is necessary.

Rosacea: When "Acne" Isn't Really Acne

When Debbie walked in my office, she was close to tears. "I really hope you can help me," she whispered. "I've tried everything to get rid of my acne, and it just keeps getting worse!"

A fair-skinned redhead in her 40s, Debbie's face was covered with tiny red pimples. What's more, she had a red flush that extended from cheek to cheek and over her chin. She had tried numerous treatments, both over the counter and prescription, but to no avail. As I examined her, I noticed that despite all the bumps, she had no blackheads at all. In response to my questions, she admitted the redness and pimples got worse whenever she ate spicy foods, drank hot coffee, or had a glass of red wine.

Debbie, it turned out, did not have acne at all. Instead she had *rosacea*, a skin condition most often seen in fair-skinned women who tend to flush and blush. Many people with rosacea don't know they have it; they assume it's acne because it starts with tiny

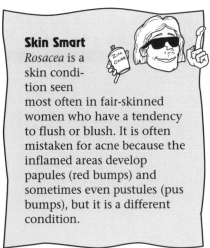

Skin Smart
Rosacea is a skin condition seen most often in fair-skinned women who have a tendency to flush or blush. It is often mistaken for acne because the inflamed areas develop papules (red bumps) and sometimes even pustules (pus bumps), but it is a different condition.

pimples and red areas on the forehead, nose, cheeks, and chin. These reddish patches gradually spread and become more pimply; the surface of the skin develops thin red lines caused by enlarged blood vessels.

If left untreated, rosacea can progress. Patients may develop permanently reddened skin and dilated superficial blood vessels. In the worst cases, they may develop a condition called *rhinophyma*, in which the nose becomes thickened and bumpy. Fortunately, this condition is rare.

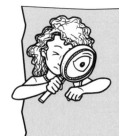

More Than Skin Deep

Some historians believe comedian W. C. Fields suffered from severe rosacea. In his case, the untreated condition led to a permanently ruddy complexion and a condition called *rhinophyma*, in which the nose becomes bulbous from excess tissue. Rhinophyma rarely occurs in women with rosacea.

Rosacea is most common in fair-skinned adults, especially women from 30 to 50, although it can appear at any age. At first, it might seem as though you just have extremely sensitive skin or a tendency to blush easily. Like Debbie, many find the flushing gets worse when they eat spicy foods or drink alcohol and hot beverages. Very hot showers or saunas, stress, or anything else that brings a flush to the face may aggravate the condition.

We don't know what causes rosacea, but fortunately it can be treated and often reversed, especially if caught at an early stage. Topical medications should improve it within two months. Sometimes doctors recommend oral antibiotics to control skin eruptions if the topical medications are not fully effective. Permanently enlarged blood vessels can be treated with a laser or can be "zapped" with a tiny electric needle.

Saving Your Skin

Don't treat rosacea with the over-the-counter acne medications, because they may make it worse. Consult a dermatologist for accurate diagnosis and treatment.

It will also help if you avoid anything that flushes and irritates your skin. Frequent offenders include alcoholic drinks (especially red wine), hot beverages, hot spicy food, saunas and steam baths, extremely cold weather, harsh soaps, and cosmetics containing alcohol or other irritants. Exposure to sunlight can trigger rosacea outbreaks, so always wear a sunscreen of SPF 15 or higher.

The Least You Need to Know

➤ Acne develops when sebum (your natural moisturizer) gets trapped in pores or when pores rupture, releasing their contents into the surrounding skin and causing inflammation.

➤ Acne usually appears during adolescence because of a surge of androgenic hormones. Other factors that can cause acne include medications, some oral contraceptives, hot humid weather, certain chemicals, and oils.

➤ What doesn't cause acne: chocolate or other foods, dirt, and sexual activity.

➤ There are many effective treatments for acne. You can try alpha and beta hydroxy acids, benzoyl peroxide, Retin-A®, topical and oral antibiotics, or Accutane®. While extremely effective, Accutane® should be your last resort because of serious potential side effects.

➤ Some adults (especially fair-skinned women aged 30 to 50) who appear to have acne may actually have rosacea, a skin condition characterized by chronic facial redness and red bumps or pus bumps. Topical and oral treatments can improve rosacea, especially if caught at an early stage.

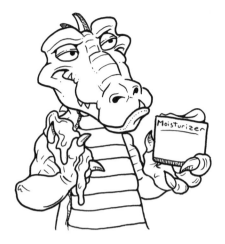

Chapter 16

Solving Common Skin Problems

In This Chapter

➤ Learn to identify common skin problems

➤ Discover easy home treatments for many of them

➤ Find out when it's time to call your doctor

➤ Learn which everyday items can cause problems for your skin

➤ Discover which conditions aren't contagious—and which ones are

➤ See why hot tubs may be dangerous to your skin

Julie's hands had recently developed a red itchy rash and tiny little blisters, and the skin was beginning to crack.

"This looks like dermatitis," I told her. "Have you been doing more wet work recently? Maybe more laundry or household chores?" "Nope," she said. "And I've been trying to take good care of my skin. As a matter of fact, I've recently started using a hand lotion on a regular basis." "When did that start?" I inquired. She thought it over. "About a week before the rash appeared," she decided. "In this case," I said, "the lotion almost certainly is the culprit. Let's take a look at the ingredients."

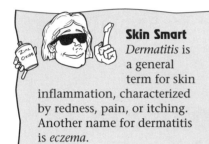

Skin Smart
Dermatitis is a general term for skin inflammation, characterized by redness, pain, or itching. Another name for dermatitis is *eczema*.

Dealing with Dermatitis

Dermatitis, also called *eczema*, is a general term meaning inflammation of the skin, characterized by redness, pain, or itching. A lot of things can lead to dermatitis, including allergies, irritation, extreme dryness, and genetic factors. In some cases, the cause is never determined.

Let's look at four common types of dermatitis: contact, atopic, seborrheic, and asteatotic.

Contact Dermatitis: Don't Touch

If your dermatitis is a reaction to a substance that touches your skin, it's called *contact dermatitis*. Your skin will become red and may swell or develop small blisters, crusts, and scales; it could also become cracked, thickened, and leathery if the dermatitis persists. If things don't begin to improve within a week, consult a dermatologist.

Contact dermatitis may result from irritation, or it could be an allergic response. Yes, there is a difference. *Irritants* are substances, such as harsh cleaning solutions and detergents, that produce a reaction on almost anyone's skin in high enough concentrations.

Allergic reactions, which are hypersensitivity reactions to a specific product, occur less frequently. The "harshness" of the product is not important, nor is the concentration. If you are allergic, you will react to extremely small amounts of the offending agent. A very common example is poison ivy; less common examples are perfume and lanolin.

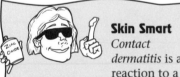

Skin Smart
Contact dermatitis is a reaction to a substance that touches your skin. The dermatitis may result from *irritants*, which are substances that produce a reaction on almost anyone's skin, or from an *allergic reaction*, which is a hypersensitive reaction to a specific substance.

How do you figure out what causes contact dermatitis? Sometimes the answer is obvious, sometimes it's not. Finding the culprit may call for some detective work, as you and your doctor eliminate various candidates to isolate the true offender. You can help by taking time before your appointment to write down your typical daily regimen and listing substances to which your skin is frequently exposed.

If your doctor suspects an allergy as opposed to an irritation reaction, he or she may do patch tests, in which small amounts of possible allergens (substances that cause allergic reactions) are applied to your skin. The sites are checked in two days and then again in four days to see whether your skin reacted. (For more information on allergies, see Chapter 3, "Common Complaints.") Your doctor will probably start by considering some of the most frequent culprits, which include the following:

➤ **Lanolin:** Lanolin, a wool derivative, is a common allergen. It is often used in moisturizers, like the one Julie had trouble with, and sometimes in soaps, cosmetics, and topical medications. If you find that several different moisturizers leave your skin red and itchy, you might be allergic to lanolin.

➤ **Rubber:** Products containing rubber may cause contact dermatitis, so rubber gloves are a problem for some people. If you sometimes develop rashes along elastic bands in clothing, underpants, or bras, you may be reacting to rubber in the elastic. Look for clothing made with spandex instead, and watch out for rubber-backed fasteners and edges.

➤ **Chromium:** Cement, chrome-tanned leather, paints, some shoe polishes, some inks, and even some matches contain chromium, and employees in the automobile, welding, foundry, railroad, and construction industries sometimes get dermatitis from on-the-job exposure. If you are allergic to chromium, talk to your doctor about all the items you should avoid.

➤ **Nickel:** The metalnickel turns up in many products, including chrome, jewelry, watch bands, and clothing accessories like buckles, zippers, clips, and buttons. Look for accessories made of nylon instead. Stainless steel also contains nickel, but it is bound so tightly that it doesn't cause problems for most nickel-sensitive types.

Earring wearers sometimes get earlobe dermatitis, which is often a reaction to nickel. Gold-plated and gold-filled jewelry may contain nickel alloys. Even 14-karat gold might contain enough nickel to cause a reaction in sensitive individuals. If your budget doesn't allow for 18-karat gold, consider earrings made of surgical steel, which tends to be well tolerated.

➤ **Hair dyes:** Some people are sensitive to an ingredient in permanent hair dyes called PPD (para-phenylenediamine), and about 25 percent of those folks also react to ingredients in semipermanent dyes. Always test a dye on a small patch of skin at least 24 hours before using it on your hair. Most PPD-allergic people can get by with temporary dyes or hair rinses; other options include a vegetable dye, such as henna, or a hair-color restorer (progressive dye).

Saving Your Skin

I've had a few patients develop mysterious rashes on their feet that turned out to be contact dermatitis. Sometimes this is a reaction to rubber or adhesives used in shoes. Another source of foot dermatitis is chromium in the chromates used to tan leather for shoes and clothing. Look for shoes and garments made of vegetable-tanned leather.

Beauty Tips

If you're plagued by earlobe dermatitis, it may be a reaction to nickel in your earrings. Ask your jeweler to coat exposed surfaces with a lacquer, plastic, or other nickel-free product. You might also apply several layers of clear nail polish to nickel-containing jewelry. (But remember, some people are sensitive to nail polish.)

185

➤ **Cosmetics and skin care products:** Fragrances and preservatives (parabens and quaternium-15, for example) are the most common cause of dermatitis from cosmetics. Look for products labeled "fragrance-free" or "without perfume"; believe it or not, items labeled "unscented" may contain perfumes to mask the smell of the chemicals. For more information on allergic reactions to skin care products, see Chapter 3.

In addition to allergies, irritation can cause contact dermatitis: soaps, detergents, solvents, household cleaners, chemicals, and even overexposure to water are frequent offenders. Irritation can develop seemingly overnight: Even if you've used a substance previously with no problems, it could start to irritate your skin. Once dermatitis sets in, your skin may become even more sensitive, and even supposedly gentle products can make things worse.

Saving Your Skin
Many things, too extensive to list here, may cause an allergic reaction. Your dermatologist can determine exactly what you are sensitive to by doing a patch test.

There are a number of things you can do to treat contact dermatitis:

➤ First, figure out what causes the dermatitis and do your best to avoid it. This may be all you need to solve the problem. In Julie's case, I advised her to avoid lanolin-containing products, as well as other wool derivatives.

➤ Don't wash affected areas with soap. Use a mild water-soluble cleanser, dry well, and then apply moisturizer.

➤ Apply topical corticosteroids to relieve inflammation. Try over-the-counter products first. If they fail, see your dermatologist for a stronger prescription product.

➤ Oral antihistamines may calm itching and help you sleep better. (You might want to use them only at night because some can make you drowsy.)

If these simple measures don't work promptly, please make an appointment to see your dermatologist. And above all, don't scratch! It will only make your skin more inflamed.

Atopic Dermatitis

Atopic dermatitis is a chronic skin inflammation in people with an inherited tendency toward allergies. Most folks with atopic dermatitis have relatives who show similar skin reactions and often have other allergy-related problems as well, such as hives, hay fever, and asthma.

Most common during childhood, atopic dermatitis is sometimes called *infantile eczema*. Often it appears as a scaly, itchy skin rash in the folds of elbows and knees, sometimes on ankles, wrists, face, neck, or upper chest too.

Treatments include the following:

➤ Corticosteroid preparations or tar creams to decrease inflammation.

➤ Oral antihistamines to control itching.

➤ Oral antibiotics. People with atopic dermatitis often harbor bacteria on their skin. To make matters worse, they have an allergic reaction to these bacteria, further aggravating their itchy, inflamed flesh. Killing these bacteria with oral antibiotics can break the cycle and provide some relief.

> **Skin Smart**
>
> *Atopic dermatitis* is a chronic skin inflammation in people with an inherited tendency toward allergies. Most of them have family members with similar skin reactions and often have other allergy-related problems, too.

Your doctor may recommend allergy testing, although it can be hard to pinpoint the cause of atopic dermatitis outbreaks. Some people experience recurrent dermatitis throughout their lives. But take heart: The condition tends to improve after childhood. Even if it doesn't go away entirely, flare-ups are likely to become less severe. If you are one of the unfortunate folks who do not outgrow atopic dermatitis, try a visit to the dermatologist. Many medical options are available for adults with this condition.

Seborrheic Dermatitis

Seborrheic dermatitis is a skin inflammation in areas with large numbers of sebum-producing (*sebaceous*) glands. The most common sites for the rash are the scalp (where it can cause an angry itchy form of dandruff), the corners of the nose, the eyebrows, behind and in the ears, the middle of the chest, and the navel. The skin looks red and scaly in these areas; the scales may be greasy and yellowish. The scaly patches could ooze or crust over; sometimes they itch, but it's usually not too uncomfortable.

> **Skin Smart**
>
> *Seborrheic dermatitis* is a reddish skin inflammation in areas with large numbers of sebum-producing (*sebaceous*) glands. It causes red skin with scales that may look yellowish and greasy.

You can develop seborrheic dermatitis at any time, but it's most common in three age groups: infancy (when it's called "cradle cap"), middle age, and the later years. It seems to run in families. We're not sure what causes it, although it may be related to a type of yeast that's often present on the skin. Some adults with seborrheic dermatitis show higher rates of immune system disorders or conditions of the central nervous system, such as Parkinson's disease. However, it does not cause any of these conditions, and most people with seborrheic dermatitis never develop them. Also, it has nothing to do with skin cancer.

Most people with seborrheic dermatitis control it easily with the following treatments:

➤ Apply an over-the-counter corticosteroid cream or lotion to the rash when it acts up. Use it as sparingly as possible.

➤ If the rash appears on your scalp, wash with a medicated shampoo containing tar, zinc pyrithione, selenium sulfide, sulfur, or salicylic acid. Try a nonprescription brand first. If it isn't strong enough, your doctor can recommend a prescription shampoo.

➤ Prescription products are available if these simple treatments don't help.

Seborrheic dermatitis may go away for years and then flare up unexpectedly. Sometimes we can trace outbreaks to stress and illness, but often the triggering factor remains unknown. Even when chronic, it's rarely serious.

Asteatotic Eczema

Sometimes skin can become so dry that it actually gets inflamed, red, and itchy just from the dryness. This condition is called *asteatotic eczema*. As you might have guessed already, alleviating the dryness helps the problem dramatically.

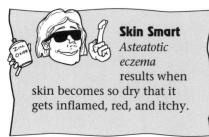

Skin Smart
Asteatotic eczema results when skin becomes so dry that it gets inflamed, red, and itchy.

If you're pestered by asteatotic eczema, I recommend taking brief showers in lukewarm (not hot) water. Use a mild water-soluble cleanser. Dry your skin and immediately apply a bland moisturizer. Moisturize your skin many times throughout the day.

If this doesn't clear up the problem, your doctor may prescribe a corticosteroid ointment, which moisturizes as it decreases inflammation.

Soothing Psoriasis

Psoriasis is a chronic skin condition in which the skin develops red thickened areas covered with silvery scales. Most often these patches appear on the knees, elbows, and scalp; more serious cases may also involve the trunk and the rest of the body.

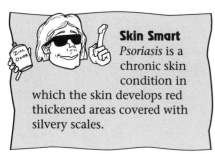

Skin Smart
Psoriasis is a chronic skin condition in which the skin develops red thickened areas covered with silvery scales.

As we saw in Chapter 2, "Your Skin: Don't Leave Home Without It," your skin constantly manufactures new cells and sheds old ones. Usually the cycle from producing a new skin cell to its shedding at the surface takes about 28 to 30 days. In psoriasis, however, this process is accelerated. Your body can't shed cells fast enough to keep up, so excess skin cells accumulate to form the characteristic scaly patches.

We're not sure what causes the condition, but it's not contagious, and there is a tendency for it to run in families.

It's equally common in men and women, and most often appears between ages 15 to 35. Some people experience their first episode about two weeks after a skin injury. This is a manifestation of the "Koebner phenomenon," in which an area that is traumatized or inflamed subsequently develops psoriasis. Flare-ups may be triggered by stress, infections, or some medications.

In some people, psoriasis is so mild they don't even realize they have it, assuming the scaly patches on their elbows or knees are just dry skin. In others, it covers most of the body. While the condition is chronic and tends to recur, you have a wide choice of treatments to control it, including:

➤ Topical medications containing cortisone, synthetic vitamin D, coal tar, anthralin (a drug that slows down the rate at which skin cells multiply), or a retinoid (vitamin A derivative). Simple topical emollients are also helpful.

➤ Medicated shampoos, oils, and scalp sprays. Many contain cortisone preparations or tars.

➤ Ultraviolet light therapy. If your psoriasis is widespread, you may benefit from treatment in a medically approved center equipped with ultraviolet light boxes. Unlike natural sunlight, the precise amount and wavelength of ultraviolet exposure in these light boxes can be controlled, allowing for the safest possible treatment. Medically controlled exposure to UVB can be a big help for people with moderate to severe psoriasis.

Saving Your Skin
Follow your doctor's instructions closely when using topical corticosteroid medications. While they are effective for many conditions, they can have serious side effects, including thinning skin, dilated blood vessels, bruising, and changes in skin color. People with psoriasis should avoid taking oral corticosteroids, because discontinuing them may cause a severe flare-up.

Severe psoriasis will probably benefit from one of the following:

➤ The Goeckerman Treatment (named for the dermatologist who developed it in the 1920s). This daily regimen, available at specialized centers, combines coal tar dressings and exposure to ultraviolet light. It is fairly time-consuming and messy, so it has largely been replaced by other treatments.

➤ PUVA (Psoralen + UVA); patients take a photosensitizing drug called *psoralen*, then undergo exposure to carefully measured amounts of UVA rays. PUVA treatments are done in a series; it usually takes about 30 to 40 treatments per year to keep psoriasis under control. Psoralen will make you sensitive to natural sunlight too, so you must wear protective sunscreens and medically approved sunglasses when you are outside. Since PUVA may cause photoaging and could increase your risk of skin cancer, please discuss these issues with your doctor.

➤ Methotrexate, an oral anti-cancer drug. While highly effective, it can have serious side effects, including nausea, dizziness, and liver and blood problems. Your doctor will recommend regular blood tests and may require liver biopsies to check for complications.

➤ Retinoids, prescription drugs related to vitamin A. We discussed one retinoid, Accutane®, in Chapter 15, "Acne: An Age-Old Problem." As mentioned there, retinoids have many side effects, including dry skin, elevated fat levels in the blood, headache, eye changes, and bone changes, among others. Retinoids can also cause birth defects, so doctors may hesitate to recommend them for women of child-bearing age.

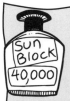

Saving Your Skin
If you undergo PUVA treatments, it's important to protect your eyes from UV. Your doctor will provide special eyegear to wear during the treatments. Ask for advice on choosing good UV-protective sunglasses to wear when you're outdoors. Generally, dark gray lenses offer the best color resolution; make sure lenses are large enough to cover your eyes.

➤ Cyclosporine. This medication is often used to prevent rejection of transplanted organs. It can be very effective for psoriasis; however, it has several possible side effects, including kidney damage. It also interacts badly with many other medications. You and your doctor will need to consider the risks carefully.

While so far there's no cure for psoriasis, researchers are constantly testing new approaches. In the meantime, one of the preceding treatments is likely to help your skin.

Impetigo: Don't Scratch

Impetigo is a skin infection caused by bacteria. Usually it shows up where skin has been injured by dermatitis or an abrasion, scratch, or insect bite. It starts as a reddish sore that oozes to form a sticky honey-colored crust. (This crust may not be visible when impetigo appears on the face, as twice-daily face washing tends to hold the crusting at bay.) The sore leaks bacteria-filled fluid that's highly contagious, and you can spread the infection to other parts of your body by scratching, or even to other people through physical contact.

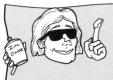

Skin Smart
Impetigo is a skin infection caused by bacteria. It's contagious and can be spread by scratching or other physical contact.

If not treated, impetigo can spread. In rare cases, the bacteria may invade underlying tissue or enter the bloodstream. These are serious problems requiring immediate medical attention. If caught early, however, impetigo is very curable. Your doctor will prescribe topical medications or oral antibiotics. Wash sores daily with antibacterial soap, and don't share clothing, towels, or razors with anyone until the infection clears.

Coping with Cold Sores

One day you feel an itchy tingling sensation at the corner of your mouth, and a cluster of tiny, clear, fluid-filled blisters forms there. After several days, the blisters break, ooze, crust over, and eventually fall off. These unwelcome visitors are *cold sores* (sometimes called *fever blisters*), a sign of infection by the herpes simplex virus.

There are two types of herpes simplex. Type 1 usually causes the cold sores that occur on the face, although sometimes they can infect genital skin or skin wounds. Most of us contract Type 1 at some point in our lives, usually from childhood contact with people who harbor the virus.

Type 2 is most often seen on the genitals. However, this distinction is not always clear-cut, and the two types of herpes simplex are actually quite similar. The greatest difference between oral and genital herpes infections is in how we view them.

Once you get the herpes simplex virus, it never leaves. Although the cold sore heals completely, the virus quietly moves to the nerve roots where it goes dormant. Many people never experience another active infection, but in others the cold sores recur every few weeks or months. Certain factors are apt to trigger them, such as illness, sun exposure, and hormonal cycles, but often they seem completely unpredictable.

While herpes infections can be serious to people with major health problems or a weakened immune system, in most cases the cold sores are simply an annoyance. Your doctor can prescribe a medication called acyclovir to control the sores; if you use it topically, apply it with a cotton swab (not your fingers), then throw the swab away. If you get cold sores frequently, your doctor may recommend taking acyclovir orally on a regular basis. Low suppressive doses are taken daily and increased at the first sign of a cold sore.

Both types of herpes simplex are highly contagious. To avoid spreading the virus, don't kiss anyone or engage in oral sex until your cold sores heal completely. (Needless to say, if you have genital sores, abstain from genital sex too; condoms offer some protection but they're not foolproof.) Don't share towels, clothing, or eating utensils. If you touch a cold sore, wash your hands (and all other areas of skin that came into contact with the sore) immediately with soap and water. Keep your hands away from your eyes, because herpes simplex can cause painful and dangerous eye infections.

Skin Smart

Cold sores (sometimes called *fever blisters*) are a sign of infection by the herpes simplex virus. They are tiny, clear, fluid-filled blisters that form singly or in clusters.

Saving Your Skin

If you touch cold sores during an active infection, wash your hands with soap afterward to avoid spreading the virus. Never touch your eyes because herpes simplex can cause eye infections. Symptoms of eye problems include pain, discharge, a gritty sensation, or sensitivity to light. If you experience any of these symptoms, call your doctor immediately.

191

Winning over Warts

Warts are skin growths caused by a viral infection in the top layer of skin or mucous membranes. The viruses responsible belong to a group called *human papillomavirus* (*HPV*). Warts are usually skin-colored and rough-textured, though some can be dark, smooth, and flat.

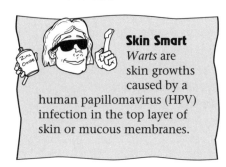

Skin Smart
Warts are skin growths caused by a human papillomavirus (HPV) infection in the top layer of skin or mucous membranes.

There are several kinds of warts, including:

➤ Hand warts, which usually grow around nails, on fingers, and on the backs of your hands.

➤ Foot (plantar) warts, generally found on the soles of the feet. Plantar warts may protrude less than hand warts because the pressure of walking flattens them. If you see small black dots in the wart, you're looking at small blockages in the tiny blood vessels that nourish the wart.

➤ Flat warts, like their name, are smooth and often smaller than other types. They tend to grow in clusters, ranging from 20 to 100 at one site. In kids, they're most often found on the face; adult men tend to have them in the beard area, and adult women, on the legs.

➤ Genital warts (condyloma) are soft growths on the external genitals, around the anus, or within the rectum; in women, they may also grow inside the vagina and cervix. Certain types of genital warts have been linked to cervical and other cancers. If you have or suspect genital warts, please discuss this with your doctor.

Are warts contagious? Yes, although it may be several months after you've been exposed before a wart gets big enough to be visible. Some people seem to catch them more easily than others. If your immune system is weakened—for instance, by illness or an organ transplant—you are more vulnerable. If you have areas of broken skin from biting fingernails or picking at hangnails, they can also provide an entry for the virus. But some people with perfectly good immune systems and intact skin just seem to be wart-prone, for unknown reasons.

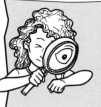

More Than Skin Deep

If you develop a genital wart, seek prompt treatment for yourself and all sexual partners. You can easily transmit or acquire genital warts through unprotected sex. If left untreated, certain types of genital warts increase the risk of cervical cancer and other genital cancers. Even after treatment, women who've had genital warts should have regular Pap tests to check for cancer.

In some lucky people, hand and foot warts may disappear on their own after several months or years. This is less common in other types of warts, and in any case, you should treat warts as soon as you notice them; otherwise they could shed tiny virus particles into surrounding skin, which will seed new growths. You might be able to destroy a wart after painting it repeatedly with a nonprescription liquid remover containing salicylic acid. (Consult your doctor first though, to make sure it's really a wart and not another skin growth requiring different treatment.) Follow package instructions and be patient, because this treatment can take weeks.

If over-the-counter preparations don't work, your doctor can apply stronger solutions in his or her office. Other treatment options include freezing the wart, burning it off with electrosurgery, removing it surgically, and treating it with a laser. Plantar warts are definitely more difficult to remove permanently than hand warts. Flat warts may also have a troublesome tendency to recur.

Genital warts can be hardest to get rid of. Several in-office treatments with acids or freezing solutions may be necessary. Large or persistent genital warts may have to be removed surgically.

Routing Ringworm

Ringworm is a skin infection caused by a fungus. Most often found on the feet, groin, scalp, nails, or trunk, the infection gets its name from characteristic ring-shaped patches of reddened, scaly skin; it has nothing to do with worms. These rings reflect the fungus's habit of spreading uniformly outward, leaving a spot of normal skin in the middle.

Most common in crowded urban areas, ringworm is contagious. You can catch it from other people; less frequently, you can get it from animals, soil, even from inanimate objects like shower stalls, furniture, or carpeting. If left untreated, scalp ringworm infections can cause bald patches. If the fungus gets into nails, the nail plate may become discolored and deformed.

Fungi thrive in moist environments, which is why they like moldy showers, humid locker rooms, and sweaty feet. To rout ringworm and reduce your risk of getting it in the first place, try the following:

➤ Wash your feet with soap at least once a day, and dry them thoroughly before putting your socks on. Don't forget to dry between your toes!

➤ Wear loose-fitting absorbent socks, and shoes made of breathable materials like leather (not vinyl). If your feet tend to perspire heavily, sprinkle a little talcum powder in your socks before putting them on.

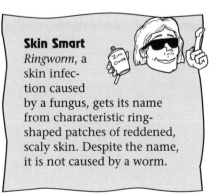

Skin Smart

Ringworm, a skin infection caused by a fungus, gets its name from characteristic ring-shaped patches of reddened, scaly skin. Despite the name, it is not caused by a worm.

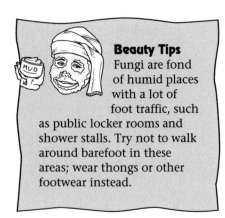

Beauty Tips
Fungi are fond of humid places with a lot of foot traffic, such as public locker rooms and shower stalls. Try not to walk around barefoot in these areas; wear thongs or other footwear instead.

➤ Change towels, washcloths, and clothing frequently.

➤ If ringworm strikes, and the infection is small and doesn't include scalp or nails, try an over-the-counter fungicidal cream. If your skin does not improve after two weeks, consult your doctor. He or she can prescribe stronger topical drugs and oral medications.

➤ For scalp and nail infections, call your doctor immediately. These fungus infections are notoriously stubborn, and nonprescription treatments probably won't work. What's more, untreated scalp infections may result in permanently scarred bald patches.

Properly treated, scalp infections should clear within two months. Fungal infections of the nails are more complicated, so you might need to take a medicine for up to three months. However, remember that toenails can take 12 to 18 months to grow out. Even though you've effectively gotten rid of the fungus, your nails won't look perfectly normal again until all the old infected nail has grown out.

Fending Off Folliculitis

In Chapter 7, "Beautiful Hair and Nails," we looked at hair follicles, tiny complex structures, buried in the dermis or subcutaneous layer, which manufacture specialized cells that grow into hair strands. *Folliculitis* is an infection of one or more hair follicles, usually caused by bacteria, less often by fungi. Often it looks like a scattering of small, white-headed pimples or red bumps around the follicles.

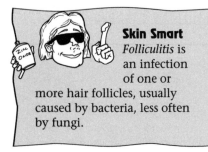

Skin Smart
Folliculitis is an infection of one or more hair follicles, usually caused by bacteria, less often by fungi.

You can get folliculitis anywhere you have hair follicles, which means everywhere except your mouth, palms, and the soles of your feet. (You have 80,000 to 120,000 hair follicles on your scalp alone.) Often folliculitis results from follicle inflammation from abrasion of the skin in the vicinity of the inflamed follicles, caused by shaving, skin injury, or friction from tight clothing. The specific cause varies, depending on where the infection is located.

Common types of folliculitis include the following:

➤ **Barber's itch:** So-called because it's an infection of the hair follicles in the beard area, especially the upper lip. It is usually caused by bacteria, but sometimes by a fungus. The pimples are generally pinhead-sized, and the area may itch for a day or two before they erupt.

➤ **Hot tub folliculitis (pseudomonas folliculitis):** This is a condition I'm seeing a lot more of as hot tubs and whirlpool baths become increasingly popular. If they don't contain enough chlorine, pseudomonas bacteria can multiply rapidly and leave you with an unpleasant souvenir of your relaxing soak one to five days later. Hot tub folliculitis may erupt as itchy little red bumps on any skin exposed to the water; I've also had patients contract it from contaminated loofahs and washcloths.

➤ **Gram-negative folliculitis:** A facial infection most common in people who take oral antibiotics over a long period to treat acne. (Its name comes from the group of bacteria that cause it.)

➤ **Pseudofolliculitis barbae:** This condition appears in people with curly hair, particularly African-Americans, whose shaved hair tip grows back into the skin rather than passing through the pore to the surface. This causes an inflammation of the skin near the hair follicle, instead of a true infection.

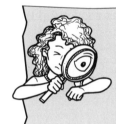

More Than Skin Deep

If you patronize public hot tubs or swimming pools, ask the management how the facilities are maintained. The chlorine level should be kept above 0.5 milligrams per liter, and the pH below 8. Otherwise, pseudomonas bacteria can multiply to infectious levels.

You can treat most cases of mild folliculitis yourself. Try the following:

➤ Wash affected areas twice daily with antibacterial soap. Dry your skin gently but thoroughly with a clean towel, and apply antibacterial ointment.

➤ Avoid wearing tight clothing or undergarments. Clothing friction could inflame hair follicles.

➤ Always use a clean sharp razor when shaving, and apply shaving cream or gel first to soften the hair. Shave in the direction of hair growth, not against it. (For more suggestions on shaving and other options for safely getting rid of hair, see Chapter 7, "Beautiful Hair and Nails.")

Most cases of mild folliculitis respond well to topical antibiotics, but more serious outbreaks might need oral antibiotic therapy. Before prescribing a drug, your doctor may order lab tests to identify the organism responsible.

The Least You Need to Know

➤ Dermatitis, or eczema, is a general term for skin inflammation. In contact dermatitis, your skin reacts to something that touches it; atopic dermatitis often reflects a family history of allergic sensitivity. Seborrheic dermatitis affects areas of skin with a lot of sebaceous glands, and asteatotic eczema is caused by extreme dryness.

➤ In psoriasis, the body produces new skin cells faster than normal, and patches of silvery scales on red skin develop. The condition is chronic, but many treatments are available.

➤ Impetigo, a contagious bacterial infection, should be treated promptly. Don't scratch, because this will spread it.

➤ Cold sores result from an infection by the herpes simplex virus. The virus remains in your body after the initial infection, which explains why cold sores have a tendency to recur. If recurrences are frequent, suppressive medications are available.

➤ Warts are caused by an HPV (human papillomavirus) infection. Genital warts are usually sexually transmitted and some types may increase your risk of cervical and other genital cancers; women who've had genital warts should get regular Pap tests to screen for cancer. Remove all warts promptly before the virus can shed into surrounding skin and seed new growths.

➤ Ringworm is a fungal infection, and has nothing to do with worms. Scalp and nail infections require prescription treatment. Mild infections elsewhere on the body may respond to over-the-counter creams.

➤ Folliculitis, infection of the hair follicles, is often caused by shaving, long-term antibiotic therapy, or even soaking in hot tubs.

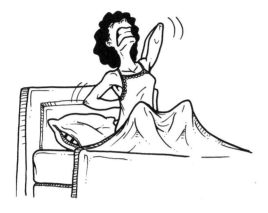

Chapter 17

Other Things That Go Itch in the Night

In This Chapter

➤ Learn to recognize the enemy: poison ivy, oak, and sumac

➤ Find out what to do if they get you

➤ Discover how to recognize and treat bites and stings

➤ Learn the safe way to get rid of ticks and deal with chiggers

➤ Protect yourself against poisonous spiders and bee stings

Joe looked sheepish. "Well, I guess I finally found out what poison ivy's like," he said ruefully. "I was cleaning out a bunch of undergrowth in my yard last week, and now look at me!"

He had an itchy red skin rash that stretched the entire length of his right arm. The rash had already spread to angry patches on his face and left arm. "Have you been scratching it?" I asked.

Joe looked more sheepish still. "I really don't mean to," he said. "I know you're not supposed to, but it just itches so much! The worst of it is, I've never had poison ivy before. I always thought I was immune. Now I know what all the fuss is about!"

Poison Ivy, Oak, and Sumac

In the previous chapter, we talked about contact dermatitis, an inflammatory reaction to a substance that touches your skin. The rash that's making Joe so uncomfortable is actually a type of allergic contact dermatitis popularly known as "poison ivy."

Come to think of it, "popularly" may be the wrong term; at least 85 percent of the U.S. population can develop dermatitis from poison ivy, making it the single most common cause of allergic reactions in North America. Every year it makes anywhere from 10 to 50 million of us miserable.

Recognizing the Enemy

This all-too-familiar rash is a reaction to any one of three closely related plants: *poison ivy*, *poison oak*, or *poison sumac* (see illustrations).

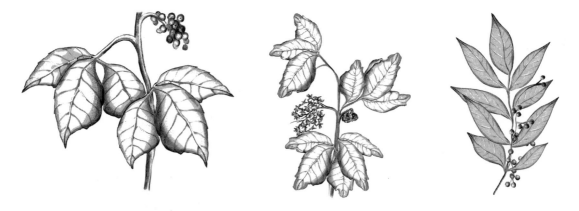

Left to right: Poison ivy, poison oak, and poison sumac, three closely related species, are the single most common cause of allergic reactions in North America.

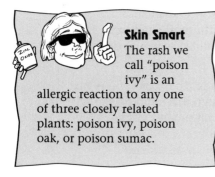

Skin Smart
The rash we call "poison ivy" is an allergic reaction to any one of three closely related plants: poison ivy, poison oak, or poison sumac.

Poison ivy grows as a wild vine in the eastern, southern, and midwestern United States, and as a shrub in the northern United States and Canada. It bears yellow-green flowers, white berries, and shiny leaves that usually grow in clusters of three, although some specimens have groups of five, seven, or nine leaves. (While the popular saying "leaves of three, let them be" is a good rule to follow, it doesn't apply to all varieties of the plant.)

Poison oak grows as a shrub in the eastern United States, and a shrub or vine in the West. It tends to be low-growing with clusters of yellow or whitish berries and leaves shaped like oak tree leaves—hence its name.

Poison sumac likes standing water; it grows in peat bogs in the North and in swampy areas in the South. It's a tall rangy shrub with cream-colored berries and anywhere from seven to 13 smooth-edged leaves.

The three species are common in North America and similar in their irritating effects. For the sake of convenience, in this chapter we will talk about poison ivy, but the discussion can apply equally to any of the three. In all three cases, the contact dermatitis we experience is a reaction to a chemical in the plants' sap called *urushiol*. If you've ever broken a poison ivy leaf or crushed a stem, you've seen urushiol; it's the oil, clear or slightly yellowish, that oozes from the plant. This sticky resin adheres to just about anything— animal fur, garden tools, lawn furniture, sports equipment, not to mention your shoes, clothing, and skin.

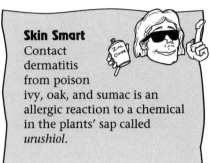

Skin Smart
Contact dermatitis from poison ivy, oak, and sumac is an allergic reaction to a chemical in the plants' sap called *urushiol*.

Recognizing the Symptoms

So potent is urushiol that it may remain viable for months, even in dead branches. It starts penetrating your skin the minute you touch it. The result is a raised, red, itchy rash that begins to appear within 12 to 48 hours after contact. Typically, the eruption has a linear streaky pattern that represents areas where the leaf or branches rubbed against the skin, but less distinctive red raised patches are common too.

Blistering is very common, and the itching can drive you crazy. New patches may appear for several days after first exposure. Sometimes these new patches are areas that received a smaller initial exposure or got a dose of urushiol secondarily by scratching. The urushiol can be spread from place to place on the body during the day of exposure or until it is washed off.

After a few days to a few weeks, the blisters become crusted and scaly. The dermatitis is most likely to hit areas with very heavy exposure or expanses of thin skin. Therefore, the eyes or genitals are often affected: Small amounts of urushiol on the hands can cause a reaction if the person rubs his or her eyes or goes to the bathroom. Thick skin, such as palms and soles, rarely develops poison ivy. Expect the rash to take two to three weeks to heal.

Urushiol does not continue to be active on the body for more than a day. Therefore, scratching days after first exposure doesn't spread it, although it can increase the risk of secondary infection or scarring. Remember that it can remain potent on inanimate objects for extended periods, however. If you put on the gloves and sweater you wore when first exposed without washing them first, you will re-expose yourself.

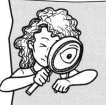

More Than Skin Deep

Droplets of urushiol can even be carried by wind and smoke. One of my patients decided to rid his yard of poison ivy by burning the vine, but paid with a red itchy facial rash that was particularly angry near the eyes. Moral of this story: Don't burn poison ivy. If you're sensitive to it, wear heavy gloves, protective clothing, and a dust mask whenever you handle it. Better still, hire someone else to clear all traces of it from your property.

We are not born allergic to poison ivy; we develop this sensitivity only after at least one run-in with the plant. Usually we encounter it as kids. The first exposure may "sensitize" us to the urushiol. That means our immune systems learn to recognize it as something we are allergic to. After that, watch out! Subsequent exposures will result in the delightful rash described above.

Interestingly, many people are more sensitive to poison ivy when they are kids and less vulnerable as they grow older. By the time we reach our 30s, researchers estimate most of us are only half as sensitive as we were. However, some people—approximately 25 to 40 million Americans—remain highly sensitive throughout their lives. If exposed at any age, they develop a terrible, itchy rash.

Never had poison ivy? You might be in the 10 to 15 percent of the U.S. population that's resistant to urushiol. However, as Joe can tell you, even if you manage to reach adulthood without an outbreak, you still have a good chance of developing the allergy if you have sufficient exposure.

Prevention: Your Best Treatment

The best way to treat poison ivy is simple: Don't get it in the first place. You can significantly reduce your risk by following a few common sense precautions:

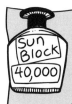

Saving Your Skin
If you've ever had a severe reaction to poison ivy, don't wait; call your doctor the minute you know you've been exposed again. He or she can prescribe corticosteroid drugs to moderate your inflammatory reaction.

➤ Learn to recognize poison ivy, oak, and sumac so you can give them a wide berth. In addition to recognizing the plants themselves, know the kind of territory they like so you can be on guard: wooded undergrowth and standing water. Don't let pets run wild because they could bring home urushiol on their fur.

➤ Eradicate poison ivy on your property with herbicides. Be sure to use them carefully, according to the manufacturer's instructions.

➤ If you must spend time in poison ivy–prone places, wear long pants, long sleeves, boots, and preferably gloves. Spring and summer are the real danger seasons because that's when the plants have the most sap with the highest urushiol content.

➤ If you think you've been exposed, be careful not to touch your face or other parts of your body until after you have washed carefully. Urushiol is almost invisible and easily spread.

➤ Wash all exposed areas with soap and water as soon as possible. You can easily spread urushiol from hands to other parts of the body on the first day of exposure until you have washed well. If possible, wash before going indoors so you don't bring urushiol in with you.

➤ Wash your clothing outdoors, with a garden hose, before going inside; then launder all clothing thoroughly. Otherwise, urushiol could rub off onto furniture and re-expose you later.

➤ While you're at it, also wash off all tools, toys, athletic equipment, lawn furniture, camping gear, and anything else that could be contaminated. Remember, urushiol stays potent for a lot longer on inanimate objects than it does on skin.

Don't Scratch!

Okay, suppose you follow all these precautions and you still develop poison ivy. What do you do now? Maddening as this dermatitis may be, it's rarely serious. Trust me, it will go away (although right now you might find that hard to believe). To help you keep your sanity, follow these tips:

➤ Don't scratch! I know, you really want to, but please don't. If you have germs under your fingernails you could infect your inflamed skin, and if you scratch vigorously, you could scar.

➤ Try a cool shower to soothe the itching, or a tepid bath filled with a solution of baking soda or oatmeal.

➤ That old standby, calamine lotion, is still helpful. This over-the-counter remedy can help a mild rash. Other over-the-counter itch remedies, many containing cooling menthol, may also help relieve your symptoms.

If the rash doesn't start improving within 10 days, or if it keeps getting worse, call your doctor.

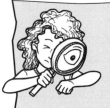

More Than Skin Deep

Immunization against poison ivy? Yes, there is such a thing. Researchers have developed a series of prescription-only pills containing graduated doses of urushiol to slowly desensitize you. The entire treatment can take up to four months before it's reasonably effective and it can have unpleasant side effects, so I recommend it only if your job or lifestyle requires constant exposure to the plant. Otherwise, it's much easier to just keep your distance.

Dodging Bites and Stings

My friend Marilyn rushed into my office with her eight-year-old son Adam. "What is this thing on his arm?" she asked, looking worried. "We tried to pull it off, but it won't budge."

Sticking to Adam's arm was a small, raised, shiny dark bump. "That's a tick," I said. "It's a good thing you didn't pull it off, because parts of it can stay in your skin and cause a reaction." "Yuck!" said Adam.

"Yuck" sums up the attitude many of us have toward ticks, chiggers, spiders, bees, and wasps. Nonetheless, their bites and stings are a reality, and it's important to learn how to recognize and treat the dangerous ones.

Ticks

Ticks are tiny eight-legged animals that attach themselves to human or animal skin to feed on blood. They're very small; most are only about one-eighth inch long or shorter, although they may swell after a generous meal.

You can pick up a tick from walking or reclining in tall grass, scrub, woods, or caves; sometimes pets bring them indoors. Once a tick gets on your skin, it bites and remains firmly attached until it has fed or you remove it. You may feel an itchy or irritated sensation when it first tries to dig in, or you might not notice it at all.

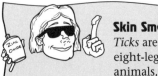

Skin Smart
Ticks are tiny eight-legged animals, only about one-eighth inch long, that attach themselves to human or animal skin to feed on blood.

While ticks aren't pleasant, the main danger comes not from the critters themselves, but from infections they can transmit via their bite. In the United States, ticks are known to spread Lyme disease, Rocky Mountain spotted fever, and tularemia. If you develop a skin eruption, fever, headache, muscle aches, or joint pain after a tick bite, call your doctor immediately.

Doctors think it takes several hours for a tick to transmit disease. This is why we recommend searching for ticks at the end of each day when you may have been exposed. (Remember to check your scalp too.)

If a tick is crawling on your skin, remove it immediately. Don't try to crush it between your fingers because the durable outer shell makes it hard to kill; drop it in a fire or flush it down the toilet. If the tick is already attached, don't pull it off! As I told Adam, this can leave pieces of its mouth in your skin—not a healthy thing.

Instead, cover the tick with a kitchen or machine oil. The oil film makes it hard for the animal to breathe, causing it to relax its jaws. When its grip loosens, remove it carefully with tweezers. Grasp the tick as closely as possible to its attachment to the skin, and pull with a slow continuous motion. After removing the tick, dispose of it as mentioned earlier, and then wash your hands and the bite area with soap.

If at all possible, you might want to have this done by a doctor who has some experience with ticks. Remember, if any portion of the animal is left under the skin, it will have to be removed by a physician who cuts it out in a minor surgical procedure. What's more, if an experienced physician removes the tick, he or she may be able to tell you if it's the type that is likely to transmit disease.

Chiggers

Chiggers are the larvae of harvest mites (also called red mites). Minute relatives of ticks, mites also have eight legs and enjoy feasting on human blood.

Summer residents of grass and weeds, chiggers are particularly common in southern states, though they range as far north as Canada. When you walk through a patch of tall brush, they attach to your skin and insert a tiny feeding tube down to a superficial blood vessel. After several hours the skin around the feeding tube starts to itch and develops a characteristic small red bump.

You're most likely to find chigger bumps on your ankles, in armpits and the crooks of elbows, and places where clothing is tight, such as the waistline and groin. If not dislodged, chiggers remain attached until they've enjoyed a full meal (anywhere from one to four days), then fall away. Sometimes you can see the tiny larvae themselves, usually in the center of bumps you haven't scratched yet, but generally people remove them unknowingly by scratching.

Unlike ticks, chigger bites aren't known to cause any diseases. However, the bumps are annoying because they can itch intensely, sometimes for several weeks. Try not to scratch, because this could infect the bite. Wash them with soap and water, and apply a soothing over-the-counter lotion. If the itching really bothers you, call your doctor. He or she can prescribe a topical corticosteroid cream or an antihistamine to use until you feel better.

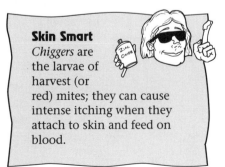

Skin Smart

Chiggers are the larvae of harvest (or red) mites; they can cause intense itching when they attach to skin and feed on blood.

Spiders

Most spiders produce venom. In fact, this is how they eat; they inject the poison through their fangs to paralyze and kill their prey. Since humans are bigger than the typical spider prey, most of the time their venom doesn't bother us. A typical spider bite registers only as a small red bump that itches for a few hours or days, and then disappears.

However, there are two spiders in the United States whose venom is potent enough to be a major health risk: the *black widow* and the *brown recluse*. Both spiders are most widespread in southern and southwestern states, although they can be found in much of North America and in other continents as well.

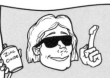

Skin Smart
Two poisonous spiders to watch out for are the *black widow* (a shiny black spider found in dark damp outdoor places) and the *brown recluse* (a brown or brownish-yellow spider that prefers dark dry environments, such as crevices in or around houses).

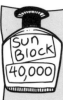

Saving Your Skin
Brown recluse spiders are fond of dark areas inside your house as well as outside. When rummaging through closets, boxes, or drawers that don't get opened often, be cautious. Shine a bright light on what you're doing, and wear gloves and protective clothing.

The black widow spider is shiny, black, and about one-half inch long, usually with an hourglass-shaped red mark on its stomach. Black widows like dark, damp outdoor environments, such as woodpiles, tree stumps, and outdoor toilets. (Every year, luckless campers get bitten on the buttocks or genitals while relieving themselves. Ouch!)

If a black widow bites you, you may feel only a pinprick, and maybe not even that. But the venom is a neurotoxin and within a few hours symptoms will appear. The bite can cause muscle spasms, stomach cramps, heavy sweating, nausea, vomiting, generalized pain, and difficulty breathing. If you experience any of these symptoms, get to a doctor as quickly as possible.

The brown recluse spider is brown or brownish-yellow, with a body about three-eighths of an inch long and long legs. The brown recluse also likes dark environments, but it prefers them dry; favorite hangouts are cracks and crevices in and around houses. Its bite is likely to be more painful than the black widow's, initially causing mild stinging followed by reddish swelling and intense pain within eight hours. A blister forms at the bite, and the skin in the area may die, becoming purple or black and then ulcerating.

While black widow and brown recluse bites are rarely fatal for healthy adults, they can be dangerous, especially for children and frail people. If you develop a worrisome reaction to any spider bite, call your doctor immediately. Some other tips:

➤ Try to identify what bit you. If that's not possible, describe to your doctor where you were and what you were doing when you think the bite occurred. This information will help your doctor identify and treat the bite.

➤ If the culprit was a black widow spider, your doctor may prescribe antivenin, a treatment to neutralize the venom. An injection of calcium gluconate can help muscle cramps.

➤ For brown recluse bites, ice packs and elevation may reduce swelling. Your doctor might give you antihistamines or, if symptoms are severe, corticosteroid injections.

Some spider bites, particularly from the brown recluse, heal slowly and may require surgical reconstruction to close properly. If a lot of tissue around the bite has died and ulcerated, a surgical debriding (scraping) can help the wound heal faster.

Bees and Wasps

Only a relatively few insects (bees, wasps, hornets, and yellow jackets among them) are capable of stinging us. Their venom contains inflammatory chemicals that cause painful red swellings at the site for perhaps two days. Seen any horror movies about people being killed by bees? The fact is that most healthy adults would have to be stung by hundreds of bees for the venom to be fatal.

Unless they're allergic, that is. Roughly 1 percent of North Americans are allergic to bee or wasp venom, and for them a simple bee-sting can be a life-threatening emergency.

As with all insect bites, prevention is the best form of treatment. During the spring and summer, be cautious when walking through woods and working outdoors. Bees and their stinging relatives get very upset if you prune, shake, or otherwise appear to threaten their home. You may not even see the hive or nest until it's too late. Some hornets nest in the ground, so be careful when walking or mowing in tall grass.

Saving Your Skin
Bees won't sting unless provoked. Unfortunately, what looks like provocation to them could look like a simple yard chore to you. When working outside, I recommend leaving the closest door unlocked so you always have an escape route.

People who are extremely allergic to insect venom experience a severe reaction called *anaphylaxis (anaphylactic shock)* after being bitten or stung. Symptoms of anaphylaxis include warm skin, redness or hives, wheezing and difficulty breathing, muscle cramps, and fainting. Call an ambulance immediately or rush the person to an emergency room, because anaphylaxis can be rapidly fatal. Patients who know they have this reaction should carry an emergency kit with them which contains a self-injecting hypodermic syringe filled with epinephrine. Use it immediately while awaiting medical care.

If the stinger is still in the skin, removing it is a good idea. This must be done properly because the embedded stinger can squeeze more venom into the wound. The stinger should be scraped away. A doctor may do this with a sterile scalpel blade. In an emergency, try scraping the stinger away with a credit card. Do not grasp the stinger to pull it

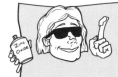

Skin Smart

Anaphylaxis (anaphylactic shock) is a severe allergic reaction. Symptoms of anaphylaxis include warm skin, redness or hives, wheezing and difficulty breathing, muscle cramps, and fainting.

out because that will cause the release of more venom from the sacs. Apply ice or a cold wet cloth to the site. If the person stops breathing, perform mouth-to-mouth resuscitation.

If you've been stung by a bee or wasp, here are some guidelines to follow:

> ➤ Is the stinger still in your skin? Try to scrape it away if you can. Don't use tweezers because the stinger may be attached to a poison sac, and you could accidentally squeeze more venom into the wound.

➤ If you cannot remove the stinger I would suggest you ask a trained professional such as an emergency room nurse or doctor to remove it.

➤ Wash the area thoroughly with soap. An ice pack will help keep swelling down.

➤ Over-the-counter hydrocortisone creams or calamine lotion can soothe itching and inflammation.

If the sting doesn't feel better within 24 hours, or if it gets worse, call your doctor. Describe the insect if you can. Your doctor will give you painkillers and other medications to forestall complications. Antibiotics may be needed if the area has become infected.

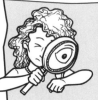

More Than Skin Deep

If you know you have anaphylactic reactions, keep an emergency kit on hand to prevent severe episodes. These kits are available by prescription and contain a self-injecting hypodermic syringe filled with epinephrine, a drug that increases the speed and force of the heartbeat. Epinephrine can cause all sorts of side effects, such as heart palpitations, anxiety, and even chest pain. But in the life-threatening situation of anaphylaxis, these kits can save lives if the epinephrine is administered properly and promptly. This is something to discuss with your doctor.

The Least You Need to Know

> ➤ The rash we call "poison ivy" is a contact dermatitis triggered by the sap of three closely related plants: poison ivy, poison oak, and poison sumac. Even dry branches contain enough sap to cause a rash.

➤ Your best bet is to prevent poison ivy in the first place. Wear protective clothing and promptly wash off your skin, clothes, and everything else that could have gotten sap on it. If you get a rash, don't scratch. Use calamine lotion and soothe itching with oatmeal or baking soda baths.

➤ If a tick digs in, don't pull it off; part of its mouth could remain in your skin. Instead, consult your doctor for help with removing it. If you can't reach your doctor, coat the tick with oil, grasp it with tweezers close to the attachment point, and pull with a smooth continuous motion. Afterward, wash the area with soap.

➤ Ice packs and over-the-counter medications effectively treat most bites and stings. Bites from two spiders, the black widow and brown recluse, can be especially serious and require medical attention. If you are severely allergic to bees, always keep an emergency kit on hand.

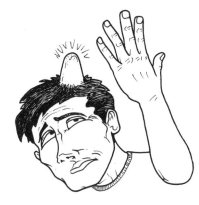

Chapter 18

Benign Bumps

In This Chapter

➤ Learn which skin growths are dangerous, and which aren't

➤ Find out what a "normal" mole looks like

➤ Discover two types of moles more likely to turn cancerous

➤ Learn to recognize hemangiomas

➤ Find out how to get rid of port wine stains and other birthmarks

---

Agnes looked both uncomfortable and worried, not a fun combination. "This may all be about nothing, and I feel silly even bringing it up," she said haltingly. "It's just you read so much about skin cancer in all the magazines. I know I've spent a lot of time in the sun in my day—really more than I should, but I love being outdoors so much! Now I'm worried it may have caught up with me."

"You see," she continued, "I have this mole and I worry that it could be cancer . . ." Her voice trailed off.

"Has it changed in any way?" I asked. "Not really," she answered. "It's just so large and dark. Also, it's right on my leg where I hit it when I'm shaving. A couple of times I've even made it bleed. Is that dangerous?"

Those Marks Called Moles

Like Agnes, many of my patients worry about various growths on their skin. Often these marks are *moles*, benign (noncancerous) skin growths that are collections of pigment cells. (The medical term for a mole is *nevus*, plural *nevi*.) Moles are extremely common. Nearly all of us have at least one, and some people may have as many as 40 or more.

> **Skin Smart**
>
> *Moles* are noncancerous (benign) skin growths that are collections of pigment cells. The medical term for a mole is *nevus* (plural *nevi*).

What do normal moles look like? They run the gamut. Let me set the record straight: There is no such thing as an "ideal" mole. Healthy moles can be flesh-colored, brown, pink, tan, or even bluish. (More than one of these colors in a mole may be a sign of trouble, however. See Chapter 19, "Skin Cancer: The Dark Side of the Sun.") They may be tiny, large, or anywhere in between, raised or flat, single or clustered. Some contain hairs, others don't.

Where Do These Things Come From?

Some moles you're born with, and others show up after birth, usually before age 20. Researchers think their number and distribution are largely determined genetically, regardless of when they first appear. Hormones may also play a role since new marks frequently appear during adolescence and pregnancy.

Did you know that even normal moles can grow and change? Most start out flat and brown, like a freckle. They tend to have a homogeneous brown color and a regular, symmetrical, oval, or round border. In time, through a perfectly normal maturation process, some moles become raised. They still have a regular border, but they now are dome-shaped. At first they stay brown, but in time, they may fade to skin color.

How do you know which changes in a mole are okay and which are dangerous? This is not an easy question to answer, and I want to emphasize that if you have the slightest suspicion about a mole, please ask your dermatologist to examine it. I would rather check on benign moles all day long than let a dangerous mark go without treatment because it wasn't brought to my attention.

One good rule of thumb: Generally, benign moles are symmetrical. If you drew an imaginary line down their middle, one-half would look very much like the other half. They also tend to have a uniform color. If there is a mottling of color, it will probably be symmetrically distributed. Lastly, they tend to be approximately the size of a pencil eraser or smaller. Many larger moles are benign, but these larger moles should be checked by a dermatologist.

What if you have a mole that is not perfectly symmetrical, or that has an irregular border or color distribution? Don't panic. Nature is not perfect, and your mole may be totally benign. However, do have it checked by your dermatologist.

Another thing to look for: Change. Yes, even healthy moles change, as mentioned before. But we're talking a very slow pace; the life cycle of the average mole is about 50 years. If you can see your mole change over a period of weeks or months, or even a year, please get to the doctor quickly.

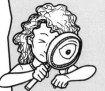

More Than Skin Deep

Don't like your moles? Today, many people don't, but they haven't always been viewed as blemishes. In eighteenth-century Europe, they were thought to enhance one's appearance. A fashionable lady would apply artificial moles or small dots of dark makeup to her face and décolletage. Some of these marks were intended to look like the real thing, but others were frankly fake, with shapes like stars and flowers. The modern term "beauty mark" is a holdover from this fad of two centuries ago.

When Should You Worry About Moles?

One question I'm asked frequently is whether moles can become cancerous. Yes, a few can, although certain kinds are more likely to do so than others. Researchers have identified two types of moles that seem more likely to develop into a serious skin cancer called *melanoma*:

➤ *Congenital nevi*, moles that are present at birth or develop during the first year. Roughly 1 percent of the population is born with congenital nevi. In adults, marks larger than 20 square centimeters seem to be especially risky (that's four centimeters by five centimeters, which is equivalent to one and a half by two inches, roughly the size of a matchbook).

   If you have one of these moles, please have it evaluated by your dermatologist. If your child has any moles that appeared during the first year of life, please have them evaluated—even if they are small. The dimensions stated here are for adults.

➤ *Atypical* (*dysplastic*) *nevi*, so-called because they tend to be irregularly shaped and larger than the typical mole (which usually means bigger than a pencil eraser).

   They may also have more than one color, although the color configuration tends to be symmetrical. Often they are darker in the center and lighter at the periphery, in the "fried-egg pattern."

This doesn't mean that if you have congenital or atypical moles, you're doomed to get cancer. Most of them never cause trouble. However, if you do have any congenital or atypical nevi, please have them evaluated by your dermatologist.

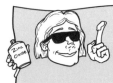

Skin Smart
Two types of moles that are more likely to become cancerous are *congenital nevi*, which are present at birth or shortly after, and *atypical (dysplastic) nevi*, which tend to be irregularly shaped and larger than average.

Be aware that, while congenital and atypical nevi seem to be higher-risk, any mole has the potential to become malignant. What turns moles cancerous? We don't know all the answers, but certainly sun exposure plays a major role. People who patronize tanning salons regularly or who suffer severe blistering sunburns, especially in childhood, have a higher risk of melanoma. Also, in rare cases, there appears to be a genetic tendency toward increased risk for melanoma. If one or more first-degree relatives have melanoma, get into the habit of examining your skin, and have a dermatologist look at your moles regularly.

In short, it's important to keep an eye on all moles. I recommend monthly self-examinations. Start from the top of your body and work your way down, using mirrors when necessary to see your back. (For more guidelines on a fast, easy way to screen your skin, see Chapter 19, "Skin Cancer: The Dark Side of the Sun.")

What should you look for? In a word, change. Not the gradual, 50-year evolution of a normal mole, but changes that occur over a span of weeks to months to a few years.

Pay attention if a mole:

➤ Grows larger

➤ Develops variations in color

➤ Starts bleeding

➤ Develops an irregular or notched border

➤ First appears after age 25

In short, if any mole doesn't look quite like its old self, in any way, call it to your doctor's attention. He or she can remove it to be examined under a microscope. If the growth contains any unusual-looking cells, more skin may be removed to get rid of all abnormal cells (see the following "Getting Rid of Moles"). Skin cancer has a very high cure rate if caught early, so removing the mole will probably take care of it. If the mole shows signs that it has not been caught early (these clues are generally visible with the microscope), your doctor will explain other treatments that can help. (For more specifics on how to recognize warning signs of skin cancer, see Chapter 19.)

Saving Your Skin
Incidentally, skin cancer doesn't have to develop from a mole; it can arise from previously normal, unmarked skin. Any new marks that appear in adulthood should be viewed with caution. Certainly most will not be cancer, but please, have them checked anyway. It's much better to be safe!

So please, if you're puzzled about any skin growths, go ahead and ask. Don't feel self-conscious. As a doctor, I love it when patients take an active interest in their own health care, and feel comfortable enough with me to ask questions and air their concerns. When it comes to your health, there's no such thing as a silly question!

Getting Rid of Moles

Fortunately I was able to reassure Agnes about her mole, which despite its size and color was a perfectly normal benign growth. Like her, many people worry that shaving over a mole or making it bleed could turn it into skin cancer. While I certainly don't recommend making any part of your skin bleed, occasionally irritating a mole will not make it become cancerous. (As you will see in Chapter 19, growths that repeatedly bleed with very minor trauma, or areas that do not heal, may represent a different kind of skin cancer.)

If a mole isn't changing and it doesn't bother you, there's probably no reason to bother it. However, you don't have to put up with a mole you don't like, since most can easily be removed. Usually, this procedure is done in the doctor's office by shaving away the mole, or by excising it and repairing the skin with small stitches.

If a mole contains hairs that annoy you, shave them gently away or clip them close to the skin surface. Another option is removing the hair permanently, perhaps with electrolysis. Be sure to have the mole evaluated and okayed by your dermatologist before you undergo the procedure. (For more on electrolysis and other methods of hair removal, see Chapter 7, "Beautiful Hair and Nails.")

Saving Your Skin
Moles that have been shaved away occasionally recur because some of the mole remained below the skin surface. However, if any mole that's been removed seems to be growing back, consult your doctor.

Seborrheic Keratoses

Seborrheic keratoses are benign growths that are extremely common in middle-aged and older people. Like moles, they are tan to dark brown in color, but unlike moles, they have a greasy or crusty surface. Sometimes they look as if you can almost peel them off. In fact, sometimes they do peel off! This is not a dangerous event, but it has scared many of my patients.

Seborrheic keratoses are benign, so they don't have to be removed. However, because they may have irregular borders and can grow quite large, I am often asked to look at them. As I've said before, if you are unsure about any mark or growth, please have your dermatologist examine it.

Skin Smart
Seborrheic keratoses are benign growths, common in people middle-aged and older. Like moles, they're tan to dark brown in color, but unlike moles, their surface may feel greasy or crusty.

Although they're harmless, many people want seborrheic keratoses removed. Some find the growths unsightly; others complain they get irritated from rubbing on waistbands or bras. Getting rid of seborrheic keratoses involves a simple office procedure. Your doctor can burn, freeze, or scrape them away.

Skin Tags

Another benign bump that worries some patients is a *skin tag*, a small growth that protrudes from your skin on a narrow stalk. (Your doctor may refer to it as an *acrochordon*.) Skin tags are soft and usually flesh-colored, although sometimes darker than surrounding skin.

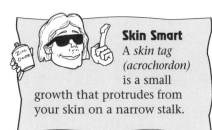

Skin Smart
A *skin tag* (acrochordon) is a small growth that protrudes from your skin on a narrow stalk.

Skin tags are common, and get even more so as we get older. Unlike moles, they often appear after age 30; while they may be a cosmetic concern, they don't appear to pose a health risk. Doctors aren't sure why they develop, but they are not cancerous.

It's not necessary to have skin tags removed; however, like moles, if they bother you, that's reason enough. Your doctor can easily remove them in the office, by burning them off with electrosurgery or snipping them with a fine scissors.

Vascular Lesions "Birthmarks"

Sometimes patients ask me to evaluate various kinds of birthmarks—reddish or purple areas of skin that are made of blood vessels. Where do these marks come from? We're not sure. Most aren't inherited, nor do they seem to be related to the mother's health or anything that happens during pregnancy.

Should you be concerned about birthmarks? In most cases, no. However, occasionally certain types can become a health risk, so it's important to have your doctor check them out. Some of my patients choose to have birthmarks removed, even when harmless, simply because they're tired of looking at them.

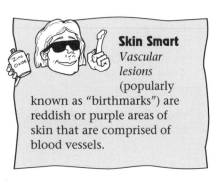

Skin Smart
Vascular lesions (popularly known as "birthmarks") are reddish or purple areas of skin that are comprised of blood vessels.

By the way, doctors do not use the term "birthmark." Medically speaking, it's imprecise: while some "birthmarks" are indeed visible at birth, others don't appear until later in life. Also, it's vague, since it could include any mark you're born with, such as congenital nevi and freckles. Since these purple and red discolorations involve blood vessels, doctors prefer to call them *vascular lesions*. ("Lesion" is a general medical term for any type of unusual localized development in skin tissues.) So next, let's take a look at three common kinds of vascular lesions: capillary hemangiomas, cavernous hemangiomas, and port wine stains.

Capillary (Strawberry) Hemangiomas

A *hemangioma* is a reddish-purple collection of blood vessels in the skin. Doctors distinguish between two types:

➤ *Capillary hemangiomas* (also called *strawberry hemangiomas*), which are raised and bright red because the blood vessels are small and are just underneath the skin surface.

➤ *Cavernous hemangiomas*, which are purplish-blue and often spongy because the blood vessels are larger and are located deeper beneath the skin.

Capillary hemangiomas usually appear by the time a baby is six weeks old. Generally, a child has only one, but some babies have two or three. If many are noted, your doctor will check to be sure there is blood vessel problem in the baby's internal organs.

Often capillary hemangiomas start growing during infancy and continue to expand for roughly a year. Generally they stay under two or three inches in diameter, although some may grow larger. Capillary hemangiomas are unpredictable; it's impossible to foretell at birth how large one will become or whether it will be one of the relatively few that outlast childhood. By age one or two, most stop growing, begin to turn pale, and slowly start to shrink. By age five, 50 percent are flat; by the time the child reaches age 10, 90 percent have flattened. Ultimately most fade, possibly leaving a faint pink or irregularly textured reminder of their presence.

> **Skin Smart**
>
> A *hemangioma* is a reddish-purple collection of blood vessels in the skin. There are two types: *capillary* (*strawberry*) *hemangiomas*, which are raised and bright red, and *cavernous hemangiomas*, which are purplish-blue and often spongy because the blood vessels are larger and are located deeper under the skin.

If your child has a hemangioma that grows, is this a problem? Sometimes. Call your doctor if you notice any of the following:

➤ **Sores or skin ulcers:** Sometimes hemangiomas that grow quickly may ulcerate and leave a painful sore that can become infected. Dressings and antibiotic creams can help.

➤ **Extremely rapid growth:** In rare cases, a hemangioma may grow so fast that it changes within one or two days. This could be the beginning of a dangerous but treatable situation. Call your doctor immediately.

➤ **Bruising:** If a bruise develops around the hemangioma, either slowly or rapidly, it deserves attention.

➤ **Persistent bleeding:** Capillary hemangiomas look like they could bleed if you just look at them, but really they shouldn't be much more delicate than any other area of your skin. If you accidentally nick or scrape one, you should expect to bleed; this is normal. But if the bleeding doesn't stop within five to 10 minutes, or if it recurs, this may be a concern.

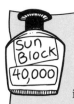

Saving Your Skin
If a hemangioma starts to bleed, treat it like any other skin injury: wash it with soap and water, and apply a bandage if necessary. Press firmly against the area for 10 minutes. If the bleeding doesn't stop, call your doctor.

➤ **Obstruction of vision or a vital organ:** If an enlarging capillary hemangioma begins to obstruct a child's field of vision or a vital organ, such as the airway, please call your doctor immediately.

Most capillary hemangiomas require no treatment, and they tend to leave the best cosmetic result if allowed to shrink on their own. However, if one starts to grow too rapidly, your doctor may recommend corticosteroid drugs, either injected or taken orally. Sometimes it's necessary to take corticosteroids for a long time, or to repeat the treatment if the hemangioma starts expanding again. Sometimes interferon is used in this situation. In cases where the hemangioma is obstructing vision or an airway, you doctor might recommend treatment by laser, excision, or other means.

Cavernous Hemangiomas

Cavernous hemangiomas, the second type of hemangioma, appear during infancy. Unlike their capillary cousins, they have a purplish-blue color and a spongy consistency, and they don't change in size appreciably. They may be large or small, but they tend to remain approximately the same size for life.

Usually, cavernous hemangiomas are nothing to worry about, except that they may bleed freely if injured. However, occasionally they could indicate an underlying health problem. For this reason, I recommend having all cavernous hemangiomas checked by a doctor.

Port Wine Stains

A *port wine stain* is a flat pink or purple discoloration in the skin, found most often on the face, neck, or extremities. Appearing at birth, port wine stains can be any size.

One type of port wine stain, usually seen on the back of the neck or scalp, commonly called a "stork bite," has a tendency to fade over the years, although sometimes it does persist. However, it's harmless and requires no treatment. Other port wine stains stay with you throughout your lifetime. Over time, their texture may change slightly, as they thicken and become more bumpy.

Skin Smart
A *port wine stain* is a flat pink or purple discoloration in the skin, found most often on the face, neck, or extremities.

Usually port wine stains are more of a cosmetic concern than a health risk. However, some people with facial port wine stains (especially on the forehead and eyelids) may have deeper vascular problems that could affect the brain, leading to seizures, and the eyes, possibly leading to glaucoma.

Occasionally, port wine stains on the arm or leg can also indicate deeper vascular problems, and the tissues surrounding these vessels may grow a little faster and larger than normal.

Needless to say, these situations need to be followed up by your doctor. Children with stains on the arms and legs should be monitored for growth problems. Children and adults with facial port wine stains should undergo complete physical exams and eye exams at least once a year.

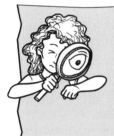

More Than Skin Deep

In glaucoma, pressure inside the eyeball increases and damages the optic nerve. If not treated, it gradually restricts peripheral vision and eventually causes blindness. Glaucoma has no symptoms, and many people don't realize they have it until they've already lost some vision. However, medications are available to control it and save your sight.

Laser treatments are available to remove port wine stains. These are outpatient procedures, usually done in a series of treatments one to two months apart. Begin laser therapy as soon as possible, preferably in infancy; the younger you start, the better it works.

Laser treatments are generally effective. At least 70 percent of patients notice a visible improvement, and in 25 percent of cases, the treatments remove the stain completely. Occasionally, they can leave tan or white patches on the skin, but this result is usually minimal compared to the original port wine stain.

Cherry Angiomas: Cherry Red and Harmless

A *cherry angioma* is a small, smooth, benign, cherry-red bump. It is a harmless growth that appears most often after age 40, and can vary in size from a pinhead to a quarter-inch. Cherry angiomas are most common on the torso but can show up anywhere on the body.

If a cherry angioma doesn't bother you, there's no health-related reason to have it removed. However, if you want to get rid of it for cosmetic purposes, your doctor can easily burn it off with electrosurgery, a minor in-office procedure.

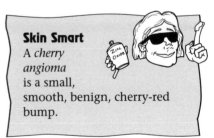

Skin Smart
A *cherry angioma* is a small, smooth, benign, cherry-red bump.

The Least You Need to Know

➤ Moles come in a wide variety of sizes and shapes. The vast majority are not cancerous and never will be. But if your mole is irregular or changing, please have it checked by a dermatologist. It is always best to be cautious with moles.

➤ Skin tags are small growths that protrude from your skin on a narrow stalk. Cherry angiomas are small, smooth, cherry-red bumps. Both are harmless and more common after age 40. If you want to remove them for cosmetic reasons, your doctor can easily burn them off.

➤ Hemangiomas are reddish-purple collections of blood vessels. Capillary (strawberry) hemangiomas appear in infancy, grow for about a year, and then begin to shrink. Call your doctor if a capillary hemangioma grows rapidly, bleeds repeatedly, or ulcerates. Cavernous hemangiomas tend to stay the same size. They are sometimes associated with underlying health problems, so check with your doctor.

➤ While generally more of a cosmetic concern, some port wine stains carry a risk of underlying problems that can lead to seizures, glaucoma, or tissue enlargement. Laser treatments are the best treatment for port wine stains, and in most cases can remove or fade them.

➤ Remember, when it comes to your health, there's no such thing as a silly question. If you are concerned about anything on your skin, go ahead and ask your doctor. The key is to watch for any change in a mole or other skin growth.

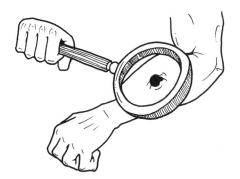

Chapter 19

Skin Cancer: The Dark Side of the Sun

In This Chapter

➤ Find out who's at risk for skin cancer

➤ Learn to screen your skin—it's fast, painless, and free

➤ Discover how to recognize precancerous and cancerous growths

➤ Learn to identify melanoma, the deadliest skin cancer

➤ Assess your options for getting rid of cancer

Joanna hadn't come to my office to consult me; she stopped by merely to say hello and pick up a prescription for her daughter. As we shook hands, though, I noticed a mark on her cheek.

"Excuse me," I said, "but I think you should have that looked at." "What, this?" she asked, fingering the pinkish, scaly patch of skin. "But it's just a rash of some kind, isn't it? Although come to think of it, it's been there for a long time. I keep rubbing moisturizer on it but it hasn't gone away."

"I'm not trying to scare you, but it could be precancerous," I told her. "The safest course of action would be to remove it."

Skin Cancer: The Unofficial Epidemic

Suppose you're a researcher who learns of a certain health condition. Every year an estimated one million Americans develop it, making it the most common form of cancer in the United States. In fact, it accounts for half of all new cancer cases diagnosed each year. Left untreated, some types can kill.

Wouldn't you call that an epidemic? While skin cancer hasn't been declared an official epidemic, it certainly sounds like one.

Skin cancer, a malignant tumor in the skin, can take several forms. The bad news, as you've seen, is that it's very common. But here's the good news: It's also very curable. Cure rates run as high as 95 percent when it's caught at an early stage, and even recurrences of most skin cancers are treatable. Another plus: By its nature, skin cancer is easy to detect and treat in these early stages, before it has time to progress and become serious.

The term *skin cancer* actually includes several types of cancers. In this chapter, I'll discuss the three most common: basal cell, squamous cell, and malignant melanoma. I'll explain how to recognize each one and how to identify precancerous signs that could signal impending trouble.

Many people are terrified by the prospect of cancer and hesitate to bring up their fears with their doctor. Don't be! Skin cancer is usually easy to treat, and we'll finish the chapter by looking at how you can get rid of it.

Skin Smart

Skin cancer, a malignant tumor in the skin, has cure rates as high as 95 percent when caught at an early stage. Even recurrences of most skin cancers are treatable.

Who's at Risk?

Lifestyle is the villain behind most cases of skin cancer: in particular, exposure to sunlight. As you saw in Chapter 10, "The Sun Is No Fun," ultraviolet (UV) rays cause an almost immediate inflammatory response in your skin. As exposure continues, the rays damage the DNA in skin cells.

After skin cells endure this abuse many times over a period of several years, they may go haywire. Abnormal cells develop and proliferate, leading to the growths we call cancer.

Who's at risk for skin cancer? All of us, as we get older. UV damage is cumulative, and by the time we reach our middle years many of us have sustained a lot of it. Certain factors do increase your vulnerability, however, including the following:

➤ **History of sunlight exposure:** People who spend a lot of time outdoors, whether working or playing, are more likely to get basal cell or squamous cell skin cancer. A history of numerous sunburns, especially blistering sunburns, is especially dangerous for the development of melanoma.

➤ **Fair skin:** Skin cancer is far more common in Caucasians (whose pale skins produce less protective melanin) than in Asians or African Americans. Even among Caucasians, risk varies with skin tone; fair-complexioned blondes and redheads are twice as likely to develop malignancies as brunettes with olive complexions. (This doesn't mean dark-skinned people don't get skin cancer; they can and do. It just means that you should be especially careful if you're pale.)

➤ **Where you live:** People in southern parts of the United States have higher rates of skin tumors than their northern neighbors because the sunlight is more intense.

Other factors are less influential than UV damage but can increase your risk:

➤ **Suppressed immunity:** People whose immune systems have been impaired in certain ways seem to be less able to fight off malignancies. This includes organ transplant recipients and some survivors of other types of cancer who have undergone radiation or chemotherapy.

➤ **Repeated exposure to X-rays:** I see this most commonly in people who underwent X-ray treatments for acne in the past.

➤ **Occupational exposure to certain chemicals, such as coal and arsenic:** Coal is used commercially as a fuel and in the production of other industrial products like coal-tar and coke. Inorganic arsenics were used in medical treatments before 1970 and are still found in some herbicides.

➤ **Scarring from diseases or severe burns:** Chronic scarring of the skin may in rare cases disrupt normal cell growth and lead to the development of skin cancer.

➤ **History of skin cancer:** If you've already had a skin tumor, you might have an increased risk for the development of new skin cancers.

As with many health conditions, family history plays a role. If your parents, siblings, or children develop skin cancer, you might, too.

Screening Your Skin

Fortunately, skin cancer is an easy disease to find. The American Academy of Dermatology recommends screening yourself regularly for the warning signs—monthly is ideal. It's easy, painless, and absolutely free!

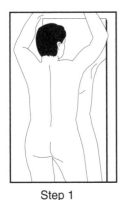
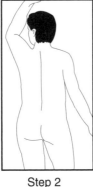
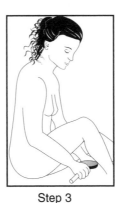
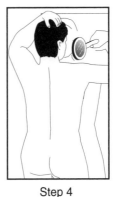
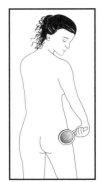

| Step 1 | Step 2 | Step 3 | Step 4 | Step 5 |

The American Academy of Dermatology recommends this five-step screening process for skin cancer. It's easy, painless, and absolutely free.

Here is a quick five-step process you can do in the privacy of your own home. All you need is a full-length mirror, a hand mirror, and a well-lit room.

1. First, raise your arms and examine your body in the mirror—front and back, right and left sides. Include your underarms.

2. Next, bend your elbows and examine your forearms, hands, and upper arms.

3. Look at the front and back of your legs and feet. Sit down and examine the soles of your feet and the spaces between your toes.

4. Using the hand mirror, examine your scalp and the back of your neck. Part and lift your hair for a closer look.

5. Finally, use the hand mirror to check your back and buttocks.

If you develop another routine you like better, great. What's important is to perform your screening exam once each month and check *all skin surfaces*. Become friends with your skin; get to know your individual pattern of moles, freckles, skin tags, and so forth.

Many of my patients ask what they should look for when examining their skin. To recap my remarks in the previous chapter: Change. If you notice any changes of any kind, anywhere on your skin, call your doctor promptly! By screening your skin on a regular basis, you will be able to recognize new developments early. As you will see, most skin cancers (although not all) develop in areas that have endured heavy sun exposure. Pay particular attention to any part of you that's gotten a lot of sun through the years.

Precancerous Growths to Watch For

One particular precancerous development to watch for: *actinic keratoses*, small scaly spots most commonly found on skin that's had a lot of sun exposure, like your face and the backs of your hands. Their color may range from gray to pink, and they have a sandpaper-like roughness that sometimes you can feel more than see.

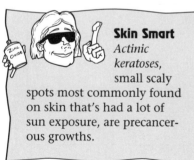

Skin Smart
Actinic keratoses, small scaly spots most commonly found on skin that's had a lot of sun exposure, are precancerous growths.

Many actinic keratoses don't develop further; in fact, as many as 40 percent may regress without any treatment. In time, some do degenerate into the squamous cell type of cancer, but removing them early stops them in their tracks.

These are the marks I noticed on Joanna's face. She immediately made an appointment for later that week, and I removed the suspicious lesions. I also reminded her to protect herself from the sun. Today her skin is clear, with no signs of precancerous or cancerous changes.

Basal Cell Cancer

The most common form of skin cancer is *basal cell cancer*, usually a bump or nodule that is pink or skin-colored, often round, with a "pearly" smooth texture. It may crust and bleed spontaneously or with minor trauma. Basal cell cancer usually shows up on sun-exposed areas like the head and neck, less often on the trunk. The over-whelming majority appear in Caucasians, especially blondes or redheads with fair skin and light-colored eyes.

Basal cell growths develop very slowly; it might take years for one to grow as wide as one-half inch. Periodi-cally, it may bleed and crust over, from minor trauma or for no apparent reason. Basal cell tumors almost never *metastasize* (spread to other parts of the body), but remain localized where they originally appeared. However, that doesn't mean you should ignore them. Eventually, if left untreated, they can grow into the tissues underneath your skin and spread to bone or other structures.

These growths respond well to treatment. Cure rates are at least 95 percent, and recurrences can almost always be treated too.

Squamous Cell Cancer

The second most common type of skin cancer is *squamous cell cancer*, red nodules or raised pink scaly patches typically found on the ears, face, and hands. Sometimes they ulcerate and crust.

When actinic keratoses turn cancerous, they develop into squamous cell tumors. If you have a history of actinic keratoses, keep an eye on them.

Unlike basal cell cancers, untreated squamous cell tumors can eventually spread to other tissues such as lymph nodes or internal organs. Every year about 2,000 people die from them. The key is early detection; when caught early, the cure rate is more than 95 percent. Most recurrences are curable, too.

Melanoma: The Deadliest Skin Cancer

Melanoma, the most dangerous form of skin cancer, can be deadly if not caught and removed promptly.

Skin Smart
The most common form of skin cancer is *basal cell cancer*, a pink or skin-colored bump or nodule that often has a "pearly" smooth surface. It usually appears on sun-exposed areas, such as the head and neck, and, less often, on the trunk.

Skin Smart
The second most common type of skin cancer is *squamous cell cancer*, red nodules or raised pink scaly patches, typically found on the ears, face, and hands, that may ulcerate and crust.

Saving Your Skin
It's never too late to start protecting yourself from the sun and wearing sunscreen. Even if you've already had a brush with skin cancer, wearing sunscreen every day, summer and winter, and avoiding too much sun exposure can help prevent recurrences.

Melanoma begins in the melanocytes, skin cells that produce the protective pigment melanin. Yes, melanoma may start in or near a mole, a tendency that appears to run in some families. If a mole enlarges, changes color, becomes irregular in its border or contour, or starts to itch or bleed spontaneously, call your doctor.

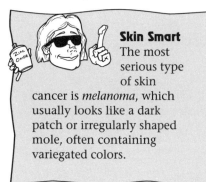

Skin Smart
The most serious type of skin cancer is *melanoma*, which usually looks like a dark patch or irregularly shaped mole, often containing variegated colors.

But be aware that melanoma doesn't have to grow from a mole; it can also seem to appear from nowhere. Since the melanocytes usually continue to make pigment, melanoma tumors frequently look like dark patches or enlarging moles and often contain variegated colors.

If you've already had one bout with melanoma, you have a nine-times-greater risk of developing it again. Another risk factor is excessive sun exposure and, in particular, a history of severe blistering burns before age 15.

Here are the warning signs of melanoma. Doctors refer to them as melanoma's "ABCDs":

➤ Asymmetry: One half of the lesion doesn't look like the other.

➤ Border is irregular: The outline is notched, uneven, scalloped, or poorly defined.

➤ Color is varied: Melanoma tumors are often dark and usually contain mixed shades of tan, brown, black, even blue, red, or white.

➤ Diameter is larger than six millimeters (roughly the size of a pencil eraser): The larger the tumor, the more dangerous it may be. However, if even a small growth shows any of these characteristics, bring it to your doctor's attention immediately.

Watch for the ABCDs of melanoma, the deadliest form of skin cancer: Asymmetry, Border irregularity, Color variety, and Diameter larger than a pencil eraser.

Melanoma is far more aggressive than basal and squamous cell cancers, and unfortunately, its rate of occurrence is increasing and has been for many years. Its incidence has doubled in the United States over the past 20 years, perhaps because people are spending more time outdoors (although other unknown factors may also play a role). On a more positive note, this skin cancer can usually be caught early, when it is curable, if people check their moles regularly and report any changes to the dermatologist immediately.

Some of my patients with congenital or atypical moles ask whether they should have them removed, before they can turn malignant. Doctors are divided on this issue. The decision on congenital moles generally depends on their size and location, so discuss this issue with your doctor. Atypical moles can be present in large numbers (some people have a hundred or more), so preventive removal could be expensive and leave scars. If the moles don't change or cause problems, it's probably not necessary to get rid of them all, but do monitor them for any suspicious developments. If the moles do change, they must be evaluated by a dermatologist promptly.

Incidentally, while melanoma (like all skin cancers) is more common in Caucasians, dark-skinned people are not immune. I've seen it in patients of all races. In African Americans, many reports suggest that the most frequent sites for melanoma are the palms of the hands, soles of the feet, under the nails, and on the mucous membranes, such as the mouth.

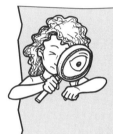

More Than Skin Deep

If you have many atypical moles, you might want to have medical photographs taken of them to help you and your dermatologist determine if any are changing. If a mole is in an awkward spot that tends to rub on clothing, interfere with shaving, or otherwise get in your way, consider having it removed.

Treating Skin Cancer

I've said it before, but it's worth repeating: If you are concerned about any mark or change in your skin, tell your doctor. This is not a time to be timid. Many skin cancers are first discovered by friends, relatives, or the patients themselves. When in doubt, go ahead and ask; it's definitely better to err on the side of caution, and the sooner you have suspicious growths removed, the better. Skin cancers are the easiest of all malignancies to treat, so by all means put medical science to work for you.

Treatment of any skin cancer depends on its type, the size of the tumor, its location, and the depth to which it has penetrated the skin. For melanoma in particular, there is a direct correlation between the thickness of the tumor and the survival rate of the patient.

The first step is to remove the growth or a sample of tissue from it, and examine it under a microscope for the presence of unusual cells. Doctors classify cancerous cells into various categories depending on their type and how aggressively they spread. If there's any chance the growth has metastasized, you may have other tests done, including x-rays, sampling tissue from nearby lymph nodes, or blood tests.

If your doctor decides to remove the growth, treatment options depend on the type of cancer or precancer and include the following:

➤ Topical chemotherapy

➤ Curettage and electrodesiccation

➤ Surgical excision

➤ Cryosurgery

➤ Mohs' surgery

➤ Radiation therapy

Let's look at each option in the following sections.

Topical Chemotherapy

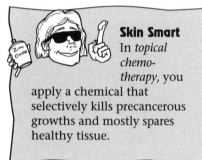

Skin Smart
In *topical chemotherapy*, you apply a chemical that selectively kills precancerous growths and mostly spares healthy tissue.

In *topical chemotherapy*, you apply chemical such as 5-fluorouracil (5-FU, for short) to your skin to kill the precancerous growths called actinic keratoses. The drug comes in lotion or cream form, and is applied for six weeks. It acts selectively to destroy abnormal tissue and mostly spares healthy skin.

It's effective, but be warned: You won't like the way it looks. For several weeks, your skin will be red, sore, and crusty. Hang in there, though, because after you stop using it, your skin will improve and the worrisome lesions should be gone.

Curettage and Electrodesiccation

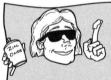

Skin Smart
Curettage involves using a sharp instrument (a curette) to scrape away cancerous cells. *Electrodesiccation* (the use of electric current to destroy tissue by heat) destroys more cells, stops bleeding, and cauterizes tissue.

Curettage involves using a sharp instrument (a curette) to scrape away cancerous cells. *Electrodesiccation* (the use of electric current to destroy tissue by heat) is done to finish the job, stop bleeding, and cauterize an area of normal tissue around the tumor site. The sequence will be repeated three times in the same session. This method may be used for basal cell cancers and sometimes for squamous cell cancers, but not for melanoma.

This approach is relatively inexpensive, easy to perform, and effective. It's also quick (a typical session takes about 15 minutes). However, it can leave a round scar, so save it for areas of skin where appearance is not an issue.

Surgical Excision

If you opt for *surgical excision*, your doctor will cut into the skin around the growth with a surgical instrument, remove the tumor, and close the wound with stitches. The tumor will probably be sent to a lab for evaluation under a microscope. If examination shows a clear margin of healthy skin cells surrounding the tumor, it's likely that all cancerous cells have been removed. If there is any doubt about this, your doctor will discuss further testing and follow up with you.

Excision takes longer than curettage/electrodesiccation (perhaps an hour), and is more expensive. You'll also have to make a repeat visit to have the stitches removed. However, if you're concerned about scars, it may be your best choice because it generally leaves only a thin line. Strategic cutting near a wrinkle or natural skin fold will make the scar even less noticeable.

> **Skin Smart**
>
> *Surgical excision* involves having your doctor cut into the skin around the growth with a surgical instrument, remove the tumor, and close the wound with stitches.

Cryosurgery

Cryosurgery (or *cryotherapy*) involves freezing the tumor site by spraying or applying liquid nitrogen directly to the skin. Your doctor will freeze the area, let it thaw, and then freeze it again.

Freezing is very effective for precancerous cells (actinic keratoses) and can effectively kill cancer cells with minimal bleeding. However, for basal cell and squamous cell cancers, many doctors recommend cryosurgery only for people who are poor candidates for other removal techniques. Freezing can cause extreme inflammation and swelling, and the area may take a long time to heal. This method is not used for melanoma.

> **Skin Smart**
>
> In *cryosurgery* (*cryotherapy*), your doctor will freeze the tumor site by spraying or applying liquid nitrogen directly to the skin.

Mohs' Surgery

If your basal cell or squamous cell cancer is large, if it keeps returning, or if it is near an important structure, such as an eye, your doctor may recommend a more complicated procedure called Mohs' surgery (named for the man who developed it). *Mohs' surgery* is a microscopically controlled excision in which each bit of tissue is mapped and examined under a microscope for cancerous cells before more tissue is removed.

> **Skin Smart**
>
> *Mohs' surgery* is a microscopically controlled excision in which small amounts of tissue are mapped and examined under a microscope for cancerous cells before more tissue is removed.

This approach is expensive and time-consuming but highly accurate because it ensures that the "bad" cells are being removed without sacrificing healthy tissue unnecessarily. It probably isn't necessary for most cases of skin cancer, but it offers an extra degree of confidence for high-risk tumors.

There are relatively few doctors trained to do the Mohs' technique. If you decide to try it, make sure your surgeon is a fellow of the American College of Mohs' Micrographic Surgery and has finished training in the technique.

Radiation Therapy

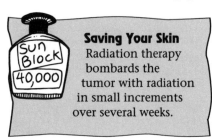

Saving Your Skin
Radiation therapy bombards the tumor with radiation in small increments over several weeks.

If you are a poor candidate for surgery, perhaps because of other health conditions, consider *radiation therapy*, which bombards the tumor with radiation in small increments over several weeks. This approach is time-consuming because it may require a series of 10 to 15 treatments.

Radiation is highly effective on basal and squamous cell cancers, and generally has few side effects (although the tumor site might feel sore). You'll probably be left with a scar. Be aware that radiation scars often get more noticeable as time goes by.

The Least You Need to Know

➤ Sunlight exposure is the single biggest risk factor for all forms of skin cancer, especially if you're fair-skinned. At lesser risk are people with bad scarring or suppressed immune systems, and those who've been exposed to many x-rays for the treatment of acne and other skin disorders and to industrial chemicals such as coal and arsenic. If you've had skin cancer once, it could reappear.

➤ Screen your skin every month for suspicious marks. This is an easy five-step process that requires only a full-length mirror, a hand mirror, and a well-lit room. Pay particular attention to the parts of you that get a lot of sun.

➤ Look for small scaly spots and patches, pearly pink or skin-colored bumps, reddish nodules, crusted areas, or areas that bleed spontaneously or with minor trauma. They could be actinic keratoses (precancerous growths) or basal or squamous cell cancers. They rarely spread, but should be removed promptly before they cause problems.

➤ Also check for the warning ABCDs of melanoma, the most serious skin malignancy: Asymmetry, Border irregularity, Color variety, and Diameter larger than a pencil eraser.

➤ If a growth does turn out to be cancer, you have a lot of treatment options. Topical chemotherapy is available for precancerous growths. Surgical excision may yield the best results on tumors but is expensive; curettage/electrodesiccation is cheaper but could leave a more noticeable scar. It is not used for melanoma. Mohs' surgery is reserved for high-risk tumors. Cryosurgery and radiation therapy are recommended for people with basal cell or squamous cell cancers who can't tolerate other treatments. Cryosurgery is effective for actinic keratoses.

Part 4
Getting Gorgeous Skin: Serious Beauty Treatments

Throughout this book, I've emphasized the importance of being an informed consumer. In no aspect of skin care is this more critical than cosmetic procedures and plastic surgery.

I've titled Part 4 "Serious Beauty Treatments," and indeed they are. Consider that, for a chemical peel, you're hiring someone to paint caustic chemicals on your face. If you choose laser therapy, you ask a doctor to burn away part of your skin. Other treatments—sclerotherapy to get rid of spider veins, collagen or fat implants to fill in wrinkles—require injections that must be carefully and skillfully placed. And plastic surgery, no matter how beautiful the result, is still surgery.

I'm not saying this to discourage you. Certainly, the treatments covered here can do wonderful things for your appearance and self-image. My point is, don't get scared; get smart! In this last section of the book, you'll learn how to choose the best procedures and practitioners.

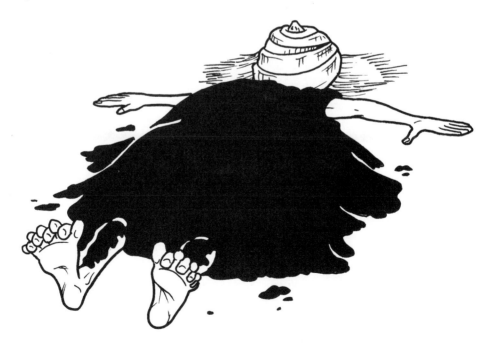

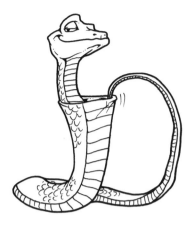

Chapter 20

Make Your Skin More A-Peeling

In This Chapter

➤ Discover what a chemical peel can do for you

➤ Find out about the different kinds of peels: superficial, medium, and deep

➤ Learn if peels are safe

➤ See who shouldn't have a peel

➤ Discover when to choose dermabrasion instead

"Well," said Sharon, "I know I want to do something. I just don't know what!"

She was sitting in my office and thinking out loud. "I have these little wrinkles and I'm getting age spots—and why not? I'm 45 and I've earned them," she mused. "I know I want to do something about them, but I'm scared. I mean, you read about so many treatments in the magazines. Peels, lasers, collagen injections, all that stuff. But at the same time, I hear horror stories about women who have chemical peels and end up with horrible burns and scars. Are peels safe? And do they really make a difference?"

What Can Chemical Peels Do for You?

Sharon is smart to consider all her options. Many people consult me about having a *chemical peel*, which involves painting the skin—usually your face—with a gel or liquid acid solution that exfoliates a layer of skin. Depending on the type of acid, the strength of the solution (and sometimes, frankly, the skill of the practitioner!), the resulting exfoliation can take off a little skin, a lot, or somewhere in between.

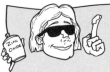

Skin Smart

A *chemical peel* involves painting the skin—usually your face—with a gel or liquid acid solution that exfoliates a layer of skin. The depth of exfoliation depends on the type and strength of the solution.

As Sharon asks, can chemical peels make a visible difference? Yes, if done correctly. We saw in Chapters 12, "Help from Hydroxy Acids," and 13, "Tretinoin and Antioxidants: The Age-Tamers?" that exfoliation can improve the appearance of your skin by peeling away outer layers of cells. In the right hands, a peel can minimize fine lines and make areas of darker pigmentation, such as freckles and so-called age spots, less noticeable. It may also get rid of shallow scars and faint acne pocks.

If done incorrectly, a peel can still make a visible difference, but it might not be one you like! This is a time to flex your comparative shopping skills. There are three categories of peels and several peeling agents. Unfortunately, since these procedures have become so popular, there are also a number of less-qualified practitioners hoping to peel your cash from your bank account. Be an informed consumer.

Common peeling agents include the following:

➤ Alpha hydroxy acids (glycolic acid, lactic acid, and others). As discussed in Chapter 12, you can buy AHAs in over-the-counter products at percentages of 1 to about 15 percent, with 4 percent being the minimum for noticeable exfoliation. Chemical AHA peels are stronger solutions, usually ranging from 20 to 70 percent.

➤ Trichloroacetic acid (TCA). TCA penetrates more deeply than AHA, so you get more effect from the peel. It comes in many different strengths, which cause differing depths of exfoliation. It's the most common agent used in medium peels.

➤ Jessner's solution (a mix of resorcinol, lactic acid, and salicylic acid, a beta hydroxy acid).

➤ Phenol, a coal tar derivative, most commonly used in deep peels. As we'll see, it may be risky if too much is absorbed through the skin.

Many superficial peels use AHAs, and a lot of my patients prefer this approach.

How Low Do You Want to Go?

Peels are classified according to the depth to which they exfoliate: superficial (or light), medium, and deep. Which is best for you? The answer depends on your skin type, the condition of your skin, how big a change you're looking for, and how long a recovery period you can tolerate.

Another consideration: your budget. The deeper the peel, the higher the price. A superficial peel may cost around $100 to $200, a deep peel could run $3,000 or more, with medium peels somewhere in between. Health insurance rarely covers a skin peel (although you might be able to get coverage if it's done to remove a precancerous growth, so ask your doctor and insurance agent).

Regardless of the type of peel you choose, your doctor may advise you to use tretinoin or an alpha hydroxy acid product on your face for at least two weeks ahead of time. The smoother and cleaner your skin, the less risk of the acid solution pooling and causing uneven results. Also, tretinoin may speed the recovery period after medium or deep peels.

Superficial Peels: The "Lunchtime Peel"

If your skin shows mild photoaging, such as fine wrinkles and slightly darker spots or patches, or you have faint scars you'd like to minimize, consider a *superficial peel*. These peels remove the horny layer (the layer of dead cells on the skin surface) and the upper-most part of the epidermis underneath. (Some doctors distinguish between this and a *very superficial peel*, which removes the horny layer only.)

A big advantage of superficial peels is their speed (the acid solution stays on your face for only a few minutes) and the minimal recovery time—hence their nickname "the lunchtime peel." Many of my patients literally stop by during their lunch hour, and then return to work. They lose no time from their jobs, and no one has to know they had anything done.

During the procedure, you'll be asked to lie down comfortably in your doctor's office. Your eyes may be covered, usually with a gauze pad, to make sure no acid drips into them, or you might simply be asked to keep them closed. Then the doctor or an assistant will cleanse your face thoroughly. I recommend not wearing any makeup that day, but if you do, it must all be completely removed before the peel. Any substance on your skin that blocks even penetration of the acid could leave blotchy results.

Then a solution—either liquid or gel—will be applied to your face. A superficial peel shouldn't be extremely painful. Your face may sting or itch while the solution is in place: "It feels like a rug burn," comments one of my patients. After a carefully measured period of time, usually just a few minutes, a neutralizer will be applied to your skin to stop the action of the acid, or the acid will simply be wiped or rinsed off with water.

After a superficial peel, your skin may look a bit pink, like a very mild sunburn. It might also feel slightly sensitive and a little swollen (although not badly so; the effect will be to plump out lines). After a few days, you may notice some flaking. This will be mild and generally looks no more flaky than dry skin.

> **Skin Smart**
>
> A *superficial peel* removes the horny layer (the layer of dead cells on the skin surface) and the uppermost part of the epidermis underneath. Some doctors distinguish between this and a *very superficial peel*, which removes the horny layer only.

> **Beauty Tips**
>
> Skin peels, even if superficial, make your skin more sensitive to the sun. Always wear a sunscreen with an SPF of at least 15, stay out of the sun as much as possible, and avoid tanning salons and sunlamps. There's no point in paying to minimize your wrinkles, only to increase your risk of more wrinkles later!

235

My patients feel their lunchtime peels give a glowing, rejuvenated appearance. They also do a good job of fading pigment irregularities. The drawback is that the benefits of each individual peel are subtle. It's a tradeoff: A peel that's superficial enough for no one to know it's happening is not going to yield dramatic improvements in one session.

These peels generally need to be done in a series. I tell my patients to plan on a total of six peels done every two to three weeks. Some patients require fewer, some require more, to get the results they want. What's more, even after a nice result, time does march on. The benefits of the peels are not permanent. Many people return for periodic "lunchtime peels" to refresh their complexions.

Medium Peels: Going Deeper

If your skin's problems are more extensive—precancerous spots, darker brown spots, shallow scars, crow's feet around eyes, mild to moderate wrinkles—you might want to consider a *medium peel*, which removes the horny layer, epidermis, and upper layers of the dermis. This involves using a stronger solution than a superficial peel, and the liquid may stay on your face longer.

As with a superficial peel, you'll lie down and have a thorough face-cleansing first. Some doctors then apply a cold carbon dioxide preparation or a weak acid solution, to prepare your skin, before applying the main peeling agent.

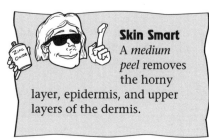

Skin Smart
A *medium peel* removes the horny layer, epidermis, and upper layers of the dermis.

More painful than its superficial cousins, a medium peel will definitely remind you there's acid on your skin. Most doctors don't provide sedatives or topical anesthetics during this procedure, although they will apply cool compresses and sometimes a fan to make a breeze on the patient's face afterward to soothe the discomfort. If you think you would like a sedative or painkiller, bring it up ahead of time. (If you do opt for sedation, be sure to bring someone who can drive you home afterward.)

Later, when you look in a mirror—well, frankly, you might be a bit taken aback. At first, your skin will have a whitish hue, which fades in a few minutes to a few hours, depending on your skin and the exact depth of the peel. After that, your skin will look red and somewhat swollen. If acid was applied near your eyes or on your forehead, your lids may be swollen shut. In a few days, your skin may develop scales and scabs. It will also develop a dry, dark membranous appearance, much as skin looks a few days after a very bad sunburn. The recovery process generally takes one to two weeks, and you will probably want to take time off work.

Eventually, though, your skin will crack and peel, exposing smoother, clearer, softer skin underneath. While the damage is more extensive than a superficial peel, the improvement in your appearance is also likely to be more noticeable. Some people feel the discomfort and inconvenience are worth it, because they end up with more visible results for the time and money spent.

Medium peels do carry a higher risk of side effects and adverse results than superficial procedures. This is, after all, a burn, albeit under controlled conditions. If your skin tends to darken after injury, you could end up with dark splotches on your face. (This is more common in people with dark complexions.) There's also a small risk of scarring. Your dermatologist will consider these risks when assessing you for a medium-depth peel.

I always do a test application of the acid, in a spot on the forehead covered by the hair, to determine how well the patient heals. This test area also allows patients to observe the healing process and decide if it is something they want to experience over the entire face.

If you are considering a medium peel, you might want to have a superficial peel first to see how your skin reacts. Another option is to have a series of superficial peels, starting with low strengths of acid solutions and gradually increasing the concentration or application time. This approach may achieve some of the same benefits with less risk.

Medium peels represent a range of depths. If a patient is undergoing his or her first medium peel, I generally do it more superficially. If a patient has already had a medium peel, healed well, knows what to expect, and wants me to go a little deeper, I can do a slightly deeper procedure.

Deep Peels: Approach with Caution

A *deep peel*, more radical still, strips off the horny layer, epidermis, and more of the dermis. We're talking a serious burn here, with proportionately more pain, longer recovery time, and greater risk of problems.

If you decide to go through with it, your doctor should do a complete preoperative exam before the procedure. Be sure to mention any health conditions and allergies at this time. You'll be given painkillers and a sedative for this peel. You may not sleep through the procedure, but you will be groggy, so make arrangements for getting home afterward.

> **Skin Smart**
> A *deep peel* strips off the horny layer, epidermis, and more of the dermis. This is a serious procedure, appropriate only in selected cases.

Often the chemical used for deep peels is phenol, a strong solution that has been reported to occasionally cause irregular heartbeats if enough is absorbed through the skin. For this reason, deep peels should be done in an office or operating room where medical equipment is available. Complications are most frequent if more than half of the face is treated in less than 30 minutes.

After your face is cleaned, your doctor will apply the peeling solution. This application is done in stages over different portions of the face, until the entire face is treated. It is likely to hurt in spite of the sedation and painkillers. Your doctor might then place a mask or dressing over your face so the solution will penetrate even deeper. The dressing is left in place for one to two days, which makes the whole process even more uncomfortable, but may enhance the results.

Beauty Tips
Two or three days after a deep peel, you probably can start to wash away peeling skin. Use a mild soap and be careful not to pull or tug at your skin, because it will bleed easily and may scar if traumatized. Ask your doctor for detailed skin care instructions.

For several days afterward, your face will be red, swollen, crusted, and peeling. You may bleed and develop oozing blisters. Most of the peeling should stop after a week and a half to two weeks, but your face will still be red, and it could take weeks or months for the red to fade completely.

Why would anyone go through this voluntarily? When all goes well, as it usually does, deep peels can lead to a definite improvement in appearance. Facial wrinkles, some scars, and some pigmentary problems, like "age spots" or melasma, can be markedly improved. At the same time, however, there's a greater risk of scarring. Some patients develop small bumps called *milia* that can be removed by a doctor; others develop skin thinning (called *atrophy*); still others find their faces left perpetually shiny.

There's also a risk of permanent changes in skin color. Patients may find their faces left lighter than the rest of their body. Unfortunately, this is not uncommon with phenol peels. Or, less often, they might have a problem with the development of darker pigmentation (called *hyperpigmentation*). Prompt treatment often improves hyperpigmentation, so call your doctor immediately if you notice any dark areas.

In some people, the initial redness is very slow to fade. And, of course, there is always a risk of scarring when peeling the skin. The deeper the peel, the greater the risk. Even in people who are excellent peel candidates and with experienced doctors, sometimes scarring does occur. Again, in many cases prompt treatment makes a big difference and can dramatically reduce scarring. For this reason, most doctors schedule frequent follow-up visits after deep peels.

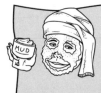

Beauty Tips
Chemical peels make your skin more vulnerable to sun-induced pigmentary changes. While the sun can cause blotchy dark marks in anyone, people who have recently undergone a peel are especially predisposed. Avoid the sun (and, of course, tanning booths) as much as possible after a peel.

For all these reasons, deep peels are rarely done. They're appropriate only if your skin shows extensive sun damage (moderate wrinkling, "smoker's lines" around the mouth, definite variations in skin color). Even then, be sure to consider all your options before deciding on a deep peel. Deep scars might be treated with dermabrasion; wrinkles may respond to collagen injections (see Chapter 21, "Injection Treatments: Shots You Could Get to Like"); pigment spots may do better with lasers (Chapter 23, "Better Looking with Lasers").

If you have any marks that could be cancerous, surgical excision or other treatments will be more effective. And remember, if you do have any spots that could be malignant, they should be evaluated carefully, not simply exfoliated. (For more on identifying and treating skin cancer, see

Chapter 19, "Skin Cancer: The Dark Side of the Sun.") Think twice—no, make that four or five times—before subjecting yourself to a deep peel, and make sure you've thought through all the potential risks.

What Won't Peels Do?

You might see ads that tout chemical peels as "nonsurgical facelifts." Sorry, but there's no such thing. Peels can minimize fine lines and differences in skin color. They may give your skin a smoother, more glowing appearance. Deep peels may even smooth out deeper wrinkles (and garner rave reviews from friends and family). However, they will not do the following:

➤ Tighten excessively sagging skin or excess skin folds

➤ Shrink pores

➤ Eradicate broken blood vessels (some laser treatments can help with this; see Chapter 23)

➤ Wipe out deep scars or acne pocks

If what you really seek is a face-lift, plastic surgery remains your best friend. (For more tips on plastic surgery, see Chapters 24, "Should You Try Plastic Surgery?" and 25, "Popular Choices in Plastic Surgery.")

Who Shouldn't Have a Peel?

Superficial peels are relatively low-risk, and most of us can enjoy them trouble-free. However, some people are definitely better candidates than others for chemical peels. For instance:

➤ If your complexion is dark, even if it's just olive, you run a risk of uneven pigmentation after peels. Many doctors advise against them for people of African-American, Native-American, Asian, Hispanic, or Mediterranean ancestry.

➤ If you scar easily or have a tendency to form keloids (raised hard scars), your skin could react to the acids by forming thickened scars. I've never seen this with superficial peels, but it has been reported infrequently with medium peels. If you are prone to thick scars or keloids, my opinion is that deep peels are just too risky.

➤ If you have a heart or kidney condition, stay away from any peel using phenol. This chemical

Saving Your Skin
In my practice, I have generally found that superficial peels are safe for most darker skin types. However, I advise people with darker complexions to avoid medium peels because of the potential pigmentary problems, and, in my opinion, deep peels are definitely not a good option for them.

may cause irregular heartbeats; if you absorb enough of it through the skin or cannot rid your system of it through the kidneys, it could be dangerous. Likewise, people with liver problems should probably avoid phenol peels.

➤ If your job requires you to spend a lot of time outdoors, the photosensitizing effects of a peel could be dangerous—not to mention making you miserable with repeated sunburns. Also, sun exposure after a peel increases your risk of post-peel pigmentary problems.

Here's one more thing to consider: If you have a history of cold sores, be sure to discuss this with your doctor. The trauma of a facial peel may cause a cold sore to appear. Then, potentially, the cold sore virus could spread across your face where the skin has been left vulnerable by the peel, causing extensive scarring. However, you can avoid this by taking a medication that your doctor can prescribe.

Dermabrasion: Sand Those Scars Away

Some scars may be too deep or extensive to be handled effectively with chemical peels. In this case, your doctor might suggest *dermabrasion*, removal of the surface layer of skin with high-speed sanding. A rapidly rotating wheel or circular brush abrades the skin, literally scraping away tissue. While most often used on scars, sometimes dermabrasion can remove wrinkles, tattoos, and small benign or precancerous growths.

Skin Smart
Dermabrasion removes the surface layer of skin with high-speed sanding by a rapidly rotating wheel or circular brush.

While it usually doesn't "erase" scars, dermabrasion smoothes irregularities in skin texture and makes them less noticeable. If your scars are very deep, your doctor may suggest so-called punch grafts followed by dermabrasion. In this technique, the deep scars are cut away and the resulting holes filled in with healthy skin, usually taken from behind the ear. After this heals, the entire area is dermabraded to smooth it out and obscure the "punch graft" sites.

Dermabrasion isn't for everyone. Like chemical peels, if you are dark-skinned it can leave you with patches of uneven or dark pigmentation, and if you scar easily, the dermabraded area could heal with a thickened scar. It could improve appearance by anywhere from 20 to 75 percent, but rarely by 100 percent; it won't erase marks entirely or produce baby-smooth skin.

Saving Your Skin
If you have taken Accutane® for acne, wait at least one year before trying dermabrasion, because the drug can affect your skin's ability to heal. Some physicians suggest waiting even longer. Please discuss this with your doctor.

It's crucial to select a practitioner who has training in and experience with dermabrasion. Uneven pressure or a too-heavy hand could leave you with worse scars than before! If your dermatologist does not perform dermabrasion, ask him or her for a referral. One other word of warning: If you take Accutane® for acne, you must stop taking it for at least a year before undergoing dermabrasion. Accutane® can interfere with your skin's ability to heal. Be sure to discuss this with your doctor.

Dermabrasion is generally done on an outpatient basis, either in a surgery center or the doctor's office. You'll be given sedation and local anesthetics, but usually not general anesthesia. In the past, after you were numb the doctor would spray a cold substance onto the skin to stiffen the tissue and make it easier to get uniform results. These refrigerants are no longer available because of fears that they may damage the ozone layer.

These days, other techniques are used to stiffen the skin, such as injecting fluid and local anesthetic medications. Then your doctor will carefully sand the area with the rotating wheel, and follow up with a topical antibiotic cream and maybe a topical anesthetic. The final touch is a mask-like dressing that stays on your face for one or two days.

When you remove the mask, be warned: Your face will look red, moist, swollen, and crusty. The worst of it should clear up within one and a half to three weeks, although your skin may still have reddish patches for six weeks to a few months. Most dermabrasion patients are back at work within three weeks.

Enjoying the Benefits, Minimizing the Risks

As you can see, dermabrasion and chemical peels require considerable skill. Consider that they amount to deliberate destruction of skin cells, either by burning or scraping them away. Uneven or sloppy technique can produce terrible results. Even superficial peels can have complications. Just ask Carol.

An olive-skinned brunette and enthusiastic sunbather, Carol decided to have a chemical peel to get rid of her sun-induced freckles. "I chose a salon in a mall near my house," she recalls. "I stopped by for an interview and talked with the cosmetologist, who used terms like 'facial rejuvenation' and 'instant facelift.' I decided to go through with it, and went back two days later."

"Afterward," she continues, "my face became dry and looked like it would start peeling, just as I expected. Then suddenly, before that happened, the skin on my left cheek began to swell and get red. It started to drain a yellowish fluid and developed an ugly yellow crust. Pretty soon this spread all over the left side of my face. It was really tender—and really scary!"

Carol had developed a secondary bacterial infection, called *impetigo*, in the peeled skin. I treated it with antibiotics, and fortunately she recovered without permanent scars.

Sadly, Carol's experience isn't unique. The deeper peels, of course, are more likely to cause problems. In a recent survey of 588 plastic surgeons, two-thirds of them reported at least some problems with skin pigmentation after phenol peels. Twenty-one percent—a smaller number, but still significant—have noticed problems with scarring, especially around the chin and mouth. Strong TCA solutions also present a risk of scarring.

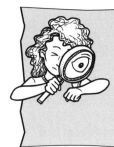

More Than Skin Deep

How can you reduce the risks of skin peels while maximizing the benefits? Choose a qualified professional. Licensed aestheticians and cosmetologists may do superficial chemical peels, but physicians can perform superficial, medium, and deep peels. Physicians are better equipped to handle complications if they should occur.

However, as Carol's experience shows, in rare cases complications may occur even in superficial peels. Keep in mind that these are acids you're putting on your face: strong solutions with the potential for burns and other skin reactions, including secondary infections. The FDA is especially concerned about the health risks of mail-order skin-peel kits and procedures performed in salons with no physician present. I share these concerns.

How can you protect yourself? I favor having even superficial peels performed by a doctor or by an aesthetician who works closely with a doctor. Certainly, many qualified cosmetologists and aestheticians do beautiful peels, but it may be safer to be under the supervision of a physician with specialized training in skin-related issues and concerns. Furthermore, in the unlikely event of a complication, a doctor can write the prescriptions necessary to treat it.

If you do decide to have an aesthetician perform your superficial peel, at least be sure that he or she is operating under the supervision of a physician, or that a doctor is readily available if a complication should occur. Deeper peels must be done by trained physicians who can handle any possible problem. As for do-it-yourself home-peel kits: please do not!

Furthermore, you don't just want to be safe; you also want to be beautiful. Legally, any physician with a valid medical license can perform these procedures, but I recommend selecting a specialist who is trained in doing cosmetic work. Usually this means a dermatologist or plastic surgeon. There are also a few ENT (ear, nose, and throat) doctors who specialize in facial cosmetic procedures. For more tips on choosing a qualified professional, see Chapter 21.

Saving Your Skin

I don't recommend using mail-order skin peelers. It takes skill and experience to perform a smooth, uniform peel on someone else; it's even harder to do on yourself. Also, there's a chance you could get acid in your eyes.

Keep in mind that you might not feel presentable immediately after any skin peel. With a superficial procedure, you may have some minor skin flaking. This shouldn't be a serious problem. With dermabrasion or deeper peels, however, it could take weeks before you feel like going out in public again. Schedule your procedure carefully for a time when you can be off work and have no pressing social engagements.

The Least You Need to Know

➤ Peels are classified according to how deeply they exfoliate: superficial, medium, or deep. Superficial peels are fast, with minimal side effects (hence their nickname "the lunchtime peel"). A medium peel goes deeper to remove the horny layer, epidermis, and upper layers of the dermis. A deep peel is more risky, and should be used only in carefully selected cases.

➤ All peels, even the most superficial, make you more sun-sensitive. Always wear sunscreen, and avoid sunlamps and tanning salons.

➤ Dermabrasion (removal of the surface layer of skin with high-speed sanding) is another approach, usually used for scars that are too deep to be removed with peels. While dermabrasion generally doesn't erase scars entirely, it can smooth irregularities in skin texture and make them less noticeable.

➤ If you have dark skin or a tendency to scar, you may not respond well to dermabrasion or chemical peels. Many doctors advise against medium or deep peels for people of African-American, Native-American, Asian, Hispanic, or Mediterranean ancestry.

➤ Chemical peels can minimize fine wrinkles, slight differences in skin pigmentation, shallow scars, and faint acne pocks. They are not "nonsurgical face-lifts."

➤ Choose a qualified professional to do your dermabrasion or peel—a dermatologist, a plastic surgeon, or an ENT doctor who specializes in cosmetic procedures.

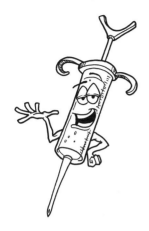

Chapter 21

Injection Treatments: Shots You Could Get to Like

In This Chapter

➤ See why collagen injections provide instant gratification

➤ Find out how a cow's collagen can help you

➤ Learn about transplanting your own fat: great idea, but nothing's perfect

➤ Discover how botulinum toxin can be your friend

➤ Get tips on finding the best doctor to perform a safe procedure

Remember Sharon, the patient who wondered about chemical peels in the last chapter? After returning for several superficial peels, she made another appointment with me. "I like the texture of my skin a lot better now," she said, "and the age spots have disappeared. But what about the deeper wrinkles? In particular, these ugly frown lines between my eyebrows. And I'm not crazy about these folds from my nostrils to the corners of my mouth, either. I know you warned me that superficial peels wouldn't get rid of them. Is there anything else I can try?"

Collagen Injections: Instant Gratification

Getting rid of wrinkles: This issue is on a lot of people's minds these days. One option you might want to consider—collagen injections.

Collagen, you'll recall from Chapter 2, "Your Skin: Don't Leave Home Without It," is a supportive protein in the dermis that gives skin its firm, supple feeling. Other animals besides humans have collagen in their skin. As I explained to Sharon, the most commonly used material for filling minor skin depressions (such as wrinkles or small scars) is *bovine collagen.*

"Bovine, as in cow collagen?" asked Sharon. "Now, this I want to hear about!"

Collagen injections are indeed made from a purified form of bovine collagen derived from cow skin. It is produced by the Collagen Corporation, which makes two general categories of collagen for injection: Zyderm™ and Zyplast™. There are two types of Zyderm™—Zyderm™ I and II. The Zyderms™ are usually used for the most superficial wrinkles; the main difference is that Zyderm™ II has a higher concentration of collagen. Zyplast™ is used for deeper wrinkles and folds.

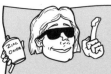

Skin Smart
The most commonly used material for filling minor skin depressions (such as wrinkles or superficial scars) is purified *bovine collagen,* derived from cow skin.

Saving Your Skin
Some people get impatient when I suggest having two test shots of collagen. "But that means waiting six weeks for my treatments!" they protest. There's a valid reason for waiting, however: An allergic reaction to injected collagen could last as long as the collagen stays in your skin, which means months. It's worth taking a little extra time to avoid persistent (and unsightly) reactions on your face.

Although bovine collagen is chemically altered in a laboratory to make it similar to human collagen, some people still experience problems with it. Roughly 3 percent of the population develops allergic reactions (sometimes to the chemicals used to alter the collagen, not the collagen itself), so it's important to make sure you're not one of them.

Before you undergo any treatments, your doctor should test your skin by injecting a small amount of collagen into your forearm and waiting four weeks. In some cases, reactions occur on a delayed basis, so even if your first test is fine, I recommend having a second test at about week three and then watching both test sites for three more weeks just to make sure. If any redness, swelling, itching, or other sign of inflammation develops in a test site, show your doctor. This reaction means you probably are not a candidate for collagen.

The collagen comes packaged as an injectable gel in premeasured syringes. The injections also contain a local anesthetic, which helps to reduce the discomfort from the shots. If you're nervous about pain from the injections, you can be given a topical anesthetic by your doctor to apply before the procedure. Then, your doctor will clean the site carefully. He or she will inject the gel just under the skin, directly into the wrinkle or whatever area of skin needs filling.

Syringes come in a variety of sizes. It takes roughly 1/2 to 1 cc (a cubic centimeter, roughly 1/30 of an ounce) to fill a single nose-to-mouth wrinkle, depending on how deep it is. (Often, but not exclusively, Zyplast™ is used in this location.) It takes a little less, approximately 1/4 cc, to fill the frown line between the eyes (Zyderm™ should be used here).

Afterward, the area is likely to be a bit red and swollen, especially if Zyderm™ is used. Why? Zyderm™ contains some water and is injected closer to the skin surface. Your doctor will take the water into account and inject a little extra collagen. This causes the initial swelling. Then when the water reabsorbs, usually overnight, the area will be perfectly filled in.

Zyplast™ treatments rarely cause much swelling. People who receive only Zyplast™ injections can usually apply a little powder (gently!) and leave the office without any noticeable marks.

I enjoy giving collagen treatments. They offer instant gratification; my patients can perceive an immediate improvement in their appearance and they're delighted. It works right away, and, in most cases, they can look better in time for dinner that evening. Meanwhile, I feel like a sculptor who has successfully repaired a slight flaw in a statue and made it beautiful again.

Beauty Tips
Rarely, some people develop a slight bruise if a small capillary has bled during a collagen treatment. This should disappear within a week. If you wish, you can cover the bruise with flesh-colored foundation.

Collagen: The Good News, the Bad News

Great as they are, do realize that collagen injections have their downside. The effects are temporary because after several months, your body will break down the substance. Gradually, those pesky wrinkles will reappear, at which point you may want to have another injection.

How long do the benefits last? This depends on the type and amount of collagen used, the depth of your wrinkles, your own individual body chemistry, and how perfect a result you desire. I advise my patients that touch-up injections every three months or so are the norm. Some come in as often as every six weeks, while others stop by once or twice per year. At more than $400 per syringe, this can get expensive. However, many of my patients find the cost is worth it. For some people, skilled collagen injections can actually replace plastic surgery (a far most costly and invasive proposition), or at any rate delay it for many years.

Notice I said "skilled." This is an area where you definitely want to locate a dermatologist or plastic surgeon who has both training and extensive experience. Some of my patients have told me stories about collagen injections they've received from less experienced physicians. If too much collagen is used or it is incorrectly placed, the collagen can form a bump that persists for weeks to months until it breaks down. If too little is used or it's too deeply placed, there won't be much improvement and the visit will be a waste of time and money. And rarely, if collagen is accidentally injected into a small blood vessel, it can obstruct blood flow through the vessel.

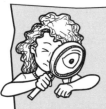

More Than Skin Deep

The FDA requires makers of injectable collagen to include label warnings about reports of a possible link with two rare connective tissue disorders called *polymyositis* and *dermatomyositis* (*PM/DM*). The link is controversial at best. As the warning says, "A causal relationship between collagen injections and the onset of PM/DM, or the other connective tissue diseases listed, has not been established." To be on the safe side, though, collagen injections are not advised for people who have already been diagnosed with connective tissue disease, such as PM/DM, lupus, or rheumatoid arthritis.

Autologous Collagen: Supplying Your Own

If you're one of the few who can't tolerate bovine collagen, another option to consider is *autologous collagen*, in which you donate your own collagen for transplant to another part of your body. This requires surgery to remove collagen-containing skin, usually from the buttocks or thighs, sometimes from excess skin removed after a face-lift or other surgical procedure. The collagen tissue is cleaned and processed; then, like the bovine variety, it is injected directly into wrinkles or other areas to plump them out. If you think autologous collagen is the answer for you, ask your doctor about the details of this technique.

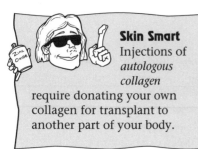

Skin Smart
Injections of *autologous collagen* require donating your own collagen for transplant to another part of your body.

The advantage of autologous collagen is that, since it's your own tissue, you won't get annoying allergic reactions. While this is great, the transplanted collagen still breaks down over time and has to be replaced periodically. Remember, this means further surgery to harvest the necessary collagen.

Scientists are working on new and improved methods for transplanting and implanting collagen tissue. Until a perfect solution is found, the truth is that most of my patients prefer bovine collagen injections.

Surprise! Fat Can Be Helpful

Ever wished you could subtract fat tissue from places where you don't want it—like your hips and thighs—and use it somewhere else to plump out wrinkles? This is the idea behind *autologous fat transplants*. Like autologous collagen, this means donating your own tissue to be transplanted somewhere else on your body.

Sometimes fat transplants are done along with *liposuction*, a procedure in which fat tissue is sucked out of subcutaneous spaces (see Chapter 25, "Popular Choices in Plastic Surgery"). At other times, your doctor will simply withdraw a syringe-full of fat, rinse and treat it, then re-inject it directly into the wrinkle, just below the skin. You may be given local anesthetic.

The plumping effects of the transplanted fat show up right away, and create an immediate improvement in appearance. As with any injection, you could have a little redness and swelling at the injection site, but it should dissipate within a day. There may also be a little bruising, which should fade within a week.

In theory fat transplants sound wonderful, but the reality is less attractive. First of all, autologous fat transplants are meant for deep folds and wrinkles. They are not very helpful for mild superficial wrinkling, nor are they useful for the more superficial components of deep wrinkles. Therefore, many people need to have bovine collagen placed on top of fat transplants to achieve the desired result.

Then there is the issue of reabsorption. Different doctors report different experiences, but it appears that no more than about 10 percent of each fat injection "takes." The body reabsorbs the rest. One study found that only 30 percent of the fat tissue injected into wrinkles survived one year, so again, you will need repeated treatments.

Many doctors harvest "fresh fat" for each procedure. These procedures tend to run from $700 to $1,500 per treatment. Others harvest fat periodically and then store it for you. They will charge accordingly for the harvesting process, but are likely to charge less for subsequent injections of fat that has already been stored.

> **Skin Smart**
> *Autologous fat transplants* involve removing fatty tissue from places where you don't want it, and transplanting it somewhere else on your body to fill in deep wrinkles and skin folds.

Bo-Tox™ Injections: A New Use for Bacteria?

Maybe you've heard of botulism, a serious type of food poisoning caused by a bacterium. When ingested in improperly preserved food, this nasty organism produces a toxin that interferes with the nervous system and causes progressive muscular paralysis.

However, the toxin also has a benign side: For more than 15 years, it's been used to relieve abnormal muscle spasms in certain health conditions. Some doctors also use it to smooth facial lines, because it temporarily paralyzes the muscles responsible. If placed between the eyebrows, for example, *Bo-Tox™* (*botulinum toxin*) *injections* paralyze the corrugator muscle, making it impossible to frown for three to six months and smoothing away frown lines. If injected into the forehead, they smooth forehead wrinkles (and prevent you from being able to raise your eyebrows in surprise). If placed beyond the outer edge of the eye (toward the temple), the injections smooth out crow's feet.

> **Skin Smart**
> *Bo-Tox™* (*botulinum toxin*) *injections* temporarily paralyze selected facial muscles, making it impossible to move them and thus smoothing out lines and wrinkles.

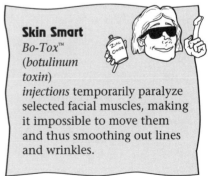

The most common side-effect of Bo-Tox™ is a temporary droop of the eyelid if the toxin filters down to the muscles that open the lid. This generally lasts two to four weeks when it occurs. Do be aware that the FDA has not yet approved Bo-Tox™ for cosmetic purposes. However, many experienced physicians are using it successfully to minimize wrinkles, and this application has become a common "off label" use for the product.

Choosing a Qualified Professional

No matter which beauty treatment you're considering, it's vital to select a well-qualified practitioner to perform it. Some pointers:

➤ Some doctors learn these techniques during their residency (postgraduate training). Others learn them from continuing education courses sponsored by various organizations. Ask your doctor what type of training she or he has had. If you have any questions about a particular organization's programs, call the Accreditation Council of Continuing Medical Education for background information (see Appendix A, "Bountiful Resources for Beautiful Skin," at the end of this book).

➤ Ask which types of procedures the doctor has performed, how many, and how often. If you want a medium peel, for instance, you may not want someone who's only done superficial peels. You don't want to be a practitioner's first dermabrasion patient or collagen injectee.

➤ Your doctor should be willing to discuss all your treatment alternatives. Maybe you'd benefit from the latest technology, or maybe you'd be better off with a simple prescription for tretinoin; there's probably more than one solution to your skin problem, and you want to make sure you choose the best. Be wary of anyone who seems eager to guide you toward a particular treatment.

> **Saving Your Skin**
> If you have a herpes simplex infection, be aware that skin irritation from injections near the mouth or chemical peels could make the virus flare up and cause an attack of cold sores. Taking the medication acyclovir before and after the procedure may prevent this, or at least moderate its severity.

➤ Before you undergo any treatment, your doctor should take a complete medical history. Don't assume that cosmetic procedures are "just a skin thing"; your overall health and lifestyle can influence how you respond during the procedure and how your skin heals afterward. Tell your doctor about all chronic health conditions and medications you take, so she or he will be forewarned if reactions occur.

➤ Your doctor should take time to describe the entire procedure (including the recovery process) with you, and be frank about possible side effects and complications. You might not enjoy hearing about them, but discussions like these are the hallmark of a caring professional who is concerned about your welfare.

➤ Do steer clear of any practitioner who makes unrealistic predictions about the results or glosses over unpleasant details like risks and adverse reactions.

As with any health-related choice, you should never feel pressured to make a decision. Don't go by price alone. Does a deal seem too good to be true? It probably is!

The Least You Need to Know

➤ The most commonly used material for filling minor skin defects is bovine collagen, derived from cow skin. Collagen injections are a tradeoff: You look better immediately, but the collagen slowly breaks down, requiring touch-up injections every few months if you want to keep your smooth skin.

➤ Although bovine collagen is purified, some people suffer allergic reactions to it. I recommend two test injections before having this procedure done on your face.

➤ It's possible to undergo autologous fat and collagen transplants, in which you donate your own tissue to be transplanted somewhere else on your body. This tissue also breaks down, and must be replaced in time.

➤ Bo-Tox™ (botulinum toxin) injections temporarily paralyze the muscles that cause frown lines, forehead wrinkles, and crow's feet. Bo-Tox™ may cause a temporary eyelid droop.

➤ Your doctor should conduct a thorough pre-procedure interview, review all your treatment options, describe the procedure, and inform you of all risks. Steer clear of anyone who glosses over the risks or seems eager to sell you on having something done.

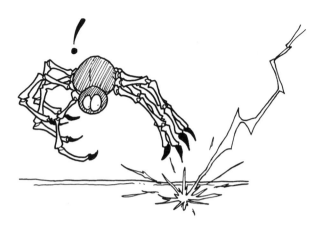

Chapter 22

Zapping Varicose and Spider Veins

In This Chapter

➤ Find out why you get varicose and spider veins

➤ Learn how to reduce the risk of developing them

➤ Recognize when these veins need medical attention

➤ Discover the therapy that's 90 percent effective for spider veins

I've never seen my friend Kay wear a skirt. The attractive 66-year-old, mother of four, was always stylishly garbed in pantsuits or jeans—outfits that didn't expose her legs.

One day I discovered why. She made an appointment and reluctantly pulled up her pants leg to show me her reason for coming: raised, bluish, bumpy veins. "For years now, I've been embarrassed to show my legs in public," she said. "Even support stockings don't push the veins in all the way. Lately they've started to itch. You know I do a lot of volunteer work, and I have to spend a lot of time on my feet those days. Seems like my legs really ache when I get home."

"I'm glad you came in, because there are effective ways to minimize them," I reassured her. "What made you decide to take action now?"

"I'll tell you what the final blow was," replied Kay. "I was baby-sitting my six-year-old grandson, and he said, 'Grandma, why are your legs so dirty?' Then and there I decided it was high time I got rid of these horrible veins!"

"Doctor, What's Wrong with My Legs?"

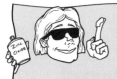

Skin Smart
Varicose veins are swollen, twisted veins just beneath the skin surface. They most often show up in the calves, thighs, vagina, and anus.

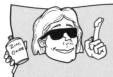

Skin Smart
Spider veins are patches of tiny red or purple blood vessels that often resemble spider webs (hence their name), but can also look like short broken lines, sunbursts, or branching trees.

Like Kay, many people are concerned about their *varicose veins*—swollen, twisted veins just beneath the skin surface. They most often show up in the calves, thighs, vagina, and anus. (Varicose veins in the lining of the anus are called hemorrhoids; see Chapter 14, "Baby and You: Your Skin During Pregnancy," for a discussion of hemorrhoid prevention and treatment.) Since most cosmetic issues relate to varicose veins in the legs, that's the type I'll focus on in this chapter.

Sometimes these blood vessels become more than just a cosmetic nuisance. As Kay can attest, they may swell or itch. Some people report an achy, tender feeling in their legs, ankles, or feet, especially after standing for long periods. In severe cases, if left untreated, varicose veins contribute to circulatory problems that could lead to skin ulcers.

Another development that drives my patients crazy: *spider veins*, patches of tiny red or purple blood vessels. Spider veins often look like spider webs (hence their name), but they can also take the form of short broken lines, sunburst patterns, or branching trees. Sometimes they're limited to a small, fairly inconspicuous area; other times they spread to cover large expanses of flesh.

Some people get varicose veins only, others develop only spider veins, and some lucky folks get both.

What Causes Varicose and Spider Veins?

Strictly speaking, varicose and spider veins are not skin conditions; they reflect developments in your blood vessels. Since they are such a frequent cosmetic concern, however, you may end up consulting a dermatologist or other cosmetically-oriented physician about getting rid of them.

Veins are blood vessels that carry deoxygenated blood on its return trip back to the heart. (Vein walls are translucent, so the bluish color you see is not the veins themselves, but the oxygen-poor blood flowing through them.) Since we spend much of our time upright, veins have to work against gravity to push blood back to the heart.

Ordinarily, muscular activity of the legs and valves inside the veins prevent blood from flowing backward. When the valves become less efficient for some reason, blood begins to "pool" in superficial veins in the legs, ankles, and feet. Over time the vein walls bulge, creating bumpy, distended varicose veins.

Why do varicose and spider veins develop? Here are several reasons:

➤ Both men and women can develop them, but they're more common in women. The hormones estrogen and progesterone may play a role, since puberty, contraceptive pills, and hormone replacement therapy after menopause seem to encourage their development.

➤ Another common cause: pregnancy. This may be due partly to hormones, partly to maternal weight gain. In particular, the weight of the abdomen might partially restrict blood return from the legs and contribute to the formation of varicose veins. (As we saw in Chapter 14, up to 40 percent of pregnant women develop them.)

➤ In general, being overweight places greater strain on leg veins. A complicating factor is that overweight people are more likely to develop other medical conditions that can impair healthy blood flow, such as high blood pressure, diabetes, and heart disease.

➤ If you stand for long periods, this increases your risk of varicose and spider veins. It's simply that much harder for your veins to fight gravity and do their job.

➤ High-heeled shoes stress leg veins further by forcing your calf muscles to stay contracted for long periods of time.

➤ A tendency to varicose and spider veins seems to run in families. If your parents and siblings develop them, you could, too.

➤ Sometimes an injury can damage veins and set the stage for later problems.

➤ Facial spider veins, especially visible in fair complexions, may be related to sun exposure in some people. Heavy alcohol drinkers and people who eat a lot of spicy or hot foods also seem more likely to develop spider veins on the face. On the other hand, many people with facial spider veins develop them even if they avoid all risk factors.

> **Beauty Tips**
> Another cause of varicose veins: Tight, constrictive clothing that restricts blood flow. This includes garters, girdles, hose with elastic leg bands, tight knee socks, poorly fitting undergarments, and pinching waistbands. Comfortable clothes don't just feel good; they're also good for you!

Both varicose and spider veins get more common as time goes by. It's estimated that up to 75 percent of Americans over age 65 have them. In most cases, varicose veins are just a cosmetic nuisance. Occasionally, though, a vein may become red, swollen, tender, and firm, which could be caused by thrombophlebitis (inflammation of the vein with secondary clot formation). If you develop these symptoms, call your doctor immediately.

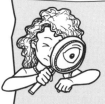

More Than Skin Deep

Sometimes spider veins on the face are a symptom of rosacea, a skin condition most often seen in fair-skinned women who have a tendency to flush. In rosacea, the face tends to become red and develops red bumps and sometimes small spider veins. If your spider veins are accompanied by outbreaks of small pimples and pinkish patches, consult your doctor. (For more on rosacea, see Chapter 15, "Acne: An Age-Old Problem.")

How Do You Get Rid of Them?

Perhaps, like Kay, you're glad to know what causes varicose and spider veins—but you're more interested in getting rid of them! Don't get discouraged, because effective treatments are available.

These veins tend to be superficial (right under the skin), and they're not the only blood vessels in the vicinity. This is fortunate because it means you can get rid of them without jeopardizing your circulation.

Sclerotherapy: Irritating Veins Into Leaving

The most common treatment for zapping spider veins is *sclerotherapy*—injecting an irritating solution that causes the lining of the vessel to swell, stick together, and shrivel. When blood can no longer pass through, the vein loses its purple color. Over several weeks, the vein turns into scar tissue that fades, eventually becoming less visible or disappearing almost entirely.

In the United States, the most frequently used sclerotherapy agent is a concentrated saline solution. Saline is effective and doesn't cause allergic reactions, but it does have a drawback: Saline injections can be painful and irritating to the skin around the injection site, and some patients get muscle cramps.

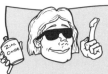

Skin Smart
The most common treatment for spider veins is *sclerotherapy*—injecting an irritating solution that causes the lining of the vessel to swell, stick together, shrivel, and eventually fade.

Sometimes other chemicals are used, such as sodium morrhuate. A chemical called Aethoxysklerol® is widely used in Europe and the United States, although it is not FDA-approved for this purpose. Other products are also available.

Superficial veins sometimes result from deeper vascular problems. Before you undergo sclerotherapy for spider veins, your doctor may evaluate your legs and look for varicose veins or other signs of deeper vein impairment. He or she might also advise you to have vascular blood flow studies performed. If a deeper problem is detected, it should be corrected before you treat the superficial vessels.

Otherwise, you may treat one set of superficial spider veins, only to find a new set crop up quickly.

If you decide to undergo sclerotherapy, your doctor will cleanse the injection site thoroughly, and then insert a very thin needle into the vein and inject a tiny amount of sclerosing solution. (One-tenth of a milliliter can be enough to zap a spider vein into oblivion.) Many doctors apply a compression dressing over the site to enhance the solution's effects and reduce leakage into surrounding skin. Wearing special compressive stockings for two days after treatment may help shut down the vessel for good.

Many people have more than one unsightly vein, and there's no reason your doctor can't treat several in one visit. Depending on the location of a vessel and how it connects to others, one strategically placed injection may be enough to get rid of several veins.

Depending on its size, a vessel might have to be injected more than once. Schedule treatments at least three to four weeks apart, giving you time to heal and your doctor time to see if further injections are necessary.

Sclerotherapy is not risk-free. Some people develop persistent brownish stains at the injection site that take six to 12 months or longer to disappear. If the solution is accidentally injected into tissues around the vein, or if it leaks from the vein, a skin ulcer and sometimes scarring could result.

Up to one-third of patients develop new groups of very tiny red blood vessels near the injection site of spider veins (especially on thighs). Most of them eventually disappear on their own, although some might need sclerotherapy, too. Complications are more common when treatment involves large vessels rather than small spider veins, so I generally avoid treating anything larger than spider veins with this method.

Generally, however, sclerotherapy is highly effective. Even if it doesn't make all the offending blood vessels vanish completely, about 90 percent of patients feel it makes them look a lot better.

Other Treatments

If the vessel is too large for sclerotherapy to be an option, your doctor may recommend surgery to tie off a vessel (a process called *ligation*) or remove it ("*stripping*" the vein). For this procedure, you will probably want to consult a specialist in vascular surgery. Usually these procedures are done only on large varicose veins that are painful, ulcerated, or apt to bleed.

Saving Your Skin
Legally, any physician can perform sclerotherapy; there is no certification or qualifying exam required. However, it takes a sure hand to inject just the right amount of solution into just the right spot. As with any cosmetic procedure, protect yourself by choosing an experienced doctor who has done many of these procedures.

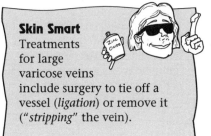

Skin Smart
Treatments for large varicose veins include surgery to tie off a vessel (*ligation*) or remove it ("*stripping*" the vein).

Facing Up to Facial Spider Veins

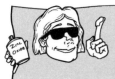

Skin Smart
Electrodesiccation, a method for treating facial spider veins, transmits an electric current through a tiny needle to destroy the vein.

I don't recommend sclerotherapy for facial veins; consider electrodesiccation or laser treatments instead. (For more on cosmetic laser treatments, see Chapter 23, "Better Looking with Lasers.")

In *electrodesiccation,* your doctor inserts a tiny needle which transmits an electric current that destroys the vessel. This procedure can be done in the doctor's office. It should not cause a scar, although sometimes it can leave a tiny depression that resembles a pore.

How to Keep Them from Coming Back

Okay, you've gone through the treatments, those ugly veins have vanished, and for the first time in a decade you're wearing shorts. Now, how can you keep them from coming back?

It's frustrating, but true: Varicose and spider veins often develop because of lifestyle factors, such as being overweight, wearing tight clothing and socks, and spending lots of time standing in one place. If these conditions still exist, be aware that more varicose and spider veins could appear. And if spider or varicose veins run in your family, your tendency to develop more of them could be higher no matter what you do.

Sometimes unhappy patients will insist that problem veins have returned after treatment. This may be true, if deeper vessels are "feeding" the more superficial ones. Often what happens is that other vessels in the area respond to the same precipitating factors, become engorged with blood, and form new varicosities.

Beauty Tips
Exercise doesn't have to be formal or arduous to benefit your blood vessels. Even walking just 10 or 15 minutes, several days a week, is a good start. For more guidelines on exercise, see Chapter 8, "Keeping That Youthful Look."

This makes prevention an important component of varicose vein therapy. For a recap of factors that encourage their development, see "What Causes Varicose and Spider Veins?" above. Other pointers:

➤ If you have any health condition (diabetes, for example) that affects your circulation, talk to your doctor about effective ways to treat it. Stabilizing your condition will promote healthy blood flow.

➤ If you're overweight, try to lose a few pounds. Any amount you can lose will make things that much easier on your leg veins.

➤ If you tend to be sedentary, consult your doctor about starting an exercise program. Regular physical activity keeps your blood moving—literally! Walking is great for leg veins. The muscular contraction and relaxation of the legs during walking and other exercise helps the blood return in the veins and improves circulation.

➤ Wear comfortable, loose-fitting clothes. Please, throw away the girdles, as well as undergarments that act like girdles but go by more elegant names: body shapers, slimmers, and so on. Anything that restricts circulation to and from your legs can contribute to the formation of varicose and spider veins.

➤ Wear comfortable, flat or low-heeled shoes that allow you to walk normally. If you must wear high heels, slip them off periodically to relax your calf muscles. Remember, repeated contraction and then relaxation of the leg muscles enhances blood return. Constant contraction doesn't.

➤ Speaking of restricted circulation, don't sit with your knees crossed or sit on your legs. This is a great way to reduce blood flow.

➤ Keep blood from pooling in your legs and feet. If you must sit for long periods, flex your feet periodically or elevate them if possible. If you can, stand up every now and then and stroll around a bit.

➤ On the other hand, if you have to stand a lot, try to contract and relax your leg muscles (which promotes circulation). Rise on your toes and come back down several times. Walk around if you can. Try to sit down and elevate your legs several times a day. If your feet swell, raising them at least 12 inches above the level of your heart can help.

➤ Ask your doctor whether you should wear support hose. It's important for them to fit well, because poorly fitting stockings can make varicose veins worse, not better.

➤ If you have severe or recurring problems with leg veins, you might even want to have support hose tailor-made so you're sure they fit. Some people need stockings that provide firm, even support over the entire leg; others do better with "graduated" hose that are tightest at the ankle and get looser as they go up the leg. For best results, put on the stockings before getting out of bed in the morning.

Beauty Tips
Hate the idea of support hose? Give them a chance. Many companies have come out with supportive stockings that are almost indistinguishable from "regular" hosiery. You can even find them in black and iridescent colors for formal wear.

The Least You Need to Know

➤ Varicose veins are swollen, twisted veins just beneath the skin surface. Spider veins are patches of tiny red or purple blood vessels. Both develop because blood tends to pool in superficial veins, often in the legs, ankles, and feet.

➤ Women are more likely to develop spider and varicose veins, probably because of hormones and pregnancy. Other risk factors include being overweight, standing for long periods, tight constrictive clothing, vein injuries, and a family history of problem vessels. Facial spider veins may be related to sun exposure, heavy drinking, or eating a lot of spicy or hot foods. Often they appear independently of these risk factors.

➤ The most common treatment for zapping spider veins is *sclerotherapy*—injecting an irritating solution that makes the vessel shrivel and fade. This is usually effective. Even if the vein doesn't disappear entirely, it will probably look better.

➤ Facial spider veins are treated with electrodesiccation or laser therapy.

➤ Even though varicose and spider veins will probably disappear after treatment, more could develop. The ideal is to reduce your risk of new varicosities by altering lifestyle factors that made them appear in the first place. Maintain a healthy weight, exercise regularly, and consider wearing support hose. If your job requires a lot of sitting, flex your feet periodically, keep your legs elevated if possible, and stand up and walk around when you can. If you have to stand a lot, try to contract and relax your muscles to promote circulation.

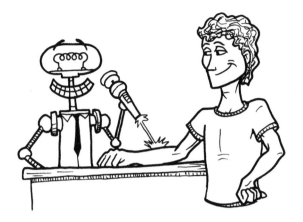

Better Looking with Lasers

When she isn't working, Vicki always seems to be outdoors: rock climbing, hiking, cycling, you name it. She has to be one of the most energetic, upbeat people I know.

So I was surprised recently when she walked into my office looking a bit depressed. "What's wrong?" I asked.

"Oh, I feel silly even mentioning this," she replied. "But it's weighing on my mind, so I decided to come see you. It's just—I love being outdoors, even though I know it's hard on my skin. Lately I've started wearing sunscreen and a hat, but I guess it's too late because I'm already getting wrinkles. Seems like my freckles keep getting darker too. I've been hearing a lot about lasers and how they can do great things for your skin. So I was wondering, well, do you think lasers could make me look better?"

Lasers: Our New Weapon Against Aging

Lasers have been getting a lot of attention in medical circles. They can produce wonderful results in many types of surgery, and these days they're being used more and more in cosmetic procedures as well. Laser technology is leading to a lot of exciting new developments that hold great promise in our quest for beautiful skin.

The word *laser* is actually an acronym; it stands for **l**ight **a**mplification by **s**timulated **e**mission of **r**adiation. (Got that?) A laser is a device that produces a concentrated beam of light; that laser beam consists of a single pure wavelength, with light waves traveling parallel to each other.

Two factors, wavelength and aim, affect the action of a laser beam. The wavelength determines how deeply the light penetrates into the skin and how it is absorbed. Aim is crucial because only cells in the beam's direct path are affected; neighboring cells are relatively unharmed.

Laser emissions vaporize the cells that absorb them. If the beam is sharply focused, high-intensity beams can slice through skin like a scalpel. (They have an important advantage over scalpels, though: As they cut, they also seal small blood vessels. Compared to conventional surgery, laser incisions are relatively bloodless.) If the beam is "defocused," vaporization of the surface skin occurs, as used in laser skin resurfacing.

> **Skin Smart**
> The word *laser* is an acronym that stands for **l**ight **a**mplification by **s**timulated **e**mission of **r**adiation. A laser is a device that produces a concentrated beam of light.

There are many types of lasers, each producing light of a characteristic wavelength and intensity. Lasers are specialized: One wavelength will work on a certain cell pigment or component, but not on others. One device can vaporize black pigment, such as a tattoo, but it won't be nearly as effective on the red pigment of a port wine stain; conversely, lasers that eradicate port wine stains might have little impact on black tattoos.

Lasers used in cosmetic procedures include the following:

➤ Carbon dioxide (CO_2) laser, which emits a colorless infrared light that is absorbed by the water in skin cells to vaporize tissue.

➤ Argonlaser, which produces a green or blue-green light that's absorbed by the red pigment in blood and by the skin's brown pigment, melanin. Argon lasers are used to treat port wine stains, spider veins, cherry angiomas, some hemangiomas, benign sun freckles, and mask of pregnancy. Since pigmented cells in the epidermis may also absorb this wavelength, the argon laser shouldn't be used on dark skin. Even in fair complexions, melanin cells could absorb the light and leave areas of lighter-pigmented skin.

➤ Argon-pumped tunable dye laser, a yellow-light device useful for treating unwanted blood vessels.

➤ Flashlamp-pumped pulsed dye laser, which shoots short pulses of yellow light that are absorbed by the red pigment in blood, destroying the blood vessel and leaving it to be reabsorbed by the body. The pumped-dye laser can remove port-wine stains, red birthmarks, hemangiomas, and enlarged blood vessels.

➤ Neodymium:Yttrium-Aluminum-Garnet laser, more commonly known as the Nd:YAG. Its light is absorbed by brown marks such as "liver spots" and freckles.

➤ Erbium:YAG (Er:YAG) laser, a newer technology that is reported to cause less heat damage and skin redness than carbon dioxide devices. Some doctors feel it may be better for performing laser resurfacing.

➤ Q-switched ruby laser, which shoots short powerful bursts of red light. It's helpful for removing tattoos and brown spots. Since the wavelength is also absorbed by pigments in the dermis and epidermis, it can sometimes leave areas that are lighter colored than before.

➤ Copper vapor laser, a yellow- or green-light device that can emit light pulses so short and rapid they appear to be continuous. It's helpful for treating benign pigmented marks.

Currently, the carbon dioxide laser is the one most often used for skin resurfacing.

Laser Peels: Resurfacing Your Skin

One of the most popular cosmetic laser procedures, and the one that interests Vicki, is *laser resurfacing* (also called a *laser peel*)—using a laser to remove superficial, and sometimes not so superficial, layers of skin. Often it is done with a pulsed-mode carbon dioxide laser.

Why are pulsed-mode lasers so popular? While conventional lasers have been used in medicine for years, their rays of continuous, highly concentrated light are so intense that they quickly burn deep into tissue. This makes them great for slicing through skin and excising tissue inside the body, but it's impractical for treating superficial conditions on the skin surface. Deep penetration quickly leads to charring, which can leave unsightly scars.

Skin Smart
Laser resurfacing, also called a *laser peel*, uses a laser to remove superficial layers of skin.

The pulsed laser, however, produces short bursts of energy, separated by pauses of less than one-thousandth of a second. Tiny though these intervals are, they make a huge difference in the amount of heat generated and transferred into adjacent tissue.

The result? Pulsed-mode lasers give the physician greater control of how deeply the beam will penetrate and how much tissue will be removed. The energy bursts vaporize target cells without significantly harming other tissues. This is handy for removing wrinkles, pigmented marks, and small scars.

Another helpful feature: the laser energy can be adjusted from about 10 to 540 pulses per second. The longer the pulses, the deeper the beam's penetration. Long pulses are effective for areas of thicker skin, such as around the lips; shorter pulses and a lighter touch work better for the thin delicate skin around the eyes.

When doctors first started doing facial laser resurfacing, they discovered an unexpected bonus: In addition to improving surface defects, the laser heat shrinks underlying collagen fibers by about one-third of their length and tightens surface skin. After a laser resurfacing, the skin isn't just smoother—it's often more taut.

Going for Your Laser Resurfacing

If you decide to try laser resurfacing, your doctor may prescribe tretinoin (see Chapter 13, "Tretinoin and Antioxidants: The Age-Tamers?") or bleaching agents for several weeks beforehand to prepare your skin. Your procedure will be done on an outpatient basis in an operating room.

First, your face will be cleaned thoroughly. You'll be given either general anesthesia or a local anesthetic, depending on the extent of the resurfacing and your preferences. Anesthetic drops may be placed in your eyes, along with special steel contact lenses to protect your eyes against the laser light. You'll be covered with a layer of dry surgical drapes, topped by wet drapes to prevent fire if the beam accidentally touches the material.

Your doctor, wearing special eye-protecting goggles, will gently move the laser across your face in a rhythmic motion, treating one area of skin at a time. Often two to three passes are made.

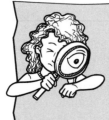

More Than Skin Deep

Most laser devices are versatile, allowing the doctor to adjust the beam multiple times during a procedure. Different energy levels and beam shapes, such as thin lines, large triangles, or small hexagons, may be used. Some lasers even shoot tiny doughnut-shaped beams to treat acne pocks.

The device is fitted with a vacuum tube that sucks in most of the vapor, although if you're awake you'll be able to smell smoke. Even with the anesthetic, you might feel slight impacts from the pulsing beam; Vicki compares it to rubber bands snapping against your skin. Depending on the equipment, the whole procedure could take anywhere from 45 minutes to two hours.

Afterward, your face won't bleed, but it will look red and raw, with shiny oozing blisters. Your doctor may offer you a choice of being bandaged or not. Each approach has its pros and cons.

If you choose to be bandaged, a dressing will be placed over your face immediately after the procedure to protect your skin from the open air. Some doctors leave the bandage in place for a few days and then have the patient apply creams to the face until it heals in about one and a half to two weeks. Other doctors keep the dressing in place for seven to 10 days. This may be inconvenient because you must keep it completely dry, which means baths instead of showers and having someone else wash your hair. However, the dressing protects your face, reduces discomfort, and shortens the healing period; you should feel able to face the public again in about 10 days.

If you leave your face unbandaged, you'll bypass the inconvenience of the dressing but the healing process will take a bit longer, perhaps two weeks, and you could experience greater discomfort. You'll have to wash your face four to 10 times per day with soap and water, and use special solutions to dissolve crusts that form. Don't pick or pull at the crusts, because this could lead to scarring. You'll be given directions to moisturize your face several times daily with Vaseline™ or another heavy lubricant.

Whether your face is bandaged or not, good oral hygiene is important to minimize infections and complications. Brush and rinse your teeth at least twice daily. Ask for instructions on how to clean your lips and the skin around your mouth.

Your doctor may recommend taking tretinoin after the procedure to help your skin heal better. Some patients also take bleaching agents to help prevent differences in skin pigmentation. Many patients' complexions have a reddish hue after laser resurfacing. It may fade promptly, but sometimes it persists for weeks or months and must be camouflaged with makeup.

Admittedly, recovering from laser resurfacing isn't fun. The fun begins after your face heals, when you start to get admiring comments from family and friends.

Saving Your Skin

If your face is bandaged following a laser resurfacing, be sure not to get any food or liquid under the dressing because it could lead to infection or irritation. Use a straw or infant "sip" cup when you take a drink.

Saving Your Skin

When moisturizing newly resurfaced skin, open a fresh new container of lubricant each time. Otherwise, you risk infecting your vulnerable flesh. Stock up ahead of time on samples and trial sizes, so you don't have to waste large (and expensive) containers.

Beauty Tips

Many patients ask when they can start using makeup again after laser resurfacing. My answer: Wait about two to two and a half weeks until the skin has fully healed and feels normal. If the makeup burns when you apply it, remove it gently and wait several more days. Your skin isn't ready yet.

The price of a laser resurfacing? Not cheap. Fees for full-face resurfacing range from about $3,000 to $5,000. If cost is an issue, you might consider a regional procedure in which just part of your face is treated; regional jobs run about $1,500 to $2,000. But remember, resurfaced areas are likely to be reddish afterward. Regional procedures could leave you with tell-tale differences in your complexion for a while.

Getting the Most from Your Laser Resurfacing

Here are some tips for making a laser resurfacing the best experience possible:

➤ Be realistic in your expectations. Laser resurfacing can give a big boost to your appearance, not to mention your ego, but please remember it isn't magic. The procedure may tighten skin, but it isn't a face-lift; it won't banish sagging necks, double chins, or very loose folds of skin. For these conditions, consider plastic surgery (see Chapters 24, "Should You Try Plastic Surgery?" and 25, "Popular Choices in Plastic Surgery").

➤ Asians, Hispanics, and African Americans are more likely to experience pigmentation problems, such as patches of lighter or darker skin, after laser resurfacing. For this reason, the procedure may not be appropriate for people with darker complexions.

➤ If you have been taking Accutane® for acne, it can affect your skin's ability to heal. Consult your doctor about how long you must be off the drug before laser resurfacing.

➤ If your skin tends to scar easily or form keloids (large raised scars), you might not respond well to the trauma of laser therapy.

➤ If you've ever had cold sores, you should take the antiviral drug acyclovir before and after the procedure. A viral infection at this vulnerable time could spread over your entire face and cause scarring.

➤ Follow your doctor's instructions carefully for pre- and post-procedure care. These details and skin-care routines are time-consuming but important; they prepare your skin for the ordeal and help it recover as soon as possible.

Saving Your Skin
Laser resurfacing makes your skin more susceptible to infection. For this reason many doctors prescribe a course of antibiotics for laser patients. Many also prescribe a course of acyclovir for all laser patients, whether they've ever had cold sores or not.

People with extremely ruddy complexions, highly sensitive skin, or numerous facial spider veins may not be good candidates for laser resurfacing. If your face shows lots of blood vessels, consider getting laser treatments for the spider veins first, before undergoing resurfacing. For more information, read on.

Zapping Spider Veins with Lasers

In the preceding chapter, we saw that sclerotherapy can be helpful when spider veins, those annoying patches of tiny red or purple blood vessels, appear on the legs and feet. Well, spider veins may appear in other places, too. On the legs and elsewhere, another treatment option is to zap them with a laser (such as the copper vapor, flashlamp-pumped pulsed dye, or other lasers). These devices heat the blood inside the veins and damage the inner wall, making the vessels shrivel and disappear.

To reduce the risk of bleeding, avoid taking aspirin, ibuprofen (such as Motrin® or Advil®), vitamin E supplements, or any blood-thinning drugs for at least two weeks before the procedure. The laser treatment normally lasts five to 15 minutes; during that time, you'll wear protective eyegear. There could be some discomfort; patients report that, like laser resurfacing, it feels like rubber bands slapping the skin.

Post-treatment, the area is likely to be pink or bruised; it should heal within two weeks. If you had leg veins treated, wear an elastic bandage or support hose for several days.

It might take more than one session to eradicate all spider veins. Even after laser treatments, sclerotherapy may still be necessary to get rid of stubborn vessels.

Post-procedure infections and scarring are rare. However, about 10 percent of patients who have spider veins treated report light- or dark-colored pigmentation changes in the area of the vessels. Usually, these changes are temporary and fade with time.

Both sclerotherapy and lasers can be effective in removing spider veins on the legs. Each method has its advantages and disadvantages, so the choice is up to you and your doctor. For eradicating spider veins on the face, lasers are far superior to sclerotherapy. In fact, I do not recommend sclerotherapy for facial veins at all.

Incidentally, as we saw in Chapter 22, "Zapping Varicose and Spider Veins," spider and varicose veins are often lifestyle related. Whether you have them removed by sclerotherapy or lasers, be aware that new vessels may take their place. See Chapter 22 for tips on preventing them.

> **Beauty Tips**
> If you're having laser treatments on your legs, wear shorts or a skirt to your appointment so the doctor can easily reach your spider veins. You may want to bring long pants to wear afterward, because your legs will probably be bruised or pink.

Getting Rid of Other Skin Marks

Lasers can minimize and possibly eradicate various types of skin marks, including tattoos, freckles, "age spots," port wine stains, hemangiomas, cherry angiomas, and mask of pregnancy. As we saw earlier, it all depends on the wavelength of the laser and how it's aimed.

The laser beam works by penetrating the skin and splitting targeted cells into tiny fragments that are then removed by the body. Several laser treatments may be necessary to eradicate marks completely. The blood vessels that form port wine stains, for example, are not uniform, so it may take more than one session to eliminate all of them. Erasing an amateur tattoo often takes about six sessions, while a professional tattoo may require 10 or more.

Occasionally, laser treatments leave a scar or an area of skin that's permanently lighter or darker. Rarely, the texture of treated skin will change and become a little more rough. In general, though, laser treatments can be a great way to get rid of many different unwanted lesions.

When Lasers Are Overkill

Beauty Tips
The least expensive way to banish a wart is to apply an over-the-counter liquid wart remover. Most contain salicylic acid, a beta hydroxy acid that slowly exfoliates the wart away. Be patient, because it can take weeks or months to see results.

Having said that, however, I do want to mention that there are times when lasers are overkill, comparable to using a machine gun on a mosquito. Consider the following instances:

➤ If you're trying to get rid of a skin tag, other options—snipping with sterile scissors or burning with an electric needle—may be just as effective, at a much lower price.

➤ If a wart is driving you crazy, try an over-the-counter wart remover. If that doesn't work, your doctor can apply stronger removers, freeze the wart, or surgically remove it.

For more ideas on getting rid of benign skin marks and bumps, see Chapters 16, "Solving Common Skin Problems," and 18, "Benign Bumps." If there is any chance that a lesion could be cancerous, it should be properly evaluated before being removed. For more on identifying and getting rid of cancerous growths, see Chapter 19, "Skin Cancer: The Dark Side of the Sun."

Are Lasers Better?

Many patients ask me whether lasers are safe, and how they compare to more established therapies, such as chemical peels and dermabrasion.

Frankly, you'll find a certain amount of disagreement, even among doctors, over which method is best, how long the benefits of laser treatments last, and what the possible risks may be. Actually, lasers, chemical peels, and dermabrasion share many of the same risks, which include the possibility of infection, scarring, and post-procedure pigment changes. With phenol peels, the risk of skin lightening is greater than with lasers, but lasers may leave more post-procedure redness.

The main advantage to lasers may be their skin-tightening effects because of the collagen shrinkage they cause. Also, with lasers (as with dermabrasion) the doctor might have a little more control over the precise depth of the procedure. However, this is not always the case. It has a lot to do with how experienced a doctor is in the procedure he or she is performing.

What about the long-term effects? Physicians have had years to follow up on the results of chemical peels and dermabrasion. Many have only recently begun to perform laser procedures, so they haven't had time to assess their patients' long-term progress.

More Than Skin Deep

A few laser manufacturers are building freestanding laser centers that offer resurfacing and other procedures. While many of these facilities are staffed by qualified doctors, some may not always have a qualified physician on the premises. My advice: Don't base your choice on location or convenience. Find a physician you trust to perform your laser procedure, and go to the facility that he or she recommends.

However, new information on lasers is coming in all the time. One study, which tracked the progress of 300 laser-resurfacing patients for 12 to 18 months after treatment, found that improvement in facial wrinkles and scars remained consistent through that time.

A joint study by dermatologists at the Medical University of South Carolina and the University of Melbourne (Australia) has identified several possible complications of laser resurfacing. All may be temporary if treated promptly. They include the following:

➤ Approximately 10 to 20 percent of laser resurfacing patients develop darker pigmented areas of skin within four weeks after the procedure. Tretinoin cream and bleaching cream can minimize these marks if applied soon after they appear. Many doctors prescribe tretinoin and bleaching agents for all their laser patients to prevent pigmentation problems in the first place.

➤ Between 1 to 6 percent of patients develop red, irritated skin creases, perhaps caused by tight adhesive bandages. Trimming off the irritated edges prevents further problems. Some doctors have stopped using these bandages.

➤ Perhaps 1 percent of all laser patients (and 4 percent of those who received more aggressive resurfacing for deeper wrinkles) get small scars. Weekly injections of steroids, if started right after scars appear, can soften the scars and may prevent them from becoming permanent.

Saving Your Skin
Like chemical peels and dermabrasion, laser resurfacing leaves your skin more vulnerable to UV. While your skin recovers, avoid direct sunlight and wear a strong sunscreen. If you're not in the habit of using sunscreen, test it before the procedure to find a product that doesn't irritate your skin. The last thing you need afterward is a skin reaction!

For moderate wrinkles and scars, laser resurfacing seems just as effective as deep chemical peels; it may even be better because of the possible skin-lightening side effects of phenol. Also, with lasers the doctor can go a little deeper in trouble spots, thus giving a more uniform result. And laser has the added benefit of possibly tightening the skin, which further helps wrinkles. For more superficial wrinkles and pigmentation problems, it's not yet clear whether lasers are better than other treatments. Ultimately, it depends on your individual situation, and this is a decision only you and your doctor can make.

Before deciding on any cosmetic procedure or plastic surgery, it's crucial to do your research, know your options, and find a well-qualified doctor. In Chapter 24, "Should You Try Plastic Surgery?" I'll discuss strategies for doing just that.

The Least You Need to Know

➤ A laser is a device that produces a concentrated beam of light. There are several types of lasers, each producing light of a characteristic wavelength and intensity. One wavelength is great for zapping spider veins, another is ideal for eliminating freckles.

➤ Laser resurfacing, usually done with a carbon dioxide laser, removes superficial layers of skin. An unexpected bonus: Laser resurfacing can shrink underlying collagen fibers by up to one-third, making skin tighter as well as smoother. After laser resurfacing, follow your doctor's skin-care instructions closely to avoid infections and complications that could cause scarring.

➤ Lasers are also an effective way to get rid of spider veins and skin marks, such as freckles, port wine stains, tattoos, "age spots," hemangiomas, cherry angiomas, and mask of pregnancy. It can take more than one laser treatment to get rid of a mark completely. Stubborn spider veins might need additional sclerotherapy.

➤ For some skin marks, such as skin tags and warts, lasers may be overkill. Consult your doctor about other, less expensive ways to get rid of them. If there is any chance a skin growth could be cancerous, it should be properly evaluated before being removed.

➤ The long-term benefits and risks of laser treatments are still being evaluated, although laser resurfacing may have some advantages over deep chemical peels. Treat all laser resurfacing complications promptly, before they become serious.

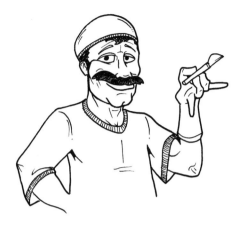

Chapter 24

Should You Try Plastic Surgery?

In This Chapter

➤ Find out if plastic surgery is for you

➤ Get the scoop on who's having what done where

➤ See if your insurance might pay for your procedure

➤ Discover how to cover up with cosmetics while you're healing

➤ Learn how to find a qualified plastic surgeon

Meredith takes excellent care of herself. She exercises regularly and eats healthfully. Sensible and analytical, she carefully researches all the skin care products that touch her face. She's definitely not one to be swayed by the latest fad.

Soon after her fifty-second birthday, she made an appointment with me. "I feel a bit silly bothering you about this," she began with uncharacteristic hesitation. "I know people come to see you all the time with real problems, and I feel like I shouldn't even mention it."

"It's just that I feel so self-conscious about my wrinkles," she continued, "not to mention this sagging stuff under my chin. My daughter videotaped my birthday party last week, and I couldn't help noticing how old I look. I worry about it, and at the same time I'm annoyed with myself for even paying attention. Fifteen years ago, I laughed at the idea of plastic surgery—and now I find myself actually considering it! Do you think plastic surgery would be a good idea?"

"You're the only one who can make that decision," I said. "But certainly a lot of people are having plastic surgery these days, and most of them get good results. Why not look into it? With your talent for doing careful research and weighing the options, I know you'll come up with the right answer."

Would You Benefit from Plastic Surgery?

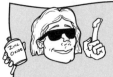

Skin Smart

Plastic surgery is a surgical specialty dedicated to the reconstruction of facial and body defects present from birth, or caused by injury, burns, disease, or aging. Procedures performed mainly to improve the appearance of a healthy person are called cosmetic surgery.

"Why is it called 'plastic' surgery?" Meredith asked me. While we associate the term *plastic* with modern man-made objects, it derives from the ancient Greek word *plastikos*, meaning "to mold or shape." *Plastic surgery* is a surgical specialty dedicated to the reconstruction of facial and body defects present from birth, or caused by injury, burns, disease, or aging. Many of the first plastic surgeries were done to close difficult wounds or replace tissue lost from trauma or cancer.

Today, many people are getting interested in plastic surgery's potential to correct those telltale signs of aging: wrinkles, sagging skin, unsightly fat. Or, they might choose surgery to correct design flaws caused by Mother Nature rather than Father Time. These endeavors fall under the heading of *cosmetic surgery*: procedures performed mainly to improve the appearance of a healthy person.

Who's Getting What Done Where?

Who's having cosmetic surgery? A lot of people! While many plastic surgeries are still done to remove tumors and repair injuries, cosmetic procedures are growing more common every day. According to the American Society of Plastic and Reconstructive Surgeons, Inc., a professional organization, the number one cosmetic procedure is liposuction, which removes unwanted fat deposits; about 110,000 are performed every year.

While many people want liposuction done on the neck, it can also trim hips, buttocks, thighs, abdomen—or just about anywhere you feel you're carrying a bit too much baggage. Other popular cosmetic surgeries include eyelid repair (more than 76,000 procedures per year), face-lifts (over 53,000), and forehead lifts (about 23,000). In Chapter 25, "Popular Choices in Plastic Surgery," I'll go into more detail about each of these.

Once limited to celebrities and other folks of high net worth, plastic surgery is getting steadily more democratic. These days 70 percent of patients have yearly incomes under $50,000; 30 percent make less than $25,000.

The trend is likely to continue. About 27 percent of cosmetic surgery patients have more than one procedure done at a time; 17 percent are repeat customers. In a recent survey, more than half of Americans said they could see the day coming when cosmetic nips and tucks would be as routine as hair dyes.

Should you jump on the plastic surgery bandwagon? Perhaps, but do remember that cosmetic surgery is still surgery. All surgery carries some risk, and it's impossible for the surgeon to absolutely guarantee the final results. Ultimately, the outcome will be determined not just by the surgeon's skill, but also by your individual anatomy, how your body reacts to surgery, and how well you heal.

Here are some pointers for maximizing your chances of a happy ending:

➤ First and foremost, be realistic. While plastic surgery can definitely improve your appearance, it won't transform you into the top model or movie star of your dreams. Also, while it may subtract years from your face, it can't stop the clock from continuing to tick. The results might look great, but they can't be permanent. Ask your surgeon what you can realistically expect from the surgery—and be willing to accept the answer.

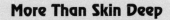

More Than Skin Deep

Most people seek plastic surgery so they can look like themselves, only better. Not so the patients of one plastic surgeon I've heard about, who specializes in helping people resemble their favorite celebrities. Elvis Presley is a particularly popular choice; this doctor has surgically crafted several clones of The King, one so successfully that the man now places highly in Elvis look-alike contests.

➤ Recognize that your concerns about your appearance are valid, and don't feel you must apologize for them—to yourself or anyone else. Like Meredith, many people feel self-conscious inquiring about plastic surgery; they worry that they're being vain and silly. However, this attitude is an impediment that will only make it more difficult to ask questions and do the research necessary to make an informed decision. Relax! It's natural to want to be attractive and make the most of yourself.

➤ Have a complete medical exam. If you have any chronic health conditions, seek treatment so they are well controlled. Be sure to give your plastic surgeon a complete health history and a list of all the medications you take, both prescription and over the counter. (This includes aspirin, which can interfere with blood clotting—an important surgical consideration, and any vitamins or herbs you may be taking.)

➤ Cosmetic surgery is most successful when your skin is elastic enough to heal well and maintain its newly crafted tautness. For this reason, many plastic surgeons recommend having procedures done in your 40s, 50s, or 60s. That doesn't mean cosmetic surgery can't be successful on 70- or 80-year-olds, because it can. However, the trend is toward having procedures done earlier rather than later.

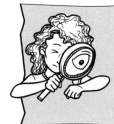

More Than Skin Deep

Smoking cigarettes greatly increases the risk of surgical complications. Some plastic surgeons refuse to perform elective cosmetic procedures on smokers. If you're having trouble quitting, here's one more good reason to do so.

➤ The best candidates are people close to their healthy weight. There's no way around it: Excess fat tissue stretches skin. If you have surgery to tighten sagging skin, but gain weight later, your skin will stretch again. Maintaining a healthy weight will help maintain the positive results of your cosmetic procedure.

➤ Remember, before the surgery makes you look better, it's going to make you look a lot worse! No one is presentable in the days following a cosmetic procedure. When you glance in a mirror, you may wonder why you did it. Ask your surgeon ahead of time what you can realistically expect in terms of discomfort and recovery time. You might even ask to see photos of patients in various stages of healing, so you'll be prepared.

Beauty Tips

I've had patients schedule plastic surgery a few weeks before a wedding or important business trip, only to be disappointed (and embarrassed) because their skin still showed signs of trauma. Schedule surgery for a time when you can be away from work and other commitments for at least two weeks. Allow six months for healing before a major event.

➤ Plan for "downtime." At the very least, you'll need someone to drive you home after the procedure. You may also need extra help around the house for days or weeks.

➤ Don't rush to sample the latest techniques. The media frequently trumpet new products and surgeries as the ultimate cure for aging. It's tempting to jump right in and try them. But remember, it could take years before side effects and complications become apparent. You don't want to be the guinea pig for an experimental procedure; opt for the tried-and-true with a known track record for improving appearance.

And here's another point: The newer the procedure, the less time surgeons have had to practice it. When it comes to something as important as your face, there's no substitute for experience.

Plastic Surgery: Not for Women Only

Traditionally, cosmetic surgery has been regarded as a "female" concern. While it's still more common among women than men, the fact is that men are catching up fast. Today almost one-quarter of U.S. cosmetic procedures involve men, a huge increase in only 10 years. Do you assume that most male patients are Hollywood types? Guess again; the majority are businessmen, aged 40 to 60.

Favorite male cosmetic procedures: hair transplants, eyelid surgery, and getting rid of undereye bags. Some guys get facelifts, others opt for liposuction. A few go for more exotic touches, such as implants to beef up buttocks, chest muscles, or calves.

While most cosmetic surgery advice pertains to both men and women, male patients do have a few issues of their own. For instance, their facial skin has a richer blood supply, so they bleed more during surgery. Men are more likely than women to develop post-surgical pooling of blood under the skin (a hematoma).

Since they don't wear makeup, men also have a harder time hiding surgical scars. If your hair is thinning, scars could be especially tricky; talk with your surgeon about the best placement of incision lines. (One plus: You won't have to shave for several weeks after surgery while your skin heals, and whiskers may help conceal telltale signs of certain surgeries.)

More Than Skin Deep

If you're considering hair-replacement surgery, be aware that it generally requires multiple procedures separated by long periods of recovery to assess how the transplants "take." A full regimen of hair transplants could last 18 months, two years, or more, and the transplant sites may be obvious to other people, especially during early stages. If this doesn't seem compatible with your job or lifestyle, ask about alternatives, such as hair weaves, scalp reduction, or minoxidil (see Chapter 7, "Beautiful Hair and Nails," for more information).

Who Pays? Probably You!

If plastic surgery is being done for reconstructive purposes (such as breast reconstruction following a mastectomy), your health insurance may pay for it. If your goals are cosmetic, however, better save up your cash. Most cosmetic cases are done on a fee-for-service basis with no health insurance coverage.

An exception might be if you can demonstrate a health-related need for the surgery. For instance, some patients get at least partial coverage for having a nose restructured by showing it will improve their breathing. Procedures to remove precancerous marks or spots may also be covered. In rare cases, surgery to raise drooping eyelids improves vision enough to qualify for insurance.

It never hurts to ask your doctor about circumstances that could provide at least some coverage. If your insurance provider does agree to chip in, get a written confirmation of what it will pay. However, in most cases, be prepared to hear that the total bill is your responsibility.

How large will the bill be? Fees for plastic surgery vary widely, depending on the procedure and the region of the country. Even within the same community, prices will differ. Surgeons' fees for a forehead lift range from $1,500 to $5,000; the national average is $2,000. (This doesn't include the costs for anesthesia, the operating room, if one is used, and other surgical expenses, which can add more than $1,000 to the bill.) Surgeons' fees for a face-lift start as "low" as $4,000 and go up to $18,000 or more; anesthesia and possibly operating room costs may tack on another $2,000 to $3,000.

Endoscopic Surgery: Small Incisions with Big Results

Endoscopic surgery involves the use of an *endoscope*, a special viewing instrument that allows a surgeon to see images of the body's internal structures through very small incisions. The endoscope is a viewing device only; a separate surgical instrument—such as scalpel, scissors, or forceps—must be inserted and manipulated, often through a different incision.

Endoscopic surgery has been around for years (for instance, to remove gallbladders and repair arthritic knee joints), but it's fairly new in plastics. The advantage? It allows the surgeon to operate through smaller incisions, which reduces the risk of scarring. Many endoscopic procedures can be performed on an outpatient basis, and recovery time tends to be shorter.

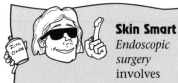

Skin Smart

Endoscopic surgery involves using an *endoscope*, a special viewing instrument that allows a surgeon to see images of the body's internal structures through very small incisions. While endoscopic surgery isn't new, it's a relatively recent technique in cosmetic surgery.

Sound enticing? It is, but be aware that endoscopic cosmetic surgery is relatively rare. Of the roughly two million plastic surgery procedures done each year, only about 21,300 are endoscopic. This option is most often offered with forehead lifts; about 50 percent are done with an endoscope. A few other procedures—breast augmentation, face-lifts, and tummy tucks (abdominoplasty)—can be done with an endoscope, but most are still done with conventional (open) surgery.

If your doctor suggests endoscopic surgery, it's important to do your research. Clearly the technique has great potential, but you need to feel comfortable with your surgeon's level of experience. The endoscopic approach has its drawbacks as well as advantages, including the risk of infection, damage to blood vessels or nerves, internal perforations, and accumulated fluid beneath the skin, which may need to be drained.

Refer to "Finding a Great Plastic Surgeon" later in this chapter for guidance. In addition, make sure your surgeon has privileges to perform both the endoscopic procedure and its conventional version at an accredited hospital. If a complication occurs during surgery, your doctor may have to switch to the open technique.

Covering the Damage: Cosmetics to the Rescue

Regardless of which procedure you choose, whether endoscopic or conventional, I can promise you one thing: You won't look your best afterward for at least several days. Almost everyone suffers temporary swelling, redness, and bruising, not to mention unappetizing incision lines. Depending on the procedure and your skin's healing ability, it may take weeks or months before you feel completely back to normal. In the meantime, a little strategic makeup can help you cover the damage and show your best face in public.

Ask your doctor for advice about the best products to buy and when you can start using them. As a general rule, look for products that are hypoallergenic, fragrance free, and irritant free. If you have stitches, hold off on makeup until the sutures have been removed and all incisions are completely closed. If you've had eyelid surgery, wait for your doctor's okay before using eyeliner.

Some tips:

➤ To mask bruised and pinkish areas, try a color corrector. These tinted cosmetics are complementary to skin tone and help neutralize it. A green color corrector can help to balance reddish patches from surgery; a pink corrector can offset green and yellow bruises.

➤ Over the corrector, apply concealer (flesh-colored and similar to foundation, but thicker and more opaque) to cover incision marks, scars, and bruises. Choose one that covers well, but with a light enough texture that you can apply it without pulling on your skin.

➤ Minimize swollen areas (such as cheeks and the sides of your nose) by shading them with a foundation slightly darker than the concealer. You may also want to highlight other areas (such as cheekbones) with a slightly paler foundation to make them more prominent. Be careful to blend everything smoothly together; you don't want to look striped!

Beauty Tips
Don't use concealer around your eyes or on wrinkled skin. It's heavy, and will collect in lines and accentuate them. Apply your regular foundation in those areas instead.

While you recover, you might find yourself applying more makeup than usual or using makeup that's thicker and more opaque than your usual brand. Be sure to remove it completely every night. For tips on effective cleansing, see Chapter 4, "Clean Living: The Best Way to Clean Your Skin."

Finding a Great Plastic Surgeon

Okay, having read this far, you've decided to keep going and consult a plastic surgeon. How can you find the one who's best for you?

As I told Meredith, this is where your research skills come in. After all, you don't want just anyone messing with your face, do you? The results of this procedure are going to be with you for a long time, and you want to make the experience as healthy, pleasant, and rewarding as possible. It's worth spending time and effort to find a plastic surgeon you trust and feel comfortable with.

Legally, any doctor can perform plastic procedures. While some of these practitioners do excellent work, others may have less experience than you would prefer.

I recommend looking for a physician who is board-certified in plastic surgery. What does board-certified mean? To earn this credential, issued by the American Board of Plastic Surgery, a doctor must have graduated from an accredited medical school, completed three or more years of residency training in general surgery or an equivalent specialty, and then completed at least two additional years of residency training in plastic surgery. After that, the surgeon must practice plastic surgery for at least two years and pass written and oral exams before being board-certified.

More Than Skin Deep

The American Society of Plastic and Reconstructive Surgeons is a professional organization that includes most board-certified plastic surgeons. The Society distributes helpful brochures describing various cosmetic surgeries; it also offers a referral service. You can get the information free by calling the Society or by downloading it from their World Wide Web site. For information on contacting the Society as well as other resources, see Appendix A, "Bountiful Resources for Beautiful Skin," at the end of this book.

Here are some good sources to check with:

➤ Your family doctor and dermatologist may be able to recommend a plastic surgeon. Ask how many people they've referred to this surgeon, whether the patients went ahead with the procedure, and what they thought of the results. Would they send a family member to this person?

➤ Call a respected local hospital and ask for a list of board-certified plastic surgeons who have "privileges" to perform the specific procedure you're considering. If a surgeon has hospital privileges, that means she or he has been officially approved to perform that type of surgery at that facility.

➤ Nurses and other operating room personnel see what goes on behind the scenes, after patients are asleep. They also have the opportunity to watch surgeons in action and observe how they respond to stress and emergencies. This can be a useful perspective. Ask who they would choose if they planned to have your surgery.

➤ If you know people who have had plastic surgery, by all means ask how they liked their surgeon and whether they'd recommend him or her. I recommend consulting the sources mentioned in this chapter in addition to your friends, however. Tempting though it may be to rely on their opinion, every patient is an individual. While you may think a pal's eyelids look great after surgery, there's no guarantee her plastic surgeon can make yours look the same. Your bone structure, skin, and health history are uniquely your own, and so are the results of your surgery.

Saving Your Skin

Even if you're not planning to have your surgery done in a hospital, make sure your plastic surgeon has hospital privileges to perform that particular procedure. There have been cases of surgeons losing hospital privileges because of negative surgical outcomes, but continuing to operate in outpatient surgery centers or their offices.

From all this information, create a list of plastic surgeons you'd like to consult. I recommend meeting with at least two or three of them to discuss your goals, the procedures that would be best for you, and the results you can realistically expect. You may find striking consensus, or you might be surprised at how different their suggestions are. The more practitioners you consult, the broader your basis for comparison will be.

You'll probably have to pay for each consultation. Yes, it hurts to spend the money, but look on it as an investment in your health (and your face). Interviewing plastic surgeons is a crucial part of your research. The more information you gather, the better informed your decision will be. Some surgeons will count the consultation fee toward your surgery, so ask about this option.

Before the appointments, read up on the procedures you are considering. If you already have a general idea of what's involved, you won't have to spend valuable time asking basic questions. Bring a written list of queries with you, so you can refer to it. As you chat, note whether the surgeons are willing to answer questions, discuss their qualifications, and explain medical information in terms you can understand. Steer clear of anyone who makes you feel silly for asking questions or worrying about risks.

Some questions to ask:

➤ Which cosmetic procedure do you recommend for me, and why? Would you have it done on yourself?

➤ How many of these procedures have you done, and how often do you do them?

➤ Are there any nonsurgical treatments that could produce similar results? (For instance, if wrinkles are the main concern, would laser resurfacing or a chemical peel be just as effective?)

➤ What are the risks and complications of this surgery? What outcome can I realistically expect? Should I expect to look younger, and if so, in what way?

➤ Can I see before-and-after photos of people who have had this procedure? (Ask if you can talk to several patients, to see how they feel about their experience.)

➤ What should I expect during the surgery? Do you recommend general or local anesthesia?

➤ How much discomfort should I expect during recovery, and how long will it take to recover? How much time should I set aside to be off work?

➤ What scars does this procedure usually leave, and how can I hide them?

➤ How long will the results last?

More Than Skin Deep

While they're recovering, plastic surgery patients look less wrinkled because their skin is swollen. As the swelling subsides, facial lines will become more visible, although they should be less obvious than before the procedure. Take this into account when viewing before-and-after photos; ask how long after the procedure the pictures were taken. Photographs of still-healing faces will look unrealistically smooth.

If you are considering more than one procedure (for instance, eyelid surgery with a facelift), ask if the surgeon would recommend doing both at the same time. This approach can save time and money because you don't have to come back for repeat surgery. On the other hand, it can also increase the risk of complications.

Be wary of surgeons who gloss over potential risks and complications. (As one of my colleagues notes, if they haven't encountered any problems, they haven't done enough surgery!) The vast majority of people who have plastic surgery are glad they did. My goal is to make sure you're among them.

The Least You Need to Know

➤ Plastic surgery is dedicated to the reconstruction of facial and body defects present from birth, or caused by injury, burns, disease, or aging. Procedures performed mainly to improve the appearance of a healthy person are called *cosmetic surgery.*

➤ To be a good candidate for cosmetic surgery: Be realistic about what you expect from it; maintain a healthy weight; be a non-smoker; have a complete medical exam first; be prepared to look worse before you look better; and opt for tried-and-true procedures over the latest fad. Cosmetic surgery is most successful on people whose skin is elastic enough to heal well and maintain its new shape.

➤ Cosmetic surgery isn't cheap, and it's rarely covered by health insurance. An exception might be if your doctor can demonstrate a health-related need for the surgery.

➤ Look for a physician who is board-certified in plastic surgery and has hospital privileges to perform your particular surgery. Get names from your family doctor, dermatologist, nurses, local hospitals, and acquaintances who have had similar procedures.

➤ Interview two or three plastic surgeons before making your decision. Find out about their qualifications and experience with this particular procedure. Ask what you can realistically expect in terms of results, risks, complications, and recovery time. Are there any nonsurgical treatments that would be just as effective?

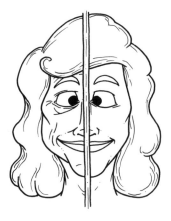

Popular Choices in Plastic Surgery

Last week I saw Meredith again. "You look great," I told her.

"I feel great!" she exclaimed. "I followed all your suggestions, found a great plastic surgeon, and decided to go ahead with it. I had a face-lift, and while I was at it, I had liposuction to get rid of my double chin. Before the surgery, I'd been dreading my high school reunion; now I'm actually looking forward to it. All my friends tell me how good I look. What an ego boost!"

"Dr. Gordon," she continued, "I can't thank you enough for the time you spent with me. Your advice was really helpful. It made all the difference in my finding a good surgeon and getting good results!"

This is the physician's best reward: a happy patient. In this chapter, I'll alert you to the latest in cosmetic surgery techniques, and show you how to make those beautiful results last as long as possible. I want you, like Meredith, to be a satisfied customer!

Liposuction: Bidding Farewell to Fat

Got any fatty tissue you don't want? (Silly question, right?) Then you might want to consider *liposuction*, which uses a tube and vacuum device to remove exercise-resistant fat deposits. (Sometimes you'll see it called *suction-assisted lipectomy*, *liposculpture*, or *lipoplasty*.) About 110,000 liposuctions are performed every year, making it the leading cosmetic procedure in the United States.

Popular sites for liposuction include chin, cheeks, neck, upper arms, above the breasts, abdomen, buttocks, hips, thighs, knees, calves, and ankles. Pockets of excess fat tissue are broken up, then vacuumed away through a small hollow tube. While liposuction isn't a substitute for overall weight loss, it can be a great way to get rid of localized padding.

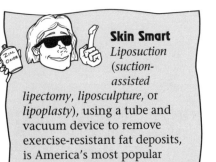

Skin Smart

Liposuction (suction-assisted lipectomy, liposculpture, or lipoplasty), using a tube and vacuum device to remove exercise-resistant fat deposits, is America's most popular cosmetic procedure.

The best candidates for this procedure are close to their healthy weight, but with pockets of unwanted fat in specific areas. Another plus: elastic skin that will adapt readily to your body's new contours. If your skin is loose, it may ripple or sag. If you've ever gained or lost significant amounts of weight, tell your surgeon because this can affect the elasticity of your skin. (In some cases, excess skin folds can be removed in a separate surgery.)

Before you undergo liposuction, have a thorough physical exam. This procedure is not recommended for people with poor circulation, heart conditions, lung disease, or a history of blood clots. It also may not be a good idea if you have varicose veins or recent surgery on the same area you want suctioned. Be sure to tell your surgeon about all health problems, even apparently minor ones. If you undergo abdominal liposuction without warning your doctor you have a hernia, for instance, it could be accidentally punctured. Some people are simply not good candidates for liposuction, so be wary of any doctor who agrees to do it without examining you first.

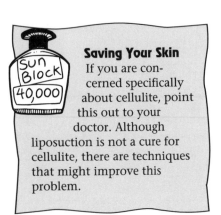

Saving Your Skin

If you are concerned specifically about cellulite, point this out to your doctor. Although liposuction is not a cure for cellulite, there are techniques that might improve this problem.

Liposuction is usually done on an outpatient basis, in the surgeon's office or a hospital or surgery center. On the day of your procedure, here's what you can expect:

➤ Before the action begins, you'll be asked to undress and stand as the surgeon marks areas of fat deposits on your body. This might seem a bit strange, but these marks provide important guidelines to follow during surgery. After you lie down, your fat tissue will settle into your body; without this "map," it would be hard to judge where and how much to suction.

➤ Your body will be painted with liquid disinfectant, and you'll lie down on the operating table. Depending on the area to be suctioned and your preferences, you'll be given either sedation, general anesthesia, or localized anesthesia to numb the lower part of your body. An IV (intravenous) line may be placed in your arm to administer medication and fluids.

➤ After you're asleep (under general anesthesia) or awake but comfortable, the surgeon makes a small incision and inserts the hollow tube into fatty tissue. By manipulating the tube, the surgeon breaks up the fat into pieces small enough to be suctioned through the tube. More than one incision may be necessary to remove all the targeted fat. Even with local anesthetic, you may feel some vibration, tugging, or stinging.

➤ The procedure can last anywhere from 30 minutes to several hours, depending on how much fat is being removed and how difficult it is to reach. While the extracted fat is sucked into a container that continuously measures how much has been removed, the surgeon must also exercise his or her own judgement by observing the amount left and comparing it to other parts of your body. (This is an art as well as a science. You can see how important it is to find an experienced surgeon!)

➤ A snug elastic dressing will be placed over the treated area; this controls swelling and compresses the incision holes. You should wear it 24 hours a day for two to three weeks, then just at night for a few weeks more, depending on your surgeon's instructions.

Saving Your Skin
If you plan to have extensive liposuction, talk to your doctor about donating blood in advance. It can be stored and held for you in case you bleed enough to need a transfusion.

Afterward, as with many cosmetic procedures, you'll probably wonder at first why you did it. In the following weeks, you won't look slim and trim. Far from it; you may even look heavier because of swelling, bruising, and the extra fluids you received during surgery. The suctioned areas will feel sore, and they may burn or feel numb.

The soreness should start to improve within a week, and normal sensation will return. Most of the swelling and bruising should resolve within two months, although some swelling could remain for six months or more. Avoid strenuous activity for two to four weeks. However, your doctor may advise you to start walking around as soon as possible to prevent blood clots from developing.

While liposuction is generally considered a relatively safe procedure, there is still a small risk of complications such as blood clots, dehydration (you lose a lot of fluid when fat tissue is suctioned), and, in rare cases, perforation of organs. If you experience any unusual symptoms during recovery, like heavy bleeding or increasing pain, call your doctor immediately.

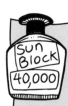

Saving Your Skin
Can liposuction be fatal? Yes, in rare cases. Of the approximately five million liposuctions done since 1983, about 15 patients have died. Many of them were probably not good candidates for the procedure to begin with. If you've been counseled not to have liposuction for health reasons, follow this sensible advice.

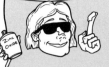

Skin Smart
In *tumescent liposuction*, the surgeon first injects targeted fat cells with an anesthetic solution that constricts blood vessels. This reduces blood loss and postoperative pain, swelling, and bruising.

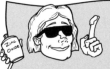

Skin Smart
Ultrasound-assisted liposuction uses ultrasound waves to emulsify fat before suctioning it out. While not a substitute for conventional liposuction, it can be effective for removing large pockets of fat or fat from fibrous body areas.

There is another risk: You might not like the results. About 10 to 20 percent of liposuction patients end up with irregular body contours noticeable enough to require touch-up liposuction. Most surgeons don't charge extra for a touch-up, but you will have to pay for the operating room, if used, and anesthesia. Wait at least three months after the procedure to decide whether you need a touch-up because you will still be swollen.

Most liposuction veterans, though, love their new body shape. How long do the results last? For many years, especially if you avoid gaining weight. A healthy diet and regular exercise are essential for maintaining your new contour.

Two newer liposuction techniques, tumescent and ultrasound, are available now and may reduce the risk of complications.

Tumescent Liposuction

In *tumescent liposuction*, the surgeon first injects targeted fat cells with an anesthetic solution that constricts blood vessels. The average liposuction patient loses more than a pint of blood during the procedure; with tumescent liposuction, blood loss drops to less than half a pint. This technique also reduces postoperative pain, swelling, and bruising.

The main advantage of tumescent liposuction is that all that local anesthetic solution reduces the amount of sedation needed and makes general anesthesia unnecessary. Another great advantage is the reduction of blood loss. Also, as the solution is injected, the fat in that area becomes swollen, firm, and pale (*tumescent* comes from the Latin word for "to swell"), making it easier to manipulate the tube with less tissue damage.

After a tumescent procedure, you can typically return to normal activity within a few weeks. After about three weeks, most of the swelling should subside; all swelling should be gone after three months.

Ultrasound-assisted Liposuction

Another promising technique is *ultrasound-assisted liposuction*, which uses ultrasound waves to emulsify the fat before suctioning it out. While not a substitute for conventional liposuction, ultrasound-assisted liposuction can be an effective tool for removing fat from fibrous body areas, such as the male breasts or the back, or for removing large pockets of fatty tissue. Sometimes the two techniques are used during the same procedure to treat different parts of the body.

Ultrasound-assisted liposuction causes less bleeding than the conventional technique, but shares many of the other risks. Plus, it's more likely to cause fluid to pool under the skin, and it's possible for the ultrasound device to burn the skin. It generally takes longer than traditional liposuction and may require the placement of drains in the skin for a few days to siphon off fluid.

Eyelid Surgery: Opening Your Eyes to the Possibilities

Maybe your upper eyelids droop more than they used to. Maybe your lower eyelids look puffy and baggy. Perhaps the whole eye area just seems wrinkly, crinkly, and tired.

For any of these reasons, you may want to consider *eyelid surgery (blepharoplasty)*, which removes fat and trims excess skin and muscle from upper and lower eyelids. Successful eyelid procedures can open up your eyes and make you look more alert and youthful; sometimes they may even help you see better. They are among the most popular facial cosmetic procedures in the United States.

Before undergoing eyelid surgery, have a complete medical exam. Occasionally, undereye bags can signal a thyroid or kidney problem. A few health conditions—including high blood pressure, heart disease, and diabetes—make eyelid procedures more risky. You should also have a thorough eye exam to check for glaucoma, a detached retina, and other eye problems that can complicate post-surgical healing.

Skin Smart

Eyelid surgery (blepharoplasty) is a procedure to remove fat and excess skin and muscle from upper and lower eyelids.

If you wear glasses or contact lenses, bring them along when you consult your surgeon. Also bring relevant information from your most recent eye exam. During this appointment, your vision and teardrop production will be evaluated. If your eyes are extremely dry and too much eyelid tissue is removed, infections or corneal damage could result.

Discuss your goals and expectations with the surgeon. Do you want to "do" just the upper eyelids, just the lower, or all four? Does one eye need more work than the other? (It's not uncommon to have asymmetrical eyes.) Do you want only the fat removed, or would you also like to see less skin? What do you want the final result to look like; would you like to preserve or change the overall shape of your eyes? Consider bringing photos of eyes you admire, or a sketch of the effect you want. Maybe you could even bring a recent photo, and mark directly on it to show how you'd like your eyes to look different. The more explicit you can be, the more satisfied you'll feel with the outcome.

If you decide to have eyelid surgery, here's what you can expect:

➤ Most often, you'll be given sedation and a local anesthetic that numbs the area around your eyes; some surgeons prefer general anesthesia. The whole process usually lasts one to three hours.

➤ Protective steel contactlenses may be placed on your eyes, your face will be cleaned with antiseptic, and sterile drapes will be placed around your eyes. The surgeon makes incisions that follow the natural curve of your eyelids, and removes underlying fatty deposits. If you have excess skin or muscle, the surgeon may trim them slightly as well before closing the incisions with tiny stitches.

➤ If you want just the lower eyelids done, to remove fat but not skin, your surgeon can make an incision inside the lower lid and remove the fat. This approach should not leave a visible scar.

➤ Afterward, your eyes will be lubricated and possibly bandaged. Your lids will feel tight and sore. The doctor will prescribe pain medication; placing cold saline compresses on your eyes will make them feel better and also reduce swelling. You'll be given instructions on how to care for your eyes, including cleaning them and using eyedrops.

➤ It's important to remain as quiet and still as possible for at least 24 hours. In rare cases (an average of four in 10,000 patients), eyelid surgery results in visual impairment or blindness. Often, this is due to bleeding behind the eyeball, caused by bending over, lifting objects, vomiting, sex, or other actions that raise blood pressure too soon after surgery. If you experience sudden pain or changes in vision, call your doctor immediately.

➤ Keep your head elevated for several days after the procedure, even when sleeping. Sleep in a reclining chair, or prop your head on extra pillows in bed. Don't lie face down for two to three weeks. If you tend to roll over onto your stomach during sleep, try sewing a large ball into the front of your nightshirt to make this position uncomfortable.

Saving Your Skin
You're likely to need some assistance after eyelid surgery; it's hard to do even routine chores with your eyes bandaged! Furthermore, bending and moving around increase your risk of complications. Arrange ahead of time to have temporary help for about three weeks.

➤ Recognize that you'll feel miserable for up to a few weeks. Your eyes will burn and feel itchy, weepy, and gummy. You'll probably be sensitive to light, and you may experience temporary visual problems like blurring or double vision. You should be able to read or watch TV after three days, but contact lens wearers will have to leave their lenses out for about two weeks.

After eyelid surgery, most people feel ready to face the world again within 14 days. However, for the next three weeks or so, you should avoid anything that raises your blood pressure, like vigorous exercise and sports. In addition, avoid things that raise pressure in the head and eye area like bending over and lifting. Your eyes may be sensitive to sunlight and wind for several weeks; wear dark sunglasses and sunscreen while you're outdoors. In most cases, you'll be left with thin scars that will eventually fade to almost invisible white lines. Often your surgeon can place the incision so these scars are hidden by the natural fold of your eyelid.

About 5 percent of eyelid patients need touch-up surgery after the first procedure, sometimes because there is more than one pocket of fat in the lids. An eyelid procedure will not completely eliminate crow's feet, lift sagging eyebrows, or get rid of dark undereye circles entirely. It can, however, give you an alert, well-rested, youthful look that may last five years, a decade, or longer.

> **Saving Your Skin**
> In rare cases, if too much skin is removed or scar tissue develops inside the lower lid, the lower lid could be pulled down after surgery. This "basset hound" look is often temporary. If it persists, further surgery can correct it.

Face-lifts: Presenting Your Best Face to the World

Hate those creases between nose and mouth? Vexed with those vertical lines on your neck? Is your jawline more jowly than it used to be? If you answered yes to any of these questions, you might want to consider another popular cosmetic procedure. A *face-lift* improves facial appearance by removing excess fat, tightening muscles, and redraping skin (the medical term is *rhytidectomy*, derived from the Greek word for "wrinkles").

A face-lift can take eight to 10 years off your appearance. It'll make you look fresher and more rested. Like Meredith, many patients find it also boosts their self-confidence and helps them achieve a more positive, outgoing attitude.

As with all cosmetic procedures, though, it's important to be realistic in your expectations. A face-lift will improve the face you already have, but it won't make you look like someone else. If you weren't born with high cheekbones or a chiseled jaw, a face-lift won't create them for you. (There are other surgical procedures that may do these things; consult your surgeon for details.)

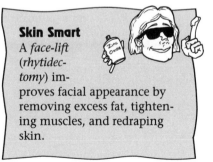

> **Skin Smart**
> A *face-lift* (*rhytidectomy*) improves facial appearance by removing excess fat, tightening muscles, and redraping skin.

This procedure does a great job of lifting sagging skin, but it has little effect on fine wrinkles, crow's feet, or lines around the mouth. (To improve small wrinkles, consider a laser or chemical peel, or a prescription for tretinoin.) A face-lift does little for the upper part of the face (forehead, eyebrows, and the area around the eyes), which is why some people combine it with a forehead lift (see the following section, "Forehead Lifts: Raising Your Eyebrows").

A face-lift is a highly individual procedure. As with eyelid surgery, it's important to discuss your desires and expectations with your plastic surgeon. Consider bringing a sketch of the effect you want, or marking directly on a recent photo. A qualified surgeon will be honest with you about the degree of improvement you can expect. At the same time, please remember that plastic surgery is an art as well as a science, and there are many variables that can affect the final outcome.

Most face-lift patients are between the ages of 40 and 60, but the procedure has been done with great success on 70- and 80-year-olds as well. To get a realistic idea of what it can do for you, lie on your back and hold a mirror above your face. This is a more reliable guide than pulling your skin back with your fingers, which distorts your face.

> **Saving Your Skin**
> In rare cases, some skin cells die after a face-lift because their blood supply is cut off by tight stretching. Smokers are 20 times more likely than nonsmokers to experience skin loss—one reason surgeons are reluctant to do face-lifts on them. Even nonsmokers should avoid secondhand smoke for at least a week after the procedure; it can irritate healing cells.

A face-lift is major surgery, with potential for serious complications. A small percentage of patients (about 1 to 2 percent) experience postoperative bleeding under the skin, which sometimes can be drained and at other times requires more surgery. And 1 to 2 percent develop infections that generally respond well to antibiotics. Another risk is damage to the nerve that controls facial muscles. About 1 to 2 percent of patients suffer nerve damage; the risk rises to 5 percent with more aggressive techniques that cut deeper into subcutaneous tissue.

How can you protect yourself against these complications? Stop smoking, and have a complete medical exam. The most common cause of postoperative bleeding is high blood pressure, so you shouldn't have a face-lift until your pressure is under control. Any health condition that impairs blood supply to the skin—such as diabetes or circulatory disorders—could retard the healing process, and people with chronic illnesses may heal more slowly.

Here's what to expect if you decide to go ahead with a face-lift:

➤ Before the surgery, your hair will be washed with antibacterial shampoo and fastened away from your face. The surgeon will mark circles on your face to delineate the fat distribution under your skin; as with liposuction, these marks serve as guideposts during surgery.

➤ Most face-lifts are done with a sedative and a local anesthetic, so you'll be awake but drowsy and numb; you may occasionally feel some tugging or discomfort. Some surgeons prefer to use general anesthesia, in which case you'll sleep through the procedure.

➤ There are several techniques for doing face-lifts, depending on your face structure and the surgeon's preference. This drawing shows a typical incision, which starts at the temple (above the hairline), extends down in front of the ear, then curves up behind the ear into the lower scalp. The surgeon separates the skin from underlying muscle and fat, and then lifts and tightens all the tissue. Excess skin is trimmed away, and excess fat trimmed or suctioned. Then the tissue is stitched into its new position.

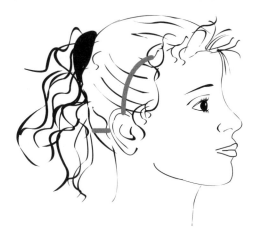

A typical incision for a face-lift starts at the temple (above the hairline), extends down in front of the ear, and then curves up behind the ear into the lower scalp.

➤ The whole procedure can take several hours. Afterward, most patients complain of numbness and tightness rather than actual pain. Your doctor will prescribe medication for the discomfort. Some numbness is normal and should disappear in a few weeks or months.

➤ Expect to see swelling, bruising, and incision lines; your features may look a bit distorted and stiff. Keep your head elevated and stay quiet for the first week or so. You can probably phase into more activity after two weeks, but consult your doctor for specific guidelines.

➤ After three weeks, you'll probably feel and look better. Most patients return to work by this point. As time goes by, the swelling will subside and you'll continue to improve. You'll always have some scars, although they will fade. In any case, generally they're hidden by your hair or the natural folds of your face and ears.

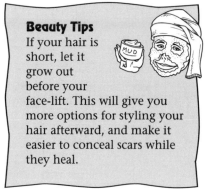

Beauty Tips
If your hair is short, let it grow out before your face-lift. This will give you more options for styling your hair afterward, and make it easier to conceal scars while they heal.

Be patient. The full benefit of your face-lift might not be apparent until months after the procedure.

Forehead Lifts: Raising Your Eyebrows

As I mentioned earlier, a face-lift can do great things for your cheeks and jawline, but little for your forehead or eye area. For this reason some people combine it with a *forehead lift* (sometimes called a *brow lift*), which removes muscle and other tissue to smooth the forehead, raise the eyebrows, and minimize frown lines. Of course, you can also have a forehead lift done by itself, or with eyelid surgery, liposuction, or almost any other cosmetic procedure. If you're tired of sagging eyebrows or stubborn forehead lines, whether horizontal or vertical, a forehead lift may be in your future.

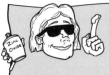

Skin Smart
A *forehead lift* (sometimes called a *brow lift*) removes muscle and other tissue to smooth the forehead, raise the eyebrows, and minimize frown lines.

Before deciding on a forehead lift, sit down with your surgeon and discuss your goals. How far above your eyes do you want your eyebrows to sit after the surgery? How much would you like them to arch? This is another case where it's a good idea to bring a recent photo and compare ideas about what's possible and desirable.

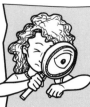

More Than Skin Deep

People can have surprisingly different notions of the perfect eyebrow. Some women favor high eyebrows, placed up to three-quarters of an inch above the brow bone. A generation ago in the United States, the trend was toward brows with a pronounced curve. Today fashion favors a lower, straighter, more natural eyebrow. Make sure your surgeon understands your preference.

Most forehead lifts are performed under sedation and local anesthesia that numbs the forehead, although some surgeons prefer general anesthesia. If you're awake, you may feel some pulling and slight discomfort, but no actual pain.

As with any cosmetic procedure, there's some risk of complications, especially postoperative bleeding under the skin, a blood clot, damage to forehead nerves, or loss of sensation along the incision line. Generally, these complications are temporary and resolve with time. Some patients experience permanent hair loss along the incision scar; further surgery can be done to remove excess scar tissue.

Up to now, we've discussed procedures done with conventional surgical techniques. A forehead lift can be done this way, or it can be performed endoscopically, using a pencil-thin viewing instrument called an *endoscope* that permits smaller incisions. For more on endoscopic surgery, see Chapter 24, "Should You Try Plastic Surgery?"

An endoscopic forehead lift leaves a few small scars, usually above the hairline, compared to an ear-to-ear scar for the conventional approach. Smaller incisions mean less risk of numbness and hair loss. However, endoscopy does carry other risks, including a greater chance of postoperative swelling under the skin and possibly more risk of nerve damage. Furthermore, since it's a newer technique, you'll have to look harder to find a plastic surgeon who's experienced with it, and fewer studies have been done on its long-term effectiveness.

Endoscopy works best on patients with relatively elastic skin, perhaps 45 and younger. Be aware that, if a problem occurs during endoscopic surgery, your surgeon may have to switch to the conventional technique to finish the procedure. The conventional approach might be better if you have loose skin and muscle because the tissue can be trimmed to tighten and smooth your forehead.

Conventional Forehead Lift

If you choose to go the conventional route, here's what you can expect:

➤ Wash your hair the morning of the surgery. Before the procedure starts, your hair will be tied back, away from the area of the incision; some hair may need to be shaved.

➤ The surgeon will make a long incision that goes literally from one ear to the other, traveling across the top of the forehead. Ideally, the incision will be above the hairline so the scar won't show. If your forehead is unusually high or rounded, it may have to be located just below the hairline.

➤ The surgeon will lift the forehead skin and expose underlying tissue. If you have deep frown lines, the surgeon may thin or remove muscle fibers to make it harder to scowl. A strip of excess skin is trimmed from the top of the forehead (perhaps one-half to three-quarters of an inch); the remaining tissue is pulled up to the incision line and stitched down.

> **Beauty Tips**
> Male patients with high or receding hairlines have a harder time concealing forehead lift scars. Consult your surgeon for suggestions; one option is a mid-scalp incision that follows the natural curve of the skull.

➤ The procedure typically lasts two to two and a half hours, longer if you're having other procedures done at the same time. Afterward you might have a headache, but the incision line itself will feel numb. Your face will be swollen, your eyelids bruised, and you may have temporarily blurred vision from the swelling. About 20 to 30 percent of patients also feel nauseated. Your doctor will prescribe medications for the pain and nausea as necessary.

The bruising and swelling will subside, and you should feel ready to face the world in 10 days to two weeks. Most visible traces of the forehead lift should vanish after three weeks. Many doctors recommend avoiding strenuous activity (exercise, heavy housework, sex, anything that raises your blood pressure) for a month or so; consult your surgeon for specific guidelines. As the nerves heal, the incision area may start to itch; the itching should disappear within six months.

Endoscopic Forehead Lift

If you opt for endoscopy, preparations for surgery will be similar to those mentioned previously. During the actual surgery, though, here's what happens:

➤ Rather than making one long incision, your surgeon will make three, four, or five short cuts, each less than an inch long, just above the hairline. The surgeon then inserts a slender endoscope through one of the incisions. The endoscope is connected to a video screen, which displays the muscles and tissues underneath the skin.

➤ Following the picture on the screen, the surgeon inserts an instrument through a different cut to lift the forehead skin and manipulate underlying tissues. As with the conventional forehead lift, muscle fibers may be thinned or removed; eyebrows may be lifted and stabilized in a new position. Then, the surgeon closes the incisions with sutures or clips.

➤ Afterward, you'll experience some numbness, soreness, and swelling around the wounds, but probably less than with the conventional technique. Endoscopic patients also seem to have less trouble with postoperative itching.

Recovery time is often faster than with the conventional forehead lift. Still, consult your doctor for guidelines about resuming normal activities and returning to work.

For detailed descriptions of forehead lifts and the other procedures discussed in this chapter, you might consult *Are You Considering Cosmetic Surgery?* by Dr. Arthur Perry and Robin Levinson. Another helpful resource is the American Society of Plastic and Reconstructive Surgeons (see Appendix A, "Bountiful Resources for Beautiful Skin," at the end of this book).

Making the Results Last

No matter which cosmetic procedure you choose, you'll probably be delighted with the outcome. Many people don't realize how their appearance has altered through the years, until they see what a wonderful difference plastic surgery can make.

Now there's this great-looking person staring back at you from the mirror. So how do you stay this way? While no cosmetic procedure can be permanent, you can do a great deal to protect your enhanced appearance and make it last as long as possible. Here are some guidelines to follow:

➤ If you smoke, stop. In addition to its other negative effects, smoking causes wrinkles and impairs circulation in facial blood vessels (see Chapter 9, "Skin No-Nos"). Many surgeons are reluctant to perform face-lifts or other cosmetic procedures on smokers because their skin takes significantly longer to heal and the results may not look as good. Give your face a break: Quit smoking. While you're at it, stay away from secondhand smoke too.

➤ Stay out of the sun as much as possible, especially during the first six months after your procedure. Sun exposure increases your risk of uneven pigmentation, and it can make scar tissue darken. Plus, as we saw in Chapter 10, "The Sun Is No Fun," ultraviolet rays damage skin cells and accelerate the aging process. This advice goes for tanning salons and sun lamps too.

Saving Your Skin
The guidelines presented in this chapter—indeed, throughout the entire book—are general principles that apply to most people. However, since every individual is unique, your situation may be different. Always consult your doctor for guidance, and ask for clarification if there's anything about a procedure you don't understand.

➤ Wear a good sunscreen—SPF 15 or higher—every day, summer and winter. Look for a moisturizing sunscreen you can wear under makeup, or a foundation with a built-in sunblock. I recommend titanium dioxide as the active ingredient. (See Chapter 11, "Fighting Back Against Photoaging," for more on sunscreens.)

➤ Follow a gentle, low-impact skin care routine; avoid irritating chemicals, harsh cleansers, and trendy treatments. Use the mildest products that are effective on your skin. Stronger isn't necessarily better!

➤ Your skin reflects your overall health, so eat a nutritious diet and get regular exercise. And please, relax every now and then.

Do these tips sound familiar? That's not surprising, because they're the same strategies that made your skin beautiful before surgery, too. Enjoy them in good health!

The Least You Need to Know

➤ Plastic surgery can make you look great, but it's still surgery, with a risk of complications. Follow your doctor's advice closely in preparing for and recovering from your procedure.

➤ Liposuction removes unwanted fat by suctioning it through a hollow tube. It is not a cure for obesity; the best candidates are people close to their healthy weight, who have fat deposits in specific areas. Two new techniques, tumescent liposuction and ultrasound-assisted liposuction, may reduce complications.

➤ Eyelid surgery removes fat and excess skin and muscle from upper and lower eyelids. Be sure to clarify your goals and expectations; you and your surgeon may have completely different ideas of how to improve your eye area.

➤ A face-lift is a great way to lift sagging skin, but it won't improve your basic features or do much for fine wrinkles, lines around the mouth, or the forehead and eye area. Again, clarify what you're looking for.

➤ Forehead lifts can be done with conventional or endoscopic surgery. Endoscopic surgery leaves smaller scars with less hair loss, but has a greater risk of postoperative swelling and possibly nerve damage; since it's newer, it may be harder to find an experienced surgeon. Endoscopic forehead lifts work best on patients with relatively elastic skin.

➤ How do you make the results of plastic surgery last? Stop smoking, avoid sunlight (natural and artificial) as much as possible, and wear a good sunscreen every day. Eat a healthy diet, exercise regularly—and relax. In short, follow the same strategies that made your skin beautiful before surgery!

Bountiful Resources for Beautiful Skin

Helpful Organizations

Accreditation Council for Continuing Medical Education
Suite 7340
515 North State Street
Chicago, IL 60610-4377
Phone: (312) 464-4377
Fax: (312) 464-2586

American Academy of Dermatology
P.O. Box 4014
930 North Meacham Road
Schaumburg, Illinois 60168-4014
Phone: (847) 330-0230
Fax: (847) 330-0050

American Association for Hand Surgery
444 East Algonquin Road
Arlington Heights, IL 60005
Phone: (847) 228-9758
Fax: (847) 228-6509

American Electrology Association
106 Oak Ridge Road
Trumbull, CT 06611
Phone: (203) 374-6667

American Society for Aesthetic Plastic Surgery
3922 Atlantic Avenue
Long Beach, CA 90807
Phone: (310) 595-4275

American Society for Reconstructive Microsurgery
444 East Algonquin Road
Suite 120
Arlington Heights, IL 60005
Phone: (847) 228-9717

American Society of Maxillofacial Surgeons
444 East Algonquin Road
Suite 120
Arlington Heights, IL 60005
Phone: (847) 228-3327

American Society of Plastic and Reconstructive Surgeons
444 East Algonquin Road
Arlington Heights, IL 60005
Phone: (847) 228-9900

American Society of Plastic Surgery
Seven Penn Center
Suite 400
1635 Market Street
Philadelphia, PA 19103
Phone: (215) 587-9322

Association of Academic Chairmen of Plastic Surgery
444 East Algonquin Road
Suite 120
Arlington Heights, IL 60005
Phone: (847) 228-8375

International Guild of Professional Electrologists
308 North Main Street
Suite A
High Point, NC 27262
Phone: (800) 830-3247 or (910) 841-6631
Fax: (336) 841-5187

Helpful Books and Articles

"Beauty by Laser." *Good Housekeeping*, Oct. 1997, p. 145.

Paula Begoun, *Blue Eyeshadow Should Absolutely Be Illegal*. Seattle: Beginning Press, 1994.

Paula Begoun, *Don't Go to the Cosmetics Counter Without Me*. Seattle: Beginning Press, 1996.

Constance Cardozo, "Coming Clean About Cleansers." *Redbook*, Oct. 1994, p. 106.

Donald Davis, "Ironies Abound." *Drug & Cosmetic Industry*, Feb. 1989, p. 21.

Roselyn Payne Epps and Susan Cobb Stewart, co-editors, *The Women's Complete Healthbook*. New York: Delacorte Press/The Philip Lief Group, 1995.

"Facial Cleansers Can Irritate Skin." *The Edell Health Letter*, March 1991, p. 1.

Laura Fraser, "The Price of a Peel." *Health*, July–August 1991, p. 30.

Lisa Fried, "The Wrinkle Report: How Boomers Feel About Getting Old." *Discount Store News*, Sept. 16, 1996, p. S21.

"Hemorrhoids: Agony Enough to Make You Want to Jump Out of Your Skin!" *Nutrition Health Review*, Spring 1992, p. 12.

Peter Jaret, "Lasers: A New Light on Wrinkles." *Health*, Jan.–Feb. 1996, p. 50.

Kathi Keville and Mindy Green, *Aromatherapy: A Complete Guide to the Healing Art*. Watsonville, California: The Crossing Press, 1995.

Michele LaRue, "Considering a Change: Is Plastic Surgery for You?" *Back Stage*, March 18, 1994, p. 34.

Norman Levine, M.D., *Skin Healthy*. Dallas: Taylor Publishing Company, 1995.

Maria Liberati, "Alpha and Beta Hydroxy Acids: The Skin-Care Revolution." *Better Nutrition*, April 1996, p. 70.

Maria Liberati, "The UV, SPF and PABA of Sun Protection." *Better Nutrition for Today's Living*, July 1995, p. 76.

Michael Mason, "Why Anti-Aging Creams Are Hot." *Health*, Oct. 1994, p. 36.

The PDR Family Guide to Nutrition and Health. Montvale, NJ: Medical Economics Company, 1995.

Arthur W. Perry, M.D., F.A.C.S., and Robin K. Levinson, *Are You Considering Cosmetic Surgery?* New York: Avon Books, 1997.

Doug Podolsky, "The Price of Vanity." *U.S. News & World Report*, Oct. 14, 1996, p. 22.

Emily Prager, "Getting Peeled: An Acid Primer." *Harper's Bazaar*, Oct. 1996, p. 270.

Allison Rao, "A-ha! AHA's: The Missing Piece Is Found." *Better Nutrition*, April 1997, p. 70.

Craig Reed, "Fending Off Chemical Photosensitivity." *Consumers' Research Magazine*, June 1996, p. 29.

Henrietta Spencer, "Topical Vitamin C for More Vibrant Skin." *Better Nutrition*, Jan. 1998, p. 30.

Dana Sullivan, "Better Diet, Healthier Skin." *Health*, Nov.–Dec. 1996, p. 44.

Karin Sullivan, "A Little Bit of Heaven at Home: Head-to-Toe Spa Treatments You Can Do Yourself." *Vegetarian Times*, Jan. 1997, p. 60.

Stephanie Tourles, *The Herbal Body Book*. Pownal, Vermont: Storey Communications, 1994.

Ellen Welty, "Could They Really Make Me Look Younger?" *Redbook*, Dec. 1995, p. 70.

Ruth Winter, "Do Anti-Aging Cosmetics Really Work?" *Consumer's Digest*, Oct. 1997, p. 28.

Technical (But Useful) Stuff

Carla Errickson and Nancy Matus, "Skin Disorders of Pregnancy." *American Family Physician*, Feb. 15, 1994, p. 605.

Albert Kligman, M.D., Ph.D., et al., "Topical Tretinoin for Photoaged Skin." *Journal of the American Academy of Dermatology*, Oct. 1986, p. 836.

"New Study Outlines Special Hazards of Indoor Tanning." *Business Wire*, July 24, 1995, p. 7241156.

Gerald Pierard, M.D., Ph.D., et al., "Effect of Hormone Replacement Therapy for Menopause on the Mechanical Properties of Skin." *Journal of the American Geriatrics Society*, June 1995, p. 662.

Henry Roenigk, Jr., M.D., "Treatment of the Aging Face." *Cosmetic Dermatology*, April 1995, p. 245.

Mark Rubin, M.D., "The Use of Chemical Peels in the Age of Lasers." *The Journal of Clinical Dermatology*, Winter 1998, p. 38.

Victoria VanderKam and Bruce Achauer, "Laser Resurfacing of the Face." *Plastic Surgical Nursing*, Fall 1997, p. 134.

Skin Care in Cyberspace

Accreditation Council for Continuing Medical Education
http://www.accme.org

AcneNet (Roche Laboratories, Inc.)
http://www.derminfo-net.com/acnenet

American Academy of Dermatology
http://www.aad.org

American Cancer Society
http://www.cancer.org

American Society for Aesthetic Plastic Surgery
http://www.surgery.org

American Society of Plastic and Reconstructive Surgeons
http://www.plasticsurgery.org

BeautyBuzz Bookstore
http://www.beautybuzz.com/bookstore.asp

Canadian Journal of Plastic Surgery
http://www.pulsus.com/plastics/home.htm

Derminfo-Net
http://www.derminfo-net.com

International Guild of Professional Electrologists
http://www.bworks.com/igpe/

MedicineNet
http://www.medicinenet.com

Misty Isle Elements Library
http://www.mistyisle.com/library.htm

Paula Begoun Cosmetic Cop Site
http://www.cosmeticscop.com

U.S. Food and Drug Administraton (FDA)
http://www.fda.gov/fdahomepage.html

Women's Link (Bristol-Meyers Squibb)
http://www.womenslink.com

Glossary of Skin Care Terms

Acne   A skin condition characterized by plugging and inflammation of pores and surrounding skin. It can take many forms, including *blackheads* (enlarged dark pores), *papules* (red bumps), *pustules* (pus bumps), or *cysts* (larger swellings beneath the skin surface). Severe cases are referred to as *cystic acne.*

Actinic keratoses   Small scaly precancerous growths, most commonly found on skin that's had a lot of sun exposure.

Allergy (allergic reaction)   An inappropriate or abnormal response by the immune system to a substance that doesn't affect most people.

Alpha hydroxy acids   Acid extracts, often from various plant sources, that act as mild exfoliants.

Anaphylaxis (anaphylactic shock)   A severe, potentially life-threatening allergic reaction. Symptoms of anaphylaxis include warm skin, redness or hives, wheezing and difficulty breathing, muscle cramps, and fainting.

Antioxidants   Chemicals that prevent or reduce the destructive effects of free radicals.

Asteatotic eczema   Type of dermatitis that results when skin becomes so dry that it gets inflamed, red, and itchy.

Atopic dermatitis   A chronic skin inflammation in people with an inherited tendency toward allergies.

Atypical (dysplastic) nevi   Benign irregularly shaped and/or colored moles that sometimes can look similar to early melanoma. They may have a slightly higher risk of becoming cancerous than other moles.

Autologous collagen injections   Injecting transplants of your own collagen tissue into another part of your body; done to fill wrinkles or scars.

Autologous fat transplants   Removing fat tissue, often from thighs or buttocks, and transplanting it somewhere else on your body to fill in wrinkles or scars.

Basal cell cancer   The most common form of skin cancer; a skin-colored or pink bump or nodule, usually with a "pearly" smooth surface, which usually appears on sun-exposed areas like the head and neck. They may crust and bleed spontaneously or with minor trauma.

Benign   Not cancerous.

Benzoyl peroxide   A drying agent and a mild antibiotic for treating acne, available both by prescription and over the counter.

Beta hydroxy acids   A class of acids, including salicylic acid, which are used as exfoliants.

Birthmark   A common term (although it has no medical meaning) for a skin mark that is present from birth or develops at a young age. See also **Vascular lesions**.

Black widow   Poisonous shiny black spider, often found in dark damp outdoor places. Its venom is a neurotoxin, rarely fatal.

Blepharoplasty   See **Eyelid surgery**.

Bo-Tox™ (botulinum toxin) injections   Injections of botulinum toxin are used to temporarily paralyze the muscles that cause frown lines. Also used for horizontal forehead lines and sometimes for crow's feet.

Bovine collagen   Collagen derived from cow skin, the most commonly used material for filling minor skin defects.

Brow lift   See **Forehead lift**.

Brown recluse   Brown or brownish-yellow poisonous spider that prefers dark dry environments, such as crevices in or around houses. The skin in a bitten area may die, becoming purple or black and then ulcerating.

Capillary (strawberry) hemangioma   Type of hemangioma (benign collection of blood vessels) which is raised and bright red.

Cavernous hemangioma   Type of hemangioma (benign collection of blood vessels) that is a purple to bluish color and often spongy.

Cellulite   A type of fatty tissue containing bands of collagen fibers. The fibers restrict cellulite's ability to stretch, which gives the skin a characteristic dimpled appearance.

Chemical peel   Painting the skin with a liquid acid solution that exfoliates the skin. The amount of skin removed depends on the type and strength of the solution.

Cherry angioma   Small, smooth, benign, cherry-red bump.

Chiggers   The larvae of harvest (or red) mites; they can cause intense itching when they attach to skin and feed on blood.

Cold sores   Tiny clear fluid-filled blisters that form singly or in clusters; sign of infection by the herpes simplex virus.

Collagen   Protein that gives skin its strength and fullness; it also helps repair injured skin by building scar tissue. See also **Bovine collagen.**

Congenital nevi   Moles that are present at birth or develop during the first year of life. They are benign, but large ones are at risk of becoming cancerous.

Contact dermatitis   A reaction to a substance that touches your skin. The dermatitis may result from *irritants,* which are substances that produce a reaction on almost anyone's skin, or from an *allergic reaction,* which is a hypersensitive reaction to a specific substance.

Cosmetic surgery   See **Plastic surgery.**

Cryosurgery (or cryotherapy)   Freezing a skin lesion by spraying or applying liquid nitrogen directly onto the skin.

Curettage   Using a sharp instrument (a curette) to scrape away skin cells.

Cystic acne   Severe acne that includes cysts (swellings beneath the skin surface).

Deep peel   A chemical peel that strips off the horny layer, epidermis, and part of the dermis; the procedure has potential risks and side effects and is appropriate only in selected cases.

Depilatories   Creams, lotions, or powders containing chemicals that split the chemical bonds in hair, breaking it off slightly below the skin surface.

Dermabrasion   Removing the surface layer of skin with high-speed sanding by a rapidly rotating wheel or circular brush.

Dermatitis   General term for skin inflammation, characterized by redness, pain, or itching; sometimes called *eczema.*

Dermis   The innermost layer of skin, located beneath the epidermis.

Dihydroxyacetone (DHA)   The active ingredient in artificial tanning products. It interacts with the proteins in superficial skin layers to darken your skin temporarily.

Dysplastic nevi   See **Atypical nevi.**

Eczema   See **Dermatitis.**

Elastin   Elastic fibers that give skin its flexibility, enabling it to stretch and contract repeatedly as you move.

305

Electrodesiccation   Use of electric current to destroy benign growths, stop bleeding, cauterize tissue, and treat facial spider veins.

Electrolysis   The only permanent way to remove hair; destroys the hair follicle by zapping it with an electrical impulse.

Endoscopic surgery   The use of an *endoscope*, a special viewing instrument that allows a surgeon to see images of the body's internal structures through very small incisions. It is sometimes used in cosmetic surgery.

Epidermis   Outer layer of skin; lays upon the dermis.

Exfoliant   Substance that sloughs off excess cells from the skin.

Extrinsic aging   Aging caused by external factors, most notably sun exposure. See also **Intrinsic aging**.

Eyelid surgery (blepharoplasty)   A procedure to remove fat and excess skin and muscle from upper and lower eyelids.

Face-lift (rhytidectomy)   Procedure that improves facial appearance by removing excess fat, tightening muscles, and redraping skin.

Fat-soluble vitamins   Vitamins that are stored in fat, so stay in our bodies longer than water-soluble vitamins. Examples: A, D, E, and K.

Fever blisters   See **Cold sores**.

Folliculitis   Infection of one or more hair follicles, usually caused by bacteria, less often by fungi.

Forehead lift (brow lift)   Procedure that removes muscle and other tissue to smooth the forehead, raise the eyebrows, and minimize frown lines.

Free radicals   Unstable high-energy molecules that damage components of the cells in our body and may play a role in the aging process.

Hemangioma   Benign reddish-purple collection of blood vessels in the skin. Two common types are *capillary (strawberry) hemangiomas*, which are raised and bright red, and *cavernous hemangiomas*, which are purplish-blue and often spongy because the blood vessels are located deeper under the skin.

Hemorrhoids   Varicose veins in the lining of the anus.

Humectant   A substance that draws water to the skin from the environment or from the dermis, helping the skin retain moisture.

Hypoallergenic   Less likely to cause an allergic reaction than comparable products. There are no legal guidelines governing which ingredients can (and cannot) be used in hypoallergenic products.

Impetigo   Skin infection caused by bacteria; contagious; can be spread by scratching or other physical contact.

Infantile eczema   Atopic dermatitis in children.

Intrinsic aging   The built-in aging changes in the body that occur over time. See also **Extrinsic aging**.

Keratin   Tough, durable protein found in the cells of hair, finger- and toenails, and the skin's horny layer.

Keratolytic drug   A preparation that loosens and removes cells in the skin's horny layer. Tretinoin is one example.

Laser   An acronym that stands for light amplification by stimulated emission of radiation. A laser is a device that produces a concentrated beam of light.

Laser resurfacing (laser peel)   Using a laser to remove superficial layers of skin.

Ligation   Surgery to tie off a structure; for example, a varicose vein.

Liposuction (suction-assisted lipectomy, liposculpture, or lipoplasty)   Using a tube and vacuum device to remove exercise-resistant fat deposits.

Mask of pregnancy (melasma or chloasma)   Increased facial pigmentation, especially in the forehead, cheek, and chin; common during pregnancy.

Medium peel   Chemical peel to remove the horny layer, epidermis, and uppermost portion of the dermis.

Melanin   The pigment that gives our skin its color and protects us against UV radiation. It is produced by specialized cells called *melanocytes*.

Melanoma   The most serious type of skin cancer; looks like a dark patch or irregularly shaped mole; often contains variegated colors.

Metastasize   Spread to other parts of the body.

Mohs' surgery   A microscopically controlled excision where each bit of tissue is mapped and examined under a microscope for cancerous cells before more tissue is removed.

Moles   Non-cancerous (benign) skin growths that are collections of pigment cells.

Nevus (plural nevi)   Medical term for a mole.

Obese   In medical terms, being 20 percent or more over your healthy weight.

Olive   Skin color with a green undertone.

pH   A measure (on a scale from 0–14) of how acid or alkaline a substance is.

Photoaging   Skin deterioration caused by exposure to sunlight.

Photosensitivity   An unusual reaction to sunlight, often in the form of a sunburn-like skin rash. Medications, dyes, perfumes, soaps, and plants can all cause photosensitive reactions.

Plastic surgery   A surgical specialty dedicated to the reconstruction of facial and body defects present from birth, or caused by injury, burns, disease, or aging. Procedures performed mainly to improve the appearance of a healthy person are called *cosmetic surgery*.

Poison ivy, poison oak, poison sumac   Three closely related plants, each of which can cause an allergic contact dermatitis rash popularly called "poison ivy."

Porcelain   Term for a pale, even-toned skin color.

Pores   Tiny openings in the skin, many of which contain hairs. Through them, perspiration and sebum empty onto the skin surface.

Port wine stain   Flat pink or purple mark in the skin, found most often on the face, neck, or extremities. May become somewhat raised over time.

Psoriasis   Chronic skin condition in which the skin develops red thickened areas covered with silvery scales.

PUPPP (pruritic urticarial papules and plaques of pregnancy)   Very itchy rash that appears during the third trimester, usually of the first pregnancy. It usually starts near stretch marks, and then may spread. It disappears harmlessly after delivery.

Rhytidectomy   See **Face-lift.**

Ringworm   Skin infection caused by a fungus; gets its name from characteristic ring-shaped patches of reddened or scaly skin. Despite the name, it has nothing to do with worms.

Rosacea   Skin condition that causes facial redness, flushing, and swelling; often mistaken for acne because the inflamed areas develop pimples.

Ruddy   Skin color with an undertone of pink or red.

Sallow   Skin color with a yellow or golden undertone.

Sclerotherapy   The most common treatment for spider veins; involves injecting an irritating solution that causes the lining of the vessel to swell, stick together, shrivel, and eventually fade.

Sebaceous glands   Glands in the skin that produce *sebum*, a lubricant that moisturizes skin.

Seborrheic dermatitis   Reddish skin inflammation in areas with large numbers of sebum-producing (*sebaceous*) glands (for example, the corners of the nose, eyebrows, ears, scalp). It causes a skin rash with yellowish, greasy scales.

Seborrheic keratoses   Benign lesions, common in people middle-aged and older. Like moles, they're tan to dark brown in color, but unlike moles, their surface may feel greasy or crusty.

Sebum   A waxy, oily substance that surfaces through pores to moisturize skin.

Skin cancer   A malignant tumor in the skin. There are three main types, basal cell cancer, squamous cell cancer, and melanoma. All have high cure rates when caught at an early stage.

Skin tag (acrochordon)   Small noncancerous growth that protrudes from the skin on a narrow stalk.

Spider angiomas   Small red dots surrounded by tiny radiating branches of blood vessels.

Spider veins   Patches of tiny red or purple blood vessels that often resemble spider webs (hence their name), but can also look like short broken lines, sunbursts, or branching trees.

Squamous cell cancer   Second most common type of skin cancer; red nodules or pink scaly patches which may ulcerate and crust; typically found on the ears, face, and hands.

Strawberry hemangioma   See **Capillary hemangioma.**

Stretch marks (striae)   Pink or violet lines that appear as the skin stretches; often noticed during the sixth or seventh month of pregnancy. They eventually flatten and fade to become shiny flesh-colored streaks.

Stripping a vein   Surgical removal of a varicose vein.

Subcutaneous layer   Extensive network of connective tissue and fat cells that lies beneath the dermis. The subcutaneous layer stabilizes the skin and insulates and protects underlying organs.

Sunburn   An inflammation of the skin caused by overexposure to the sun's UVB rays.

Sun protection factor (SPF)   In a sunscreen, measures the relative length of time you can stay exposed to the sun before you sunburn, compared to using no sunscreen. Doctors recommend using an SPF of 15 or higher.

Sunscreen   Oil, lotion, or cream containing compounds that filter out UV rays.

Superficial peel   Chemical peel that removes the horny layer and part of the epidermis underneath. Some doctors distinguish between this and a *very superficial peel*, which removes the horny layer only.

Surgical excision   Cutting into the skin around a growth with a surgical instrument to remove a lesion and closing the wound with stitches or skin clips.

Surfactants   Wetting agents that allow oil and water to mix. They are what gives soap its cleansing action.

Telangiectases   The medical term for what are sometimes called "broken" or "spider" veins. They are tiny vessels at the surface of the skin that have dilated, and are a frequent result of chronic sun exposure.

Terminal hairs   Long, coarse, pigmented hairs that form the visible "hair" of the scalp, eyebrows and eyelashes, armpits, genitals, and extremities.

Ticks   Tiny eight-legged animals that attach themselves to human or animal skin to feed on blood.

Toners   Solutions or lotions that remove soap residue and oils and refresh the skin.

Topical chemotherapy   Application of a chemical (for example, 5-fluorouracil or 5-FU) which selectively kills precancerous growths but not healthy tissue.

Tretinoin   A long-time acne drug which has become popular recently as a treatment for photoaging. Sold under the brand names Renova®, Retin-A®, and Avita®, it is classified as a *keratolytic drug*, which loosens and removes cells in the skin's horny layer.

Tumescent liposuction   Liposuction technique; the surgeon first injects targeted fatty deposits with an anesthetic solution that constricts blood vessels. This reduces blood loss and postoperative pain, swelling, and bruising.

Ultrasound assisted liposuction   Liposuction technique; uses ultrasound waves to emulsify fat before suctioning it out. While not a substitute for conventional liposuction, it can be effective for removing larger fat pockets or fat from fibrous body areas.

Ultraviolet rays   Light rays that get their name from being located next to violet light on the spectrum. *UVB* rays are largely responsible for sunburn; *UVA* rays tan skin and play a role in long-term skin aging. *UVC* rays do not reach the earth because they are absorbed by the atmosphere.

Urushiol   The chemical in the sap of poison ivy, oak, and sumac that causes allergic contact dermatitis.

Varicose veins   Swollen, twisted veins beneath the skin surface, found most often in the calves, thighs, vagina, or anus.

Vascular lesions   Reddish or purple areas of skin that involve blood vessels; popularly known as "birthmarks."

Vellus hairs   Fine, pale, downy hairs that cover much of the body.

Warts   Skin growths caused by a human papillomavirus (HPV) infection in the top layer of skin or mucous membranes.

Water-soluble cleansers   Non-soap cleansing lotions that wash off with water.

Water-soluble vitamins   Vitamins that are dissolved by water, so we eliminate them constantly in urine, sweat, and other body fluids (examples: B-complex, C, biotin, and pantothenic acid).

Wipe-off cleansers   Cleansers that are not water-soluble so must be removed by being wiped off; can leave an oily residue on the skin that may block pores and make you break out.

Xerosis   Medical term for dry skin.

Index

A

abrasive pads as exfoliant, 45
Accreditation Council for Continuing Medical Education Web site, 300
Accutane®
    acne treatment option, 178-181
    birth defects, 179
    contact lens wearers, 178
    contraindicated during pregnancies, 160
    dermabrasion treatments, 240
    hyperostosis, 178
    length of therapy, 179
    side effects, 178-179
acne, 303
    age ranges, 170-171
    Agent Orange exposure, 172
    androgen hormones, 170-171
    bumps
        cysts, 170
        papules, 170
        pustules, 170
    causes
        chemical exposure, 172
        corticosteroids, 171
        hot weather, 172
        lithium, 171

oil-based makeups, 172
    oral contraceptives, 171
formation
    adolescence, 170-171
    myths, 172-173
soaps, 39
treatment options
    Accutane®, 178-181
    benzoyl peroxide, 174-175
    hormone therapy, 178
    hydroxy acids, 174
    oral antibiotics, 176-177
    topical antibiotics, 176
    tretinoin, 175-176
AcneNet Web site, 300
actinic keratoses, 222, 227, 303
active phase, hair growth cycle, 75-77
adolescence and acne formation, 170-171
advertising
    chemical peels, hype versus reality, 239
    claims
        anti-aging creams, 6
        dermatologist-tested, 7-8
        hypoallergenic, 7
        natural ingredients, 6-7
        pore minimizers, 22
        thigh creams, 21
    cosmetics, tretinoin substitutes, 152

exfoliants, 44-45
    moisturizer claims, 52
African-Americans
    cosmetics, selecting, 66-67
    laser peels, pigmentation problems, 266
    pseudofolliculitis barbae, 195
after-sun products for suntans, 120
age, effects on hair growth, 76
Agent Orange and acne development, 172
aging
    effects on skin, 92-93
    extrinsic, 92-93
    intrinsic, 92-93
    Louis Harris & Associates poll, 5
AHAs (alpha hydroxy acids)
    chemical face peels, 143
        agents, 234
    doctor recommendations, 144
    effects on skin, 140
    forms, 144
    frequency of use, 145-146
    historical notables, 138
    mistaken compounds, 139
    percentage of active ingredients, 143
    pH level, 143
    preferred concentrations, 144

S

X – Y – Z